FIRST WORDS:
Selected Addresses from the National League for Nursing 1894–1933

FIRST WORDS:
Selected Addresses from the National League for Nursing 1894–1933

Nettie Birnbach and Sandra Lewenson

National League for Nursing Press • New York
Pub. No. 14-2410

This book was set in Garamond by Automated Graphic Systems.
The editor and designer was Allan Graubard. Automated Graphic
Systems was the printer and binder.

The cover was designed by Lillian Welsh.

Printed in the United States of America

This work could not have been completed without the full support and cooperation of the significant others in our lives. Our heartfelt thanks to Marvin Birnbach and Richard, Jennifer, and Nicole Lewenson.

About the Authors

Nettie Birnbach, EdD, RN, is Director, Center for Nursing Research and Associate Professor of Nursing, College of Nursing, State University of New York, Health Science Center at Brooklyn.

Sandra Lewenson, EdD, RN, is Assistant Professor of Nursing, College of Nursing, State University of New York, Health Science Center at Brooklyn.

Table of Contents

Section II   CONTROL OF PRACTICE

Section V   IMAGE

Foreword

The 1894 publication of "Hospitals, Dispensaries, and Nursing," an outcome of Section III of the International Congress of Charities, Correction and Philanthropy held at the 1893 World's Fair in Chicago, was cited by noted nurse historian Mary Roberts as the earliest historic publication by which the American nursing profession can measure its progress. Subsequent limited availability of that publication led the National League of Nursing Education, in 1949, to sponsor the reissuance of those parts of the original work which were most significant for nurses. That publication was entitled *Nursing of the Sick, 1893.* It, like its progenitor, presented papers and discussions reflective of the most salient turn-of-the-century nursing concerns. Through those published reports, we learned of the impetus for the formation of the American Society of Superintendents of Training Schools for Nurses later in 1893, the organization which became the National League of Nursing Education in 1912 and then the National League for Nursing in 1952.

Now, *First Words* gives readers the rare opportunity to "hear" cardinal addresses of leaders of that evolving organization between the years 1894 and 1933. Their trenchant words, ably organized in this volume by recurrent themes consistent with present-day terminology, deliver the exigent issues of the day, as then perceived, as well as the transitions that ensued. Their words give meaning to Dock's and Stewart's comment that "the Superintendent's Society was radically progressive on every line."

Through *First Words,* the reader will recognize that the seminal ideas planted in 1893 were perennially cultivated and nourished with critical and concerned care. They weathered storms, and produced harvests, while others reseeded themselves or simply lay dormant waiting for further attention. *First Words* clearly teaches us that as we travel on our professional paths, we have been sustained by what those before us have planted and tended, and that we need to sow seeds of our own for future travelers.

The history of nursing comes alive and takes form through the selectivity and insight reflected in this volume compiled by two creative nurse historians. Reading this unique collection, which is further enhanced by the authors' perceptive commentaries, will help one achieve a more comprehensive perspective on a constantly evolving nursing profession.

Eleanor K. Herrmann, EdD, RN, FAAN
Professor, University of Connecticut

Preface

As the National League for Nursing prepares to celebrate its 100th
birthday in 1993, it is fitting to reproduce selected addresses as they
were presented at the annual conventions. A review of the papers
presented indicates that they fall into themes that repeat themselves
over time. The emerging pattern reflects ideas that are useful for their
historical significance and for their relevance to today.

First Words includes selected addresses from the proceedings of the
annual conventions of the American Society of Superintendents of
Training Schools for Nurses (hereafter the Superintendents' Society),
and the National League of Nursing Education (NLNE) between 1894
and 1933. As an organizing framework, six current themes were chosen
that coincide with patterns discovered in the proceedings: education,
control of practice, recruitment, ethics, image, and power.

Educational reform during the late 19th and early 20th centuries
promoted women's education, elevated admission standards, generated
a theoretical base for nursing curricula, and incorporated pedagogical
theory in teaching and learning strategies. Control of practice was
viewed as germane to the implementation of educational reforms,
professional credentialing, and the regulation of nursing practice. Over
time, the Superintendents' Society focused its efforts on standardization
of nursing education, control of private duty registries, enactment of
registration laws, and the development of new practice settings for
nurses. The need to recruit appropriate students into nursing was a

significant professional issue. Leaders in the Superintendents' Society and NLNE recognized the importance of recruitment campaigns as the way to attract new students. They developed strategies for responding to the continually changing supply and demand for nurses and directed recruitment drives toward educated, independent women. With respect to ethics, early concerns centered on the moral integrity of the profession and the safe practice of nursing. The roots of contemporary ethical codes can be found in the early convention proceedings. Nursing's image was another issue of concern during the first 40 years of the organization. The Superintendents' Society worked to overcome the tarnished image of the untrained, unkempt, and uneducated nurse. They sought women who were willing to devote their energies to nursing study and professional growth. Power, by its very nature, has been an ongoing theme for nursing. Throughout the developmental years of the NLN, power through organization remained a central, unifying idea. As the speeches reveal, empowerment of nurses was essential to control of nursing practice, education, and ultimately health care. Leaders, well aware of the importance of power, spoke of its use and ways to attain it.

Dimensions of the six identified themes survive to the present as organized nursing continues to struggle with issues surrounding education, control of practice, recruitment, ethics, image, and power. Although the temptation of the historian is to edit or comment on words of the past, there are times when those words contain such vision and clarity that little or no comment is necessary. Thus, the speeches often speak for themselves.

This work focuses on ideas and events specific to one organization, the Superintendents' Society, which became the NLNE in 1912 and was reorganized as the National League for Nursing (NLN) in 1952. The presentations are limited to selected years and patterns that link the past with the present. The patterns recur over the 40 year period and serve as markers of change. Just as they enlighten our understanding of the past, they are our guides to the future.

Because of the enormous number of presentations in the proceedings, it became necessary to be selective and omit those that did not relate to the themes of concern. Selection criteria included the topic, the presenter, and the length. Attention to less well-known speakers entered the selection process as well. People like Agnes Brennan, Harriet Gillette, and Bertha Harmer, although not as familiar as Isabel Hampton Robb, Isabel Stewart, Adelaide Nutting and Lavinia Dock, nevertheless contributed greatly to professional ideas during their careers. The 40 selected papers, reprinted in their entirety, were written by nurses exclusively with one exception, the presentation by an important friend to nursing, Frances Payne Bolton. Several notable speeches were excluded that had been published elsewhere, such as Adelaide Nutting's, "The Outlook in Nursing," published in 1926 and republished by Garland Publishing Inc. in 1984. To allow room for publication of a wider selection of speeches, the length of each paper was a determining factor in some cases.

Many of the speeches chronicle the early history of nursing. As such, the history and purpose of the Superintendents' Society can be found in the prologue and Nutting's "Thirty Years of Nursing Progress" is part of the epilogue. However, to enable the reader to understand further the context in which the organization was formed and the speeches were made, a brief historical overview is included in the prologue.

First Words is intended for use by nursing educators. It can be used to augment nursing history content in the undergraduate and graduate nursing curricula as well as in RN completion programs. In addition, courses that target professional issues, nursing history, and women's issues would benefit from the work. The book is divided into six sections comprising the identified recurring themes. Each section is designed to stand alone and is useful to those planning workshops, seminars, and discussion groups. The preface and prologue establish the rationale and background for the work and the epilogue presents a summary of the themes including their relationship to present day concerns. Although this book is not intended to be a complete history of nursing, it is clearly evident that throughout the years highlighted the Superintendents' Society and the NLNE played a significant role in shaping the history of nursing in America.

As we approach the NLN's centennial we recognize the importance of preserving selected speeches from the annual conventions. Availability of the books that hold those speeches is limited. Books that can be accessed are yellowing and crumbling with age and will soon be lost to future generations. It is imperative that we save the words of our past to be read now and in the future. *First Words* begins this process and provides access to significant words spoken during the formative years of the NLN and the nursing profession.

Prologue

Nurses training began in America in 1873 when three Nightingale-influenced schools opened at Bellevue Training School for Nurses in New York, the Connecticut Training School for Nurses at New Haven, and the Boston Training School for Nurses at Massachusetts General Hospital. From then on, schools opened at a growing number of hospitals throughout the country. By 1880, fifteen schools had opened and graduated over 323 trained nurses; by 1900, 432 schools had opened and graduated over 11,000 nurses (Burgess, 1928). The rise of trained nursing as a profession offered opportunity to the late 19th-century "new woman." Before nurse-training schools existed, experience taught a person how to nurse. There were no standards and any woman could call herself a nurse. Following the American Civil War, the lack of trained nurses adversely affected the nation's health and reform groups advocated opening nurse-training schools. Florence Nightingale had already begun this campaign in England and greatly influenced its initiation in America.

As nurse training schools opened, the late 19th-century women's movement encouraged women to become financially self-supporting and independent. With few opportunities available for women to do this, nurses' training gave women a chance to learn a profession and support themselves. Women who entered nursing in the years following 1873, became pioneers in the development of nursing education and improvement of practice.

Pioneer nurse educators faced opposition from physicians who objected to nursing's growing self-governance. Nursing, often considered a "natural" role for women and one that women were born to, did not require formal education or training. Moreover, physicians saw trained nurses as too independent and too threatening to their own positions in the hospital. Hospital boards, however, found nurse-training schools to be a financial boon to their institutions and as such relied heavily on the services provided by the school. The educational process was secondary. Thus, nursing educators, were challenged by the need to educate nurses in a system that showed little regard for women's education, women's roles, or women's professions.

Nursing educators sought support elsewhere and gained insight into the value of organization from other late 19th-century reform movements such as the suffrage, settlement house, and labor movements. By 1889, women's councils such as the International Council of Women and the National Council of Women were formed which further exemplified the importance of unity gained through organizing. Organization was recognized as the power of the day and nurses joined together to achieve their objectives.

Nursing's leaders organized to counteract the external control exerted by those who inhibited the profession's growth. They organized so that each superintendent did not face this opposition alone. United, they worked towards standardizing nursing education. They looked at educational theories to develop curricula, integrate theory and practice, and learn how to teach. They were interested in the quality of life for students and graduates and sought better conditions for both. In keeping with their goals, nurse educators moved the nursing profession into the 20th century and made significant contributions to the American public's health and well-being.

Education provided a way to attain goals and remained the central theme of the Superintendents' Society and the NLNE between 1894 and 1933. Because of education's centrality to all of the identified issues of the time, education cannot be easily separated from any of the selected themes. However, this book is arranged in a thematic format to facilitate study of the organization's ideas and activities.

The speeches of the Superintendents' Society and the NLNE tell the story of nursing *as it was heard* at the conventions. They form patterns that not only provide a structural basis for the book, but remain a part of the contemporary landscape in nursing. What seems so new to us, the contemporary crisis of issues we face in health care today, is not without precedence in the past.

Following is the history and constitution of the NLN as written in the proceedings of the First and Second Annual Conventions of the Superintendents' Society.

Introduction

Isabel A. Hampton
Chairman Committee

The beginning of the American Society of Superintendents of Training Schools for Nurses is found in the year of the World's Fair, 1893.

Among the many international gatherings or "Congresses" held in Chicago at that time was the Hospital and Medical Congress, being a section of the Congress of Charities, Correction and Philanthropy.

The idea of having a "nursing section" in connection with it originated with Mrs. Bedford Fenwick, of London, who was in Chicago in the winter previous to the World's Fair on business connected with the English Hospital and Nursing Exhibit. The suggestion was favorably received by the organizers of the Congress, and Dr. Billings, of Washington, who had been appointed chairman of the Hospital and Medical Congress, was asked to form a sub-section on nursing. He also gave the plan cordial support, and appointed Miss Isabel Hampton, superintendent of nurses at the Johns Hopkins Hospital, chairman of the nursing sub-section.

The Nurses Congress was held in the Hall of Columbus, in June 1893, on the 15th, 16th and 17th of the month, and the records of its proceedings are elsewhere reported. It was attended by a number of superintendents of training schools for nurses, most of whom were from Canada or the United States. The Chair took this opportunity of suggesting, informally, the formation of an Association of Superintendents of Training Schools, and the idea was cordially received by those to whom it was presented. Miss K. L. Lett, of St. Luke's Hospital, invited a number to meet in her sitting room to talk it over, and it was there agreed that a general meeting be called the next morning. Accordingly, at the close of the session of the nursing sub-section on the following morning, the Chair requested all the Training School

Superintendents to remain. About eighteen were present, among whom were:

Miss Alston, Mt. Sinai Training School, New York.
Miss Betts, Homoeopathic Hospital, Brooklyn, New York.
Miss Bannister, Wisconsin Training School, Milwaukee.
Miss Darche, New York City Training School, Blackwell's Island.
Miss Dock, late of Johns Hopkins Hospital, Baltimore.
Miss Davis, University Hospital, Philadelphia.
Miss Greenwood, Jewish Hospital, Cincinnati, O.
Miss Hampton, Johns Hopkins Hospital, Baltimore.
Miss Lett, St. Luke's Hospital, Chicago.
Miss McKechnie, City Hospital, Louisville, Ky.
Miss Nourse, Michael Reese Hospital, Chicago.
Miss Palmer, Garfield Memorial Hospital, Washington, D.C.
Miss Sutliffe, New York Hospital, New York.
Miss Somerville, General Hospital, Lawrence, Mass.
Miss Wallace, Children's Hospital, San Francisco, Cal.

The Chair explained the purpose of the meeting and outlined her view on the advantages of an association. The discussion was informal and showed a unanimous feeling in favor of so uniting. A temporary organization was then effected, Miss Alston being chosen chairman, and a committee was appointed to meet at St. Luke's Hospital to frame resolutions for presentation on the day following. Members of the committee were: Miss Hampton, Miss Davis, Miss Darche, Miss Alston, Miss McKechnie, Miss Palmer, Miss Sutliffe and Miss Lett. At the meeting the next day, June 16th, they reported as follows:

The committee appointed to draft resolutions, preparatory to forming a Society of Superintendents of Training Schools for Nurses, would respectfully report—that it is considered that such an association would be desirable, and it is recommended that it be formed under the following rules and regulations:

(1) Name and object of the Society—
   This Society shall be known as The American Society of Superintendents of Training Schools for Nurses.
   Its object—
      1. To promote fellowship of members.
      2. To establish and maintain a universal standard of training.
      3. To further the best interests of the nursing profession.

(2) Qualification of members—
    (a) Members shall be graduates in good and regular standing from Training Schools connected with general hospitals, giving not less than a two years' course of instruction.
    (b) Members shall be Superintendents of Training Schools, connected with recognized general hospitals.

(3) Officers, their election and duties—
There shall be a President, First Vice-President, Second Vice-President, Secretary and Treasurer. These officers to be appointed and hold office until the next meeting.

(4) Meetings of the Society—
Meetings shall be held once a year. First meeting to be held in New York City, January 10, 1894.

(5) There shall be an Executive Committee on organization. This Committee to be composed of the officers of the Society and two other members. This committee to be appointed to prepare the Constitution and By-Laws, and to report at the first meeting in New York, January 10, 1894.

(6) There shall be a Board of Council.

(7) Dues—
Members shall pay an initiation fee of $5.00 and a yearly fee of $1.00.

(Hampton, 1897, pp. 3–5)

Section I
Education

Introduction to Education

Educational reforms introduced at the early conventions set the groundwork for the society's formative years. Superintendents outlined reforms to develop a uniform curriculum, lengthen the training period, create standardized admission requirements, and establish programs specific to their educational needs. Those reforms reinforced a commonly held idea among superintendents that not everyone had the ability to be a nurse. Defying the myth that nurses were born not made, superintendents demanded higher educational standards for their new nursing recruits.

Admission criteria established by schools depended on age, previous educational background, and personality, and varied at each institution. Schools responded to internal forces and frequently waived requirements to provide enough nursing staff. Requirements differed as a result of external forces as well. Schools lowered standards as demands for nurses rose in World War I and during the influenza epidemic. Similarly, superintendents raised standards because they needed fewer nurses during the 1930s. Variations in admission practices created inequality among graduates from school to school and much consternation within the Superintendents' Society.

The theory versus practice dichotomy, a common concern, resurfaced again and again in the discussions related to apprenticeship, vocational training, and professional education. Speeches frequently referred to this dichotomy when comparing differences between the terms nursing *education* and nursing *training.*

Finding the right balance between theory and practice in a curriculum intrigued nursing educators, but prearranged agreements with hospital boards often influenced this balance. In many hospitals, negotiated agreements confirmed that students would replace untrained nurses in exchange for starting a nurse training school. Those pledges left a legacy of student service to hospitals that too many nurses accepted for too long.

To ensure a strong theoretical base early in the curriculum, the Superintendents' Society introduced a preliminary or preparatory period before students worked on the wards. This phase lasted from three to eight months giving students time to study anatomy and physiology, dietetics, bacteriology, hygiene, practical nursing, and materia medica. When hospital schools did not have the facilities or resources to offer those courses, students went to preparatory schools affiliated with other hospitals, universities, colleges, and junior colleges. Specifically designed programs allowed students to take the required subjects before attending hospital training schools.

Scientific advances and trained nursing along with the opening of new hospitals steadily improved American health care. The Superintendents' Society and the NLNE adapted nursing curricula to prepare graduates to undertake those challenges found in the increasingly complex health care field. The Superintendents' Society and the NLNE sought better prepared teachers, practitioners, administrators, and superintendents by establishing programs and setting requirements for these positions.

Nurses learned how to teach through study and experience. They mastered pedagogical theory that prompted new teaching and learning strategies used in the classroom and clinical wards. Nurses interested in teaching prepared for new roles at several post-graduate programs begun by the organization, such as the one at Teachers' College, Columbia University, in 1899 and those at different summer institutes.

By 1910, nursing role specialization increased and included those of public health nursing and administration of schools and hospitals. New practice areas required curricula that kept pace with changes in theory and practice. Such additional responsibilities required of nurses more education than the general three-year training school could offer. Post-graduate courses flourished to meet the growing specialized needs of an emerging profession.

Superintendents focused on how students studied and applied their knowledge to patient care. They wanted these future nurses to be thinkers, not robots. Consequently, superintendents experimented with different teaching and learning strategies to promote independent thinking and independent thinkers. As new programs opened, nursing educators took the opportunity to test new ideas. Many turned to the clinical area for rich teaching experiences and used case studies, procedure cards, and instructor's records as learning tools. Successful clinical instruction, however relied on enough time for faculty supervision of students on the wards. As such, the superintendents questioned the educational value of too many hours of ward duty and the unsupervised hours on night duty. Educational experiences in clinical settings and assimilation of theoretical content in academic settings fit a progressive model of education which nurse educators embraced.

In the 1920s, the NLNE requested that outside agencies study their educational progress. Reports like the Goldmark report and those of the grading committee influenced the direction of the organization. Recommendations for more qualified teachers and better students shaped later reforms. The movement toward standardized examinations and development of pre-service and inservice programs heightened public awareness of the importance of nursing education, endowments for nursing schools, and moving nursing education into universities and colleges.

The following papers address the multiple issues that emerged in nursing education.

A Uniform Curriculum for Training Schools

By Mary Agnes Snively

Superintendent Training School, Toronto General Hospital, Toronto, Canada

At the request of my colleagues I have consented, with much reluctance and many misgivings, to present for the consideration of this association a paper on the subject of a uniform curriculum for training schools.

Notwithstanding the numerous difficulties which present themselves when we enter upon the consideration of this important subject, there is encouragement in remembering that, if we are prepared to admit the imperfections of the present system of education in our nursing schools, and the need of greater uniformity in our methods of work, we will have taken the first step towards reformation; the system will gradually evolve, and in time become complete.

We are all familiar with the proverb, "Rome was not built in a day." This means to us—be of good cheer, the world has never yet witnessed any great revolution which was not brought about gradually, sometimes almost impercetibly. In proof of this we have only to look backward over the history of our own profession. Only thirty-five years ago how degraded it was! At that time we find Florence Nightingale, and some other good and noble women, pondering the question of reform, and seeking by earnest effort and self-sacrifice, amid untold difficulties, discouragement and opposition, to introduce a system of management into one of the large London hospitals. The position which the profession of nursing occupies today, and the hundreds of training schools for nurses throughout the length and breadth of our land, tell us how well they succeeded in their work.

We stand today upon the attainments of our predecessors, and our gathering here is proof that we realize how much yet remains to be accomplished. We are living not for the present only. Be it ours so to do our part, that those following us may occupy a much higher plane than we now occupy—ours to "open into the future a better and more perfect way." With this thought in view we will consider briefly the present position of the training school system, the desirability of inaugurating uniformity of education in nursing, and some of the possible methods by which uniformity could be introduced and made practicable. Nursing, as it existed a few years ago, was simply mechanical, education of any kind not being deemed essential. Any kindly woman of ordinary ability, or intelligence, who was capable of administering medicine and nourishment according to directions, willing to cater to the whims of her patient and make herself generally useful, was considered a most valuable nurse. Later, when the practice of medicine became more scientific, came the demand for nurses so trained in the various departments, medical, surgical and gynaecological, as to be able to co-operate with the physician along scientific lines. It therefore became essential that a nurse should receive instruction in many branches once thought to be entirely out of her province and beyond her requirements, in order that the theoretical knowledge thus obtained might control, and make of the highest importance the practical part of her work. Accordingly lectures and class teaching were introduced into many of the larger schools.

The advantage afforded by this course of study soon became apparent, and medical men were not slow to observe the effect produced in reducing percentages of mortality in the various hospitals in which this higher system of nursing had been adopted.

Strange as it may appear, there are still to be found those who cry out in alarm against what they are pleased to call "an attempt to educate nurses." They object to the idea of nurses being taught the symptoms, treatment, etc., of the various diseases, and claim, on the principle that "a little knowledge is a dangerous thing," that nurses should remain in ignorance, and still go on in the mechanical fashion of a few years ago. But who will estimate the value of a nurse in charge of a case of enteric fever, for instance, who understands the ulcerated conditions of the intestines, and the importance of thorough cleanliness, ventilation and disinfection of excreta; the possible complications which may arise during the progress of the disease, such as hemorrhage, delirium, etc., and how to combat these in the absence of medical advice, or the great care which must be exercised as to diet, etc., during the period of convalescence, as compared with the ignorant, though kindly, woman, who understands none of these things, and is quite in accord with the patient when he clamors for a meal of beefsteak and potatoes, and hastens to satisfy the cravings of his appetite with what to him should be forbidden food, often proving all to clearly that it is the want of a little knowledge which is dangerous. And if in the case of medical cases so much better results have been accomplished, in surgery it is that modern medical science has achieved its most wonderful success. Daily in our large hospitals we see apparently hopeless cases in the hands of a skillful surgeon, assisted by a nurse, who thoroughly understands and applies the principles which govern aseptic surgery, and once more we behold the lame walk, and the blind receive their sight. And not only in this department of surgery, but in cases of simple fracture also, we find that "knowledge is power."

Take, for example, a case of fractured femur where extension and weight have been applied by the surgeon. The nurse who has been taught knows that extension must be maintained uniformly, if a minimum amount of shortening and union of the bone is to be looked for as a result, while the uninstructed nurse will, without hesitation, lift the weight repeatedly, all unconscious of the injury she is doing her patient. Nor will the young aspirant for fame in the region of gynaecology, who longs to rank among the sucessful operators of the day, think of engaging a nurse who is not thoroughly posted as to what constitutes the modern idea of surgical cleanliness, and is not thoroughly conversant with the technique[s] employed in the various operations in the realm of pelvic surgery. Or what obstetrician, whose proud boast heretofore has been that he has never once in his own practice been obliged to write as a cause of death, "Puerperal septicaemia," will not prefer as his co-worker in the field a nurse who understands that even mastitis can be prevented by care and cleanliness, and that phlegmasia alba dolens is possibly the result of septic absorption, and consequently preventable, rather than entrust his reputation to the time-honored family nurse, whose skill has been called into requisition repeatedly through successive generations, and who regards the before-mentioned complications as only natural, and reckons them among the ills which usually pertain to the parturient state.

Examples such as these could be furnished without number were it necessary, but fortunately for the nursing profession it is now generally conceded that a refined, conscientious, thoroughly educated nurse is one of the greatest blessings of the nineteenth century. True, there are many so-called trained nurses who cannot be regarded in this light, " 'T True, 'tis pity, and pity 'tis, 'tis true." The further consideration of this subject leads us to note the great diversity which characterizes the different nursing schools of today. Not only is this seen in the character of the education afforded, but in the length of time spent in the various departments of hospital work. Some schools have a regular and thorough course of lectures and class teaching, with annual or semi-annual examinations, and definite standards by which the proficiency of the pupils can be ascertained.

Others, again, have no course of study whatever. Possibly instruction of a varied nature may be guaranteed in the prospectus, or in the form of a printed circular, which announces in bold characters, "Course of lectures for training school for 1893–4," but beyond this the education never extends. Days and weeks lengthen into months and years—the nurse meanwhile either becoming self-educated or not educated at all, and she ultimately receives her certificate. By the way, this is not an imaginary illustration. Between these two extremes there are to be found an infinite variety of methods—or lack of method, as the case may be.

Again, some schools require two or three years spent in hospital work, while others, whose income depends largely upon the money obtained by nurses, send out their pupils to nurse in private families, often for months in succession—the nurse meanwhile under no super-vision whatever.

Again we find training schools attached not only to large and small general hospitals, but to the children's hospitals, private hospitals, hospitals for special diseases and sanitariums.

It uaturally [sic] follows, therefore, that the practical experience gained in these different institutions must of necessity be exceedingly varied both in character and amount. Strange that, after thirty-five years, so little has been accomplished in the way of organization! For our encouragement, however, let us call to mind the fact that only eighty years ago the medical profession was in the same chaotic state, as far as the education of its members was concerned. In the year 1815 preliminary examinations were instituted as the first step towards uniformity. These examinations were made compulsory, and year after year new subjects introduced, and higher percentages required, in order to demonstrate the fact that a liberal general education had been received. And it was not until twenty years after that the legal profession took similar steps to exclude the uneducated from its ranks.

The idea of uniformity of education in training schools is not by any means a new one. For many years it has engaged the attention and earnest thought of those interested in nursing, and yet little real progress has been made. Individual schools certainly have shown a progressive spirit. In these the standard of preliminary qualification has been raised, systematic teaching has taken the place of inefficient work, more subjects have been added to the curriculum, and examinations have meant more than formerly. Books, also, written both by superintendents of training schools and members of the medical profession, and published expressly for nurses, have multiplied in great profusion. These things are certainly an evidence of progress, and so far, are encouraging, but much yet remains to be done, and if other professions have succeeded in bringing order out of chaos, why should not the nursing profession? The ideal organization would call for state recognition, with its fixed curriculum, its board of examiners, appointed and paid by government, its centers, where at fixed periods examinations would be held, and degrees of qualification both in theoretical and practical work obtained. At present, however, this ideal seems beyond our reach; still by keeping the ideal before us, we will attain a higher standard than would be possible were we to rest satisfied with present methods. Meantime, let us consider how we can approximate the ideal. It remains, then, for this association, in view of the present lack of uniformity and the various degrees of knowledge which are implied in the term "trained nurse," to take some initiative action, in order to bring about, at least, a certain amount of uniformity in the various nursing schools here represented. Complete uniformity in practical work will never be attainable, nor, indeed, is it desirable. As long as doctors differ there will of necessity be diversity of training in the various hospitals and schools. Still, even in the practical part of a nurse's education, some approach to uniformity can be attained.

First of all a nurse's training should embrace medical, surgical, gynaecological, and, if possible, obstetrical nursing for a given time in each of these departments, in a hospital containing a sufficient number of beds to afford thorough, practical experience in these branches. Should the number of beds in a given hospital be considered insufficient, the term of service should be lengthened in order to make up for this deficiency; that is to say, if it were decided that in order to obtain a thorough experience in practical work a nurse must spend two years in a hospital containing not less than 150 beds, then it might be determined that in a hospital containing not less than seventy-five beds the term of service should be at least three years. This arrangement would enable many of the smaller training schools to come into the association, and would tend to equalize the uniformity in the practical part of our work. Then, as regards [to] the theoretical education, it will be necessary to decide what shall constitute preliminary qualification— whether a thorough English education shall be considered sufficient, or some knowledge of anatomy, physiology, hygiene, etc., be required, as is the case in the training school connected with the Royal Infirmary, Glasgow. Past experience teaches most clearly that in fixing the standard of preliminary qualification high, we will be working along the lines which tend perhaps more than any other to elevate the profession of nursing to its proper position.

Having arranged the standard of preliminary qualification, it will then be necessary to decide what text books shall be used, what subjects shall constitute a cirriculum, what length of time shall be spent in hospital work—whether private nursing shall be recognized as a part of nurses' training, how often examinations shall be held, whether examinations shall be written or oral, or both, and what percentage shall be recognized as a test of a nurse's knowledge in the various subjects.

Any number of training schools, therefore, attached to general hospitals, containing a sufficient number of beds necessary to furnish the requisite nursing experience, having arranged a satisfactory curriculum, and agreeing to teach the subjects, and maintain the standard of percentages mentioned in the curriculum, can, if thought advisable, agree to form an organization which shall be known as "The International Training School Association," let us say. This association can then agree to grant a certificate themselves, or endorse the certificates of such schools as belong to this association, and recognize as "trained nurses" only such as have complied with the requirements laid down by this association.

To those who may be disposed to look upon this step as a harsh measure, and one likely to embarrass training schools attached to small hospitals, hospitals for special diseases, etc., it may be explained that while those in charge of such institutions may for a time experience some difficulty in securing pupils, in the end it is calculated to benefit the nursing profession, and through them the general public. The effect will be to stimulate nurses to supplement the training they may have obtained in small hospitals, or hospitals where training in all the required branches has not been available by a further course in some other hospital—gynaecological, contagious, or maternity, as the case may be. A nurse in this way gains her experience in several institutions, and finally, by producing satisfactory evidence of her knowledge theoretical and practical, in the requisite subjects, obtains the certificate of "The International Training School Association." The smaller hospitals and institutions meanwhile receive an equal benefit, in that they would be able in this way to secure more experienced nurses than they could otherwise obtain. Later on, if thought advisable, other subjects could be added from time to time to the curriculum, and more stringency observed in the preliminary and final examinations; this, together with more and more careful training in the details of ward work and actual nursing, with careful records kept as to the essential details in individual cases, would be calculated to raise the profession of nursing in such a way as to hasten the time when the ideal should be attained, and state recognition an actual reality.

And now to sum up what has been presented: With the object of bringing about uniformity of education in the various training schools for nurses throughout the United States and Canada, the following uniform conditions are suggested:

1st. That a uniform matriculation examination be required before admission. This examination could be of an elementary character at first, and the standard raised as circumstances indicated. It is recommended, however, that preliminary qualification, such as a thorough English education and a knowledge of literature, and matters of general interest, are always desirable for those who minister to the sick.

2d. That a uniform period of training be required in certain hospitals recognized by a central committee or association.

That this training shall embrace medical, surgical, and gynaecological nursing, supplemented by a given number of lectures, etc., the character and extent of which shall be sufficient to qualify the nurse to perform the practical part of her work with intelligence and skill.

3d. That certain examinations shall be passed by a nurse subsequent to matriculation, and before receiving a certificate.

These examinations to be divided into primary and final. The primary to be held at the end of the first year, and the final at the end of the second year. These examinations could be held by individual training schools and in the event of a nurse removing to some special line of work, on presenting certificates of such training, and having passed the subjects embraced in the curriculum, such subjects could be proportioned and allowed. In this way a curriculum could be definitely established, and advanced from time to time as it was found possible or necessary to elevate or perfect the standard. Further, that such curriculum could be adopted by such an association as the present, or, if thought advisable, by an independent board of prominent medical men residing in various parts of the continent and interested in hospital work and the systematic training of nurses. I quote the following as an opinion of one of our prominent medical men:

"I feel sure that the work of trained nursing carried on in an organized manner would tend to the greatest possible benefit. It will only be a matter of comparatively short time when the medical profession and the public will know what such a certificate would mean as a qualification, and I feel sure would beget not only a great degree of confidence in the possession of it, but also a superior character of work on the part of those who are desirous of being fully qualified, and bringing the profession of trained nursing to that degree of eminence to which I feel it is fairly entitled."

As this paper is chiefly suggestive, I beg to close by recommending the appointment of a committee, with power to add to its numbers, to take the whole subject into consideration, and communicate by circular or otherwise with the members of this association some time during the year, so that we may be in a position to take some definite action at the next annual meeting of this association.

(Snively, 1897, pp. 24–30)

The Three Years' Course of Training in Connection with the Eight Hour System

By Mrs. Hunter Robb

Late Superintendent of Nurses, Johns Hopkins Hospital, Baltimore

Sometime over a year ago it was my privilege to prepare for the International Congress of Charity and Correction a paper dealing with the standards of education to be demanded of nurses, both before and after their entrance into a training school. It may be remembered by some of you who are now present that I spoke at some length of the necessity of a careful elimination of the undesirable candidates who present themselves. I insisted that not every woman who desires to take up the profession of a trained nurse has the natural capabilities or has had the educational advantages which are necessary to such a career. But I pointed out that, after obtaining suitable material, it is necessary to make the best possible use of it, and that here the second part of our duty begins.

Among other changes advocated in the paper just referred to was the extension of the course over a period of three years, with a day of practical work consisting of eight hours. At that time the reasons for these changes and suggestions as to the manner in which they could be carried out could be only broadly outlined. The object of the present paper is to consider these reasons in detail and try to arrive at some practical conclusion which will facilitate the establishment of such a course in the various training schools.

The subject should be dealt with without bias for any school in particular, but with a view to the best interests of all training schools which are able to undertake satisfactorily the important duty of training nurses. Between these schools there should exist a spirit of unity, and it should be our earnest desire to establish a standard of education that will be common to all. To bring about this should be, and I believe is, one of the chief aims of our association. And it seems to me that, just at present, no better opportunity could be afforded us to accomplish our end than in uniting in developing the three years' course of instruction, and agreeing, after due discussion, upon the adoption of some scheme which should also include (1) specifications of the necessary qualifications of applicants; (2) a curriculum for teaching and study; and (3) a proper grading in tests and in final examinations for certificates.

That some extension of the period of training is generally desired was evidenced by the informal discussion of the subject that took place in this assembly last year; by the suggestions since offered by the writers in our various magazines devoted to the subject of nursing, and by the fact that since the International Congress some one or two schools have lengthened their course so as to make it extend over three years, while others have this step under serious consideration.

A superintendent of a training school owes a duty, first, to the hospital, and secondly, to the nurses under her. These duties are of equal importance; the hospital must not be sacrificed, but neither have we any right to sacrifice the well-being of our nurses; some scheme must be adopted which shall prove advantageous to both. I shall, therefore, consider a little in detail the advantages or disadvantages to the hospital and to the nurses which may result from the adoption of the plan suggested. For the hospital the advantages are readily seen. In the first place, the hospital would have better nurses, since it would be benefited by having more experienced nurses during the third year of their course. Again, the hospital and training school would be relieved of the disadvantages of having to deal with so much raw material at such frequent intervals, and the school would be enabled to select from the candidates much more closely, and thus a higher standard could be more easily obtained.

If the third year's instruction were made to include a course for nurses who wished to prepare themselves more especially for hospital positions, the hospital would again be benefited, because, under present conditions, superintendents of schools have no opportunity of learning the administrative duties of such a position until after they have undertaken it. Our present methods of training allow but few opportunities for a woman to gain this practical knowledge; hence the success of a new superintendent of a training school must depend upon her native ability and such stray knowledge as she may have been able to pick up while occupying the position of head nurse. More than one nurse's career as a superintendent has been cut short by mistakes through ignorance in the beginning of her administration, mistakes which would never have occurred had she had an opportunity beforehand to become practically acquainted with the duties of her new position. Again, it must not be forgotten that while such a process of development is going on, and the superintendent is becoming competent, the hospital and pupils alike suffer, and the best work and the best teachings are not attainable.

A third year is also necessary in many cases to complete the training of pupils, who, while having all the requisite qualities of goodness and reliability, are not intellectually over-bright, and need an additional year to make them thoroughly competent in their profession. Then, there are others who, while exactly opposite, are bright, quick and easily taught, nevertheless lack a thorough comprehension of the dignity and responsibility which they have undertaken, and who do not fully appreciate the value of the discipline which they receive in the course of their training. For such pupils the protection, influence and teaching of the school during an additional third year are necessary before they can be safely left to their own judgment. In any case, a third year is to be regarded as a period of assimilation or digestion, without which the learning of the first two years will be far less valuable. That many nurses feel that they are not fully qualified at the end of two years is evidenced by the number of intelligent women who love their work, and who are interested in their profession, and who beg to be allowed to stay another year. By the establishment of the three years' course it is hoped that the number of such women would be much increased, since we may naturally expect and hope that the commercial woman will be excluded by the adoption of this plan, and, even if we have fewer graduate nurses, they are much more likely to be competent, and after all this is the main point. As a matter of fact, a slight diminution in number would not be an altogether unmixed evil. Just now the number of graduate nurses engaged in private nursing is, I am told, so great, and is growing so rapidly all the time, that many nurses are without patients half the time, I am informed that in the city of Philadelphia there are so many that a committee of physicians have already held a meeting in order to discuss the possibility of taking advantage of this condition, in order to reduce the remuneration for the services of graduate nurses—a somewhat unwarrantable proceeding on their part it would seem. But if this question is to be regulated by the laws of supply and demand, then a diminution in the number of graduates will insure a lucrative occupation to those who have had a thorough training, and who hold certificates of competency.

So much for the advantage of a three years' course to the hospital and to the nurses. But should this change alone be made, we would be worse off than before, and unless the day's work of practical nursing be limited to eight hours it would be better to go on as at present. The board of trustees recognize the advantages which would accrue to the hospitals from the adoption of the three years' course, and they would cheerfully add on the third year were it not for the fear of additional expense which would be incurred should the day's work be shortened to eight hours. I shall have some suggestions to make later on, which will perhaps relieve them to a great extent of anxiety on this point. But, first, I wish to bring forward a few reasons why one change necessarily involves the other. On the question of the length of the day's practical work, we superintendents of training schools ought to know more than other hospital authorities. We have been through every step of nursing work ourselves, and should be best competent to judge of what is right and expedient in the matter, and if we are convinced that a day of eight hours is sufficient, we should all agree in giving the project our warmest support. We are the representatives of the nurses, and if we do not advocate their rights and interests, we can hardly expect others to take thought of us.

As I said just now, a superintendent of training school undoubtedly has obligations to the hospital in which she works, and is in duty bound to give it her best thought, work and loyalty, but she has, at the same time, obligations and responsibilities also to the nurses who put themselves under her care.

I am sure that many of you have had some qualms of conscience at the way in which we are sometimes forced, I might almost say, to drive our pupil nurses through a two years' course. I assure you that I have had myself many anxious moments for the future of certain of my pupils, more especially as regards their health. It is well known that a combination of physical and mental labor is more exhausting than simple manual or simple mental occupation. It is true that for a time such a strain can be borne without producing any permanent injurious effects, and it is possible in most cases for women to stand the strain imposed upon them for two years, although I am afraid that not all of them come out of the trial unscathed. If, however, this high pressure is to be kept up for three years, I am sure that the health of nurses will suffer. A woman who works physically over eight hours a day is in no mental condition to profit to any extent by class instruction or lectures, and it is very questionable if a woman working ten, eleven, twelve, or more hours a day for three years will be equal to really good work during the third year, even if her health apparently holds out to the end of her time. Able-bodied laboring men are now everywhere advocating a working day consisting of eight hours. If this is a reasonable demand, then we are surely not justified by putting a harder task upon women who are not only upon their feet during the greater part of their time, but in addition have an enormous tax being constantly made upon their patience and temper, as well as being burdened with no little mental anxiety and responsibility.

From another standpoint let me ask, will the patients obtain the best nursing in this way, and is a neurasthenic nurse fit to take charge of patients?

I maintain, therefore, that the three years' course must not be considered at all unless the hours of practical work are shortened, but if the two changes can be made together, then the preservation of the health of the nurse and the extension of her education and training will be insured. This again will result in an increase in her competency, and consequently will be productive of greater benefits to the patients which come under her care during her training and after she has graduated.

I said just now that we must take into consideration certain means of meeting the extra expenses which might be incurred if the staff of nurses be increased in order that the hours of work may be shortened. I commend this problem to the ingenuity of every one of my hearers and shall be glad if the discussion evoked by this paper may bring out something better than what I myself have at the present time to propose. It seems to me that if the eight-hour system were once set in good running order, it would be found that the necessary increase in the number of nurses would be very small. The two propositions which I would submit are as follows: First, a uniform remuneration for each of the three years, instead of an increase every year, according to our present custom; second, the adoption of a three years' course, with a working day of eight hours, without remuneration.

At the present time the practice is to allow the pupil nurses eight dollars a month for the first, and twelve dollars a month for the second year. We say in our circulars that "this is in nowise intended as a salary, but is allowed for uniforms, text-books and other expenses incidental to their training." If this money is not intended as a remuneration for services rendered, why is the amount increased the second year, seeing that the expenses are in reality much greater the first year, when the probationer has to supply herself with the necessary text-books and a full set of uniforms. If the amount allowed during the first year is sufficient, then the second years' allowance is more than enough; in any case, the expenses of a third year would not be more than those of either of the other two, and the allowance need not be increased for the third year. Would it not be better to make a uniform allowance, say of ten dollars a month for all the course? The extra expense, then, to the hospital would resolve itself into the cost of maintenance of a certain number of additional nurses, together with their allowance of ten dollars a month.

The second proposition should, I think, find no objection, at least on the part of hospital trustees, and, as I shall explain later, the apparent objections from the nurses' standpoint, are not insuperable. This proposition advocates the establishment of a three years' course, with a practical working day of eight hours, on the nonpayment plan. The pupils would thus receive their uniform, board, room, laundry work and a really liberal education as an equivalent for the three years' service, as a result of which they would be qualified for lucrative posts, either as superintendents of training schools, managers of small hospitals, private nurses, assistants to practicing physicians, or, in fact, to fill any position where the knowledge and skill of a trained nurse can be fully utilized. This non-payment system would also place the schools, at once, on a scholastic basis, and be another means of attracting to them as students refined and intelligent women. In this connection, scholarships could be founded, which would be the means of helping poor but really competent women to their education. I am not sure that nurses more than any others who are preparing to enter a scientific profession should expect to be self-supporting from the very outset, and I do not believe that this arrangement would hinder any desirable additions to our numbers.

But above all, such an arrangement would leave no solid ground upon which hospital authorities could object to the two changes just advocated, since the requisite increase in members would add but little to the expense, and some of the money now devoted to the remuneration of the pupil nurses could be spent in paying a trained staff of head nurses, all of which should be graduates.

Further expense could be saved by having only one responsible head under the superintendent of the hospital for domestic management.

In fact, it is only by such an arrangement that the third year's training could be made as practical as it should be. This position should be occupied by the superintendent of nurses and principal of the training school, so that besides the responsibility of the work of the nurses in the wards she should have the care of the nurses' home, the linen room, the laundry, and the buying for the hospital. Her staff should consist of a graduate head nurse in each ward, one for the nurses' home, one for the laundry and linen room, and one for the office. Their assistants in all these departments should be drawn from the pupil nurses of the third year; the head nurse might also be a third year nurse. The division of the practical work during the three years might be somewhat as follows:

For the first two years—Four months in the medical wards; four months in the surgical wards; three months in the gynaecological wards; one month in obstetrics; two months in the children's wards; three months in the private wards; two months in the operating room; one month in the diet school; one month in the dispensary; one month on special duty; one month on vacation.

For the third year—Two months obstetrics; four months as assistant in superintendent's office; three months as assistant in laundry and linen room; three months as assistant in nurses' home.

During the six months in the superintendent's office, the assistants preparing for the hospital position would be expected to give a certain amount of class-teaching to pupils of the first and second years. Nurses preparing for private duty should spend part of their third year in the wards, but all should serve their time in the linen room, and in the performance of the housekeeping duties at the home.

The first two years' teaching would consist of classes and lectures covering about the same ground as at present. Class instruction could be given twice instead of once a week, and since the pupils would have more time and the instructors would be more numerous, the various subjects could be dealt with much more thoroughly than with our present system. For third year students, class instruction could be given once, or perhaps twice a week. The first four months of the first year could be devoted to class instruction on practical nursing and materia medica only, the second four months to human anatomy and physiology. At the end of the first year examinations might be held upon: (1) practical nursing; (2) materia medica; (3) anatomy and physiology; (4) diet. At the end of the second year: (1) children, (2) medical nursing, including massage; examination of urine and hygiene; (3) surgical nursing, including the duties of the operating room and the nurse's duty in emergencies; (4) gynaecological and obstetrical nursing.

The third year examination should include: (1) methods to be adopted in class teaching; (2) administrative duties of the superintendents of training schools; (3) practical care of the wards, the nurses' home, linen room and laundry; (4) hospital buying and supplies; (3) private nursing.

I need not say that the above is only a suggestive sketch for the third year teaching; I have only tried to indicate the leading points. It will remain for the association to draw up a schedule in which certain modifications can be made applicable to all training schools.

Among other things it will be their duty to decide upon the necessary qualifications for applicants, the standards of examination, the term of probation and to provide for other emergencies. My object at present is to put before you the leading points; when these are settled the rest can, I think, be comparatively easily arranged.

The daily division of work for the eight-hour system could be made to work very nicely and interfere little, if any, with the present hours for meals by taking as a basis the hours 4 and 4 for some of the nurses, and 6 and 2 for the remainder. For instance, in a ward of thirty patients, with six nurses, supposing the entire staff comes on at 7 a.m. Two are sent off at 11 a.m. (1st dinner) 2; same to return from 7 until 11 p.m. (1st supper) 2. Four and four hours work.

Two off from 11 until 1 p.m. (1st dinner); with same two on from 1 until 5 p.m. (1st supper). Four and four hours work.

Two on from 7 until 1 p.m. (2d dinner); same two on from 5 until 7 p.m. (2d supper). Six and two hours work.

The night nurse from 11 p.m. until 7 a.m.

In this way either of the hours 7 a.m. until 11 p.m. may be taken, or hours from 6:30 a.m. to 10:30 p.m. or hours from 6 a.m. to 10 p.m. With this plan the nurses' classes and lectures could very well be arranged, and one, two or more nurses could be sent off at once, according to the condition of the wards. In this way the full staff could be on during the busy hours of the morning, and there would always be two nurses in the ward during meal-time. The hours of the head nurse and her first assistant, or senior, who would always be a third year nurse, should be so arranged that one or the other should be in the ward at all times during the day, and that both should never be absent at the same time.

These are some of the conditions under which I think the three years' course could be successfully adopted. It would possibly not be advisable to try to alter the present condition at one stroke, but to make the change gradually, so that in the course of the next five years the new system could be adopted in all of our good schools. Another consideration in connection with the subject is the co-operation of the larger with the smaller hospitals, but this I must leave to be discussed at some other time.

In conclusion, I would suggest that a chairman and committee be appointed from the present convention to draw up a plan based somewhat upon the lines which have been suggested in this paper. That this plan, after having been duly considered, should be forwarded by the committee to the authorities of the various hospitals for their consideration and approval, and that the committee should ask that a trial of such a scheme may be permitted for a certain length of time in certain hospitals selected for that purpose in order that it may be thoroughly tested, after which some action may be taken, as the results of such trials would seem to indicate.

(Robb, 1897a, pp. 33–40)

Comparative Value of Theory and Practice in Training Nurses

By Miss Brennan

Superintendent of Bellevue Training School

Twenty-three years ago, it was said "that no refined, educated woman in this country could go through the severe practical training required to fit her to enter the profession of a trained nurse," whereas to-day in some of our schools a faint echo of the cry for higher education of women is heard. We take it as a sign of the times, but hope when taking up the higher, the *lower* education of women may not be neglected. The young woman who enters a training school, mark! it is not a school for nurses, but a *training* school for nurses, is supposed to do so for the purpose of becoming, at the end of two or three years' training, a thoroughly efficient nurse, and an intelligent assistant to the attending physician or surgeon—and the aim of all good schools is, in every way, to help, assist, and train the pupils to become such.

Now, no woman of education and refinement would spend two years in a large city hospital (and only those who have done so can understand what that means), unless she had some compensation in the form of theoretical teaching and study.

An uneducated woman may become a good nurse, but never an intelligent one; she can obey orders conscientiously and understand thoroughly a sick person's need, but should an emergency arise, where is she? She works through her feelings, and therefore lacks judgment.

In this progressive age, training schools cannot afford to stand still any more than other schools and colleges, and each year the graduates should be more skilled, more cultured, and, for this reason, more practical.

A nurse can always take better care of a patient if she understands the pathology of the disease her patient is suffering from; when typhoid, under no consideration will she allow him to help himself, neither would she, in pneumonia, turn him on his well side, etc., and I hold that all persons in charge of pupil nurses should strive to give a reason for, and explain why this is done or that is not done in each individual case.

The usual length of training is two years, and in that time how much has to be learned practically and theoretically, but we must discriminate and not sacrifice one for the other.

I have heard the study of the microscope advocated as necessary for the thorough education of the pupil nurse; I acknowledge it to be a most interesting and instructive one, but it requires a great deal of time and much patience. So, unless the hospital be a small one, and the patients few, the pupil nurse will not have the necessary time to devote to it, and would gain much more useful experience if she spent the half-hour she had to spare in studying the character of the pulse in the different patients in the ward, or finding out just why some nurses can always see at a glance that this patient requires her pillow turned, or the next one her position changed.

These are all simple things, necessary to the comfort and well-being of the patient, wherein the microscope cannot help, no matter how proficient the nurse may be in its use. And should the pupil practice her profession after graduating, she will find that even at a private case she has no time to use it, neither would the attending physician expect her to, any more than he would to diagnose the case or write prescriptions.

In the universities and colleges of the world, the intention now is to make teaching far more practical than heretofore; this is particularly so in medical colleges. We all know that the young physician (who most likely has stood first and taken all the honors of his class), when he enters the hospital as interne, is utterly unfit, in spite of his splendid theoretical knowledge, to put into practice what he can fluently discuss.

Now with the nurse it is different, and just here the point *trained* comes in (I take it for granted that all training schools have the same fundamental principles); from the very first day she enters the school, she begins with the practical, and takes up the theoretical to enable her to give intelligent care to her patients, and to expand her mind by contact with greater minds, in lectures and books, etc., not in any way to make her pedantic or superficial, but to fit her for immediate usefulness when she is graduated.

Theory in conjunction with practice is what we want, and although it is undeniable that theory has done more to elevate nursing than any amount of clinical practice *alone* could have done, still we must remember that "too much reading tends to mental confusion."

Practice helps to impress and retain in the memory the knowledge obtained by theory, otherwise forgotten without the practical application.

Any one who has been ill knows that the height of good nursing consists principally in what is done for the patient's comfort, outside of the regular orders. A theoretical nurse performs her duty in a perfunctory manner and may carry out the doctor's orders to the letter, but the patient recognizes there is something lacking, and *we* know that the skilled touch, the deft handling, the keenness to detect changes and symptoms, the ready tact, the patience, unselfishness, self-reliance, and good judgment can be acquired only by much practice, and a good nurse without these attributes, despite her wide theoretic knowledge, will never be a successful one.

Now with our superior intelligence and advantages we must not ignore the necessity of possessing a large amount of *good plain common sense* to form a basis for the education of our nurses, which will hold the theoretical and practical training in a state of equilibrium. Theory fortifies the practical, practice strengthens and retains the theoretical.

(Brennan, 1897, pp. 64–66)

Preparation of the Teacher for the Training School

By Lydia Anderson

MISS ANDERSON. Madam President, and Members of the Society. The fact that our training schools should be educational in their aims and methods, is no new conception to the minds of those vitally interested in nursing. It is a feature, however, to which attention must be drawn more insistently, and upon which greater emphasis must be laid, as our schools multiply and develop. In the evolution of the training school there have been two serious hindrances to the maintenance of high educational standards. One of these is found in the phenomenal growth of the work, and the other in the relation of the training school to the hospital.

In alluding to the growth, let me ask you to recall how, in less than a generation, the number of the schools grew from 15 to 1026, while the number of pupils increased from 300 to 26,000. This was possible, because, on the one hand, the work opened up opportunities which appealed directly to the instinctive interests of women, and, on the other hand, because of the very great demand for skilled nursing of the sick. Wherever such an imperative demand exists, before the supply is adequate, there is an inevitable lowering of the standards of quality in order to meet the need for quantity. There is little wonder that in meeting this emergency, some entered the work who were not qualified, and the amount of practical nursing to be done in the wards left little time for the systematic education of the pupil in the school. Again, although the first school, whose beginning we are now commemorating, started apart from the hospital, and under a separate board, that condition was not a lasting one. The improved methods of nursing, the character of the women who undertook the work, and the economy in thus obtaining nursing care for the patients by the pupils, all demonstrated the value of the training school to the hospital authorities, and the school was soon merged into the older and larger institution. Under these circumstances, the emphasis came almost of necessity to be laid upon the amount of work to be obtained from the pupil during her training, rather than on the amount of education she should receive for her future efficiency.

It is owing to the character of the women who have been the pioneers of our profession that these hindrances have been in measure overcome, and constant effort has been made to raise the educational standard in the training schools throughout our country. These leaders have insisted upon the education of the nurse, realizing that unless she is something more than a nurse, she will be something less than a woman. To the high ideals and unswerving devotion of our superintendents, we owe the legislation regarding nurses now found in so many of our states, state registration, constant efforts to improve the curriculum, state inspection, and state examinations, all tending to emphasize the educational requirements. Shall we be able to maintain our standards, however, by means of legislation, governing boards, inspectors, and examiners? We answer that as it has already been answered by educational authorities: "These may arrange the conditions of education, but the *teacher* directs the process." "As our ideal of education rises, we demand better teaching, and better prepared teachers." If the teacher is to direct the process of education, it becomes at once obvious that she must receive special preparation for her work.

In outlining a course of preparation for a teacher, it may prove of practical advantage to follow the general lines adopted in the course at Teachers College, that course which is an enduring monument to the far-sighted wisdom of the leading members of this Society.

The preparation should be grounded in a broad view of education in general, with special adaptation of the principles learned, to the needs of the nursing body. The student of today is taught that the aim of all education is social efficiency, an efficiency that not only adapts the individual to his own environment, but also renders him capable of effective service to society. In this connection it is inspiring to note the educative possibilities of the training school, as its aim in producing the efficient nurse runs so closely along the lines of other educational institutions. The study of the relation between theory and practice also brings some of our training school methods into prominence. True, we have doubtless erred in unduly emphasizing the practical at the expense of the theoretical teaching, but the great educational value of much of our practical teaching is not to be gainsaid. We certainly need now to turn our attention to the development of the theory, for, as Oliver Wendell Holmes has said: "We cannot successfully eliminate and teach by itself that which is purely practical. The easiest and surest way of acquiring facts is to learn them in groups, in systems, and systematized knowledge is science." The problem for the teacher is so to adjust the balance between the theory and practice that she will best secure the aim she seeks to gain.

The teacher must have a thorough preparation in the subject matter which she is to teach. Unless her knowledge is wide and comprehensive, she will fail to select that which is most essential for the use of her pupils. It is the teacher who can draw upon her own accumulated wealth who can make the wisest distribution of her knowledge.

The methods of teaching must also be included in the preparation, for, often, a teacher fails, not because she does not know her subject, but because she is unable to present it and impart her knowledge concerning it. These methods must be studied and practiced until they become in measure unconscious, else the "purpose" may be lost in the "process," and the teaching at best will be artificial and mechanical rather than simple and direct.

There must be added to these subjects a course in mind-study. No matter how wide the outlook or earnest the purpose, how comprehensive the study of the subject, how well-planned the methods of teaching, unless the teacher understands the capabilities of her pupils, unless she knows how to appeal to their interests, to awaken and hold their attention, she cannot hope to succeed. She must realize the ignorance and the limitations and, as well, the possibilities and capabilities of those whom she is instructing. From a knowledge of their natural instincts and capacities, she must learn how best to develop those habits and powers which are necessary in transforming the pupil into the efficient nurse.

The preparation must give the teacher also a knowledge of the history of nursing, and of the concrete problems connected with hospital and training school organization and administration, that she may enter upon her work equipped with sympathy and judgment gained by her study of educational questions in general, with their particular relations to those encountered in the training school.

Thus, briefly, we have alluded to the conditions in the training school making desirable the advent of the teacher, and then to the preparation considered adequate for the equipment of the teacher for the work. In closing, it may not be out of place to consider some of the qualifications essential in the woman who wishes thus to prepare herself. It is obvious to all that she must have the required education and mental grasp in order to undertake this work, but there is an equal, if not greater, necessity that she shall be possessed of—a high moral character. The conscious influence exerted by what a woman *says* and *does,* cannot compare in power or extent with that unconscious influence emanating from what she *is.* Her sympathy should be of that broad type that enables her to be of service to all the varying grades of intellect and efficiency that she will encounter in each of her classes. Professor Palmer, of Harvard, in writing of the ideal teacher, has said: "She must have a 'possibility of vicariousness,' thus putting herself into the place of each of the pupils. Her personality must inspire her pupils to learn not only the subject matter taught, but how they may enrich life by means of their knowledge. This woman who aspires to be a teacher of nurses must realize the wonderful opportunities offered in nursing for the development of the entire woman, her intellect, her emotions, and her will, and with the inspiration gained from this knowledge, she will call forth from her pupils that love and loyalty for the work itself, that will ever transcend any merely intellectual interest in it."

This gives us the picture of the woman we desire to see teaching in our training schools, her innate qualifications and her acquired equipment. Lest this enumeration should prove a source of discouragement to some one who knows how far short she falls of the standards set, may we remind ourselves that it is only as we set up high ideals, keeping them always in sight, and constantly endeavoring to approximate them, that we may have any ground for the hope of their ultimate realization. In so far as it is possible,, then, let us demand for our training schools that teaching, with its preparation, which we believe to be vital to the best interests of nurses and nursing.

(Anderson, 1910, pp. 139–144)

Report of the Committee on Education

By M. Adelaide Nutting

Chairman Committee on Education

When in November, the Committee on Education found itself without a chairman through the greatly regretted resignation of Miss Helen Scott Hay, it was felt that some one familiar with the work and plans of the Committee should be asked to take her place for the remainder of the year.

I therefore undertook to act as Chairman until the next annual meeting and upon the request of the Council to look into the matter of Preliminary Instruction, and Hours of Work and report progress in these directions. A *"questionnaire"* was sent out in April to 230 representative training schools, from which 125 replies have been received. Most of these have come too recently to be tabulated, and as there are yet many schools to hear from, it is impossible to present a really comprehensive report at this time. We have obtained however a general idea of the growth in this phase of training school work, and of the main features and tendencies in these courses as they have been developed in the various schools.

Statistics show that today, May 26th, 1911, we have a record of at least 84 training schools offering something in the way of preliminary instruction—against 43 in the year 1905. The wider acceptance of the idea for which these preliminary courses stand, viz: that in a rational scheme of education a certain minimum of theory should precede practice,—is of course shown in this increase, and that it is steadily gathering strength seems to be shown in the fact that during the last year 15 schools have established such courses—a very much larger number that any preceding single year, while more than one-third the entire number have been opened within the last three years. It appears that in the main only schools connected with fairly large hospitals are able to establish such a purely educational measure, since only one-fifth of the 84 schools offering preparatory instruction are connected with hospitals of under 100 beds, the remaining four-fifths being in hospitals of from 100 to 400 beds.

This is an advance which the very small school does not seem to be able even to consider. The great and constant difficulty in securing applicants of any kind—and in meeting the expense not only of suitable instruction, but even of adequate administration in the small hospital and school, afford some at least of their reasons for not attempting any departure from the older system.

Affiliations of schools with other institutions than hospitals for the purpose of securing better instruction are stated as existing in 4 colleges, 3 medical schools, and 2 technical schools.

The length of the Preparatory Course in the majority of schools proves to be three months, yet it is interesting to note that 18 schools go beyond that period and in 7 of them the preparatory course is 4 months long. In 11 it is 6 months long and in 1 it is 8 months. A two months' course is found in 20 schools and in a very few instances it is 6 weeks or under.

Tuition fees are charged in 5 schools, $25.00 in 3 instances, $50.00 in 1 instance. In the other instance The Childrens' Hospital, Boston, the fee of $200.00 covers not only preparatory instruction but tuition for the entire three years. It may be stated here that there is apparently no objection on the part of the student to paying such fees, when there is some genuine attempt made to give suitable and thorough instruction, and the student is afforded time to study. Uniforms and text books are very generally furnished by the students, though in 17 schools they are supplied by the Hospital. In one instance the text books are loaned the student. So much for general conditions about which information is readily given. It is when we come to seek the information about subjects which are taught in this preparatory period, the length of time given to each in hours and weeks, the number of hours of practical work demanded of the student, and vital questions of this nature, that we find ourselves seriously hampered. The replies to our questions showed many discrepancies and contradictions, and several of them had to be thrown out as unserviceable for use in this report. In many instances also the information given was surprisingly incomplete, and it is only by the most careful study that we have finally brought out certain points which enable us to present what we believe to be a fairly correct picture of the preparatory course in the essentials of theory and practice as now given in the majority of schools.

Average length of Course: three months.
In theory, average time daily, 1½ hours; weekly, 9 hours. (This is a liberal estimate.)
In practical work average time daily, 7½ hours; weekly, 52½ hours.

SUBJECTS TAUGHT WITH AVERAGE TIME FOR EACH.

Subject	No. of hours weekly	No. of weeks in course
Anatomy and Physiology, ...	2	12
Bacteriology, ...	1	6
Hygiene, ...	1	6
Materia Medica, ...	1	12
Dietetics and Cookery, ...	2	10
Practical Nursing, ...	2	12

Chemistry found in 3 schools, time not stated.

It must be understood that in several schools the amount of time devoted to theory is about double that recorded here. 21 schools record 2 hours, and 12 from 2⅛ to 3 hours for theory daily, but in the average the time is as stated. As for hours of practical work—15 schools require 8-8½ hours in wards or other departments during the Preparatory period, while 7 schools require 10 hours of work daily. When we stop to consider the purpose for which the preparatory course was originally established it seems clear that it is entirely lost sight of in these schools where such long hours of work are required. They would be too long if there were no attempt whatever made at theoretical instruction, but when the student is occupied in trying to master the elements of three or four new and difficult subjects, each of them requiring careful and serious study, such hours are manifestly absurd. In the ordinary college it is stated and expected that for every hour of lecture or laboratory the student will give 2 hours of study. How great an injustice it is then to our students to offer such instruction unless we can and will provide them with a reasonable amount of time for study. The consensus of opinion of those who have most carefully studied this preparatory period in its workings seems to be that 6 hours of practical work daily is the very maximum that should be demanded of the student during that period, and in those schools where the plan as originally conceived is most consistently carried out the hours of practical work are found to be 6 hours or even under. 12 schools have 5 to 5½ hours, while 8 have 4 to 4½ or under of practical work in wards or other departments. To keep the students entirely out of the wards and independent of hospital needs for any period whatsoever, even during a few weeks, has proved apparently a practical impossibility except in a very few instances. Our statistics say that in 71 out of the 84 preparatory courses the students are on duty in the wards daily, and we have seen that the average number of hours of such work is 7½.

If the amount of instruction in the various important subjects outlined is limited to that given in this first three months it seems quite clear that it is entirely inadequate. Not one of the subjects mentioned can be properly handled in the time given. In Anatomy and Physiology, for instance, about the least time in which even the elements of the subject could be grasped would be one hour of lecture and 2 hours of laboratory for a period of 15 weeks,—making about 45 hours in all. The same would hold true of the various other subjects, but so accustomed are we to superficial teaching in our training schools that we have as yet not been able to bring ourselves even to consider a plan of theoretical instruction in which the thorough grounding of the student is the object, and *the one* object. The whole question of the proper instruction of the pupil nurse in the preparatory period proves to be indissolubly bound up with the administrative needs of the hospital, and the plan from which much was hoped and expected has served to demonstrate more clearly than ever the futility of attempting to build up any sound educational scheme until the training school can be in some degree freed from its present almost complete subordination to hospital needs. This is of course largely an economic problem and can only be handled from that standpoint.

As for hours of work is must be confessed that it fairly staggers one to be obliged to state that out of 118 schools reporting on this question 50 state frankly that the working day of their pupils is 10 hours, while 18 go farther and announce an 11 or 12 hour day, and 83 out of 116 schools report a 12 hour night duty. It must be remembered that we are dealing with representative schools of high standing, and that out of the 230 to which we appealed for information we have found but 20 in which an 8 or 8½ hour day appears to be the rule. This whole question of hours of work needs careful and prolonged study and should be held over for another year for that purpose. What we need to get at are the reasons for these discreditably long hours, and we think we should be able to find them and present them in such a way as to have some helpful effect upon both schools and hospitals.

The Committee on Education after careful consideration of the data included in the foregoing reports feel that, notwithstanding certain improvements in teaching in our schools for nurses, in the housing of our students, and in some slight degree in the hours of duty, as well

as in other less important features, the essential factors in the whole
educational problem have not as yet been touched. These factors seem
to be bound up in the relationship which the school bears to the
hospital, a relationship of which the first and most far-reaching effect
is that which makes it necessary for the school in order to do the work
of the hospital to accept and admit in numbers candidates who do not
qualify from the standpoint of age, general education, natural ability,
and personal fitness for the difficult, responsible, and important work
of nursing.

The Committee believes that the present policy of admitting such
candidates into our schools for nurses will bring about a steady deterioration in the character of nursing in hospitals, homes, and in all the
fields of public and private work, and that this must be the inevitable
outcome of a continued policy of lowering requirements for admission
in order to secure numbers to maintain an unpaid service in the hospitals. The Committee feels that the necessity for admitting such candidates is due to a system which, though sanctioned by years of custom
and tradition, is one which is entirely capable of alteration and modification. They believe that in view of this a close, careful and exhaustive
study is now needed on the whole question of the education of the
nurse, inclusive of the fields of professional work which she occupies.

And the Committee further believes that such a study should be
made by neither hospital authorities, physicians, or nurses, but by some
scientific body able to bring an unprejudiced mind to the situation and
to study it from the point of view of the public welfare.

The Committee therefore recommends that this Society request the
Carnegie Foundation for the Advancement of Teaching to make such
a study.

(Nutting, 1911, pp. 70–75)

How to Help Pupil Nurses to Study

By Harriet Gillette

Instructor, Long Island College Hospital, Brooklyn, New York

It has been the experience of many training school instructors that a large per cent of the pupils do not know how to study so as to be most economical of time and effort, and the question has arisen, "How can we improve this condition?"

Pupils must feel their need for study before they will have any great interest in study. They must be made to realize that by learning how to study systematically they can get more with less effort and less expenditure of time. The aim they are to strive for throughout the course should be stated early and kept continually before them. It seems to me it should be every nurse's aim, "To be the best nurse it is possible for me to be." The thoughtful acceptance of this aim would be an aid in getting over into each pupil's experience the feeling of need for study.

The following are recognized as the most important factors in systematic study:

1. Recognition of the problem.
2. Gathering of data from various sources.
3. Organization of material into groups of related facts.
4. Exercise of scientific doubt or judgment as to soundness of statements.
5. Memorization.
6. Application of theory.

It is for the mastery of these activities then that we must work. I wish to suggest a few ways in which we can help the nurses to turn these important factors over into habit.

If very early in the preliminary course a lesson is given on the best methods of study, the pupils will have called to their attention points which will be of great help to them throughout the course. A lesson on habit formation would at this time help them to see the reason for always doing things the way they are taught—that only correct practice makes perfect.

These lessons would necessarily be very simple and would not require any great knowledge of psychology on the part of the teacher. Thorndike's *Elements of Psychology,* James's *Briefer Course,* Colvin's *The Learning Process,* and Parker's *Methods of Teaching in High School,* or McMurry's *How to Study,* would give, very simply, enough for the teacher to use in these lessons.

The recognition of the problem is given as the first step in purposeful study. I believe one reason why we fail so often in teaching is that we do not have definitely in mind just what we want to bring out and just why we wish to emphasize that particular thing.

When the pupils recognize what the problem is they can more easily solve it. When they do not know clearly what they are looking for it is not strange if they do not find it. After the problem has been raised it is the duty of the teacher to see that they stick to it till it is solved. Stating the problem and sticking to it are the first and most important factors in study.

It goes without saying that pupils are most interested in those problems which present situations with which they have to deal in their daily work. For this reason the teacher should know what the nurses are doing in the hospital and should relate the class work to the work they are doing in the wards as far as possible.

The assignment of the lesson may be a great help in recognizing the problems to be studied. To accomplish this end ample time must be given to this part of the work, instead of crowding it into a few seconds at the close of the period. The teacher should go over the assignment for the next lesson with the class, helping them to find the main points to be considered. To do this with the greatest economy of time, and with the best results the teacher must have prepared for this part of the work before coming to class.

Questions will come up during the class discussion which may be noted and assigned as a part of the next lesson. If these questions are sometimes assigned to individuals it gives them a sense of responsibility and in this way is an aid to interest.

All references should be noted in books kept for the purpose, and directions for written work should be clear and definite. The teacher must be most careful not to help too much as this will tend to make the pupils dependent upon her.

It is the habit of some instructors to give to their pupils, at the beginning of the course, an outline of the work to be covered with the references for each lesson. This has been most satisfactory in the cases where I have seen it tried. I can see that it would be difficult to get the outlines typewritten in some schools. This plan necessitates the careful working out of each lesson before the course starts, which is of course the approved method.

After the problems to be considered have been carefully stated the next step is the collecting of data bearing on the problems. The teacher, if the time for study is limited, may give the books with the page numbers for reference, but some references should be assigned which give only the name of the book and occasionally the pupils should be required to hunt for books bearing upon the subject. This makes them independent searchers for knowledge.

Those schools that have a good reference library are most fortunate. Those that do not will find the public libraries glad to coöperate with the training school. In some cities the public libraries send sets of twenty-five, fifty or more books to any city school that leaves an order with them, the books to be kept several weeks or months and gathered again by the city when word is left with the library that a new set is desired. I see no reason why these cities should not be willing to loan books to the training schools on the same terms.

If the pupils are taken to the nearest library and shown how to use the encyclopedias, Poole's Index, and the card catalogue, it will stimulate them to use these sources of information and this will offer a good opportunity to encourage them to take books from the library on cards of their own.

Much can be done toward awakening the interest, to gather data by keeping a careful watch of the medical and nursing journals and making assignments to different pupils, on which they are to report in class. If a card catalogue of these articles is kept they will be available for future use.

It will be found of service to appeal to the collecting instinct of the pupils and in this way get together many pamphlets, magazine articles and pictures relating to the different subjects studied.

We are all more interested in those things with which we have some first hand acquaintance. For this reason those training schools that are near milk laboratories, chemical laboratories, baby-welfare stations, and other places of interest to the nursing profession, have an excellent opportunity to broaden and intensify the interests of the nurse and help her to collect data which she will remember longer than if she had read about it in some scientific article.

After the problem has been stated and the data gathered together, the material must be well organized or the preceding work will be practically useless, for knowledge which is not organized is soon lost. Perhaps the easiest way for pupils to organize their knowledge is by means of outlines. In order to start them right in this direction the main points brought out in the class exercise should be written on the board as the lesson progresses. At the close of the recitation, if this is erased and several of the pupils asked to recall these facts, as the lesson's summary, they will be led to see the advantage of this method and also how to make a connected outline. When the assignment is made, the problems which the pupils find in it will serve as the skeleton of their topical outline on which they will elaborate as they study.

Notebooks may be a great help in organization or they may be practically useless—the value determined by the interest taken in them. If the teacher goes over the books carefully and requires the pupils to correct the mistakes made, before the end of the first year the pupils will be able to do pretty good work along this line and notebook correcting will be made easier for the following years. If this plan is followed it is best to have the original notes written on the right hand page and the left hand page reserved for the pupil's corrections.

Several dozens of notebooks occupying all the available space and staring at the tired instructor are a disagreeable reminder of more work to be done. This part of the work will be less burdensome if the loose-leaf notebook is used, for only those leaves to be examined need to be passed in, encased in a manila paper folder.

Very definite instructions should be given at the start as to the arrangement of the books, the meaning of the marks used in correcting and grading, how, when and where the notes are to be passed in; and no exceptions should be permitted without valid excuse.

The practice of writing in a few words the gist of a paragraph is not only helpful in organization of thought but in appreciation of meaning and concise expression.

When we come to the problem of teaching the nurse to exercise her judgment as to the soundness of statements, we have perhaps a more difficult task than we have yet encountered, but there are definite steps we can take that will enable her, in time, to evaluate with a good degree of accuracy.

We must show her as early as possible that the conclusions of men are continually changing on some of the most important problems, and that at no time do they all think alike. This, in our field of work, where one mode of treatment quickly follows another, each in turn based on perfectly good theory, should not be hard to do. We must teach her that the ready acceptance of everything she finds in print shows a lack of thought. This will be easily done if she is on the alert for magazine and newspaper articles bearing on her work, many of which are not in accord with our teachings.

She should be taught to verify statements by looking them up in some book of recognized authority. She should be taught to consider the author and the date of the publication, and to ask, "Will it work?"

Different members of the class may examine the same article and report independently on its merits, giving the reasons for their judgments. This gives good practice in weighing and considering the merits of statements.

So many people tell us they have poor memories and look upon that as an excuse for their lack of knowledge. But psychologists tell us that a poor memory means careless habits of study—that improving the methods of study improves the memory. There are certain practices, which if the pupil will follow, will be of service in her efforts to improve her memory.

First, there must be concentration of attention. We cannot truly study without it. The practice of trying to study with other pupils is a bad one for the attention soon wanders to some outside common interest and such study does not permit of concentration. If the nurse cannot fasten her attention on the thing to be studied when story books and letters or other interesting things are about, these things which claim attention against her will must be put out of sight. A study room has the advantage of having nothing about except the things that will help one to study.

Many pupils are apt to put off till the last minute the lesson to be learned and find that last minute taken up with some unlooked-for interruption. A most satisfactory way of overcoming this difficulty is to make out a study program, giving a definite time for study to each subject. If lived up to, this provides for the performance of each task and gives a feeling of preparedness and leisure which the pupil cannot have if every spare moment is taken up thinking, "I should study," instead of going at it and getting it done.

That study which is left till the last minute and then done under high nervous tension, may tide one over an examination but it does not add much to permanent knowledge.

The time taken for study, and the concentration of the attention are largely dependent on the will power of the nurse, but there are certain methods of study which help to economize time and effort. When the pupil settles down to study she must first get her mind directed to the subject to be studied. This can be done by thinking over any knowledge she has of the subject. After this experience has been reviewed for a few minutes she may read the assignment through rather hurriedly to get the author's idea. During a second more careful reading the main points may be selected and organized and later memorized. With the third reading the associations should be formed between the main points and whatever of the detail is to be learned.

In memorization the whole part method is considered by modern educators to be the more economical. The pupil reads the work to be memorized from beginning to end several times, then tries to recall as much as possible. Parts which are more difficult may be given a little extra study but the pupil then begins at the beginning and tries to recall the whole. I would emphasize the fact that pupils are usually too easily satisfied and stop before the lesson is perfectly learned.

It has been found by experiment that short periods of study with increasingly longer intervals between accomplish the best results in the study of any one lesson. This technique of study will aid the pupil's memory in just the proportion that she applies it. This part of the task is entirely dependent on her, except of course as the teacher frequently points out the value of it.

There are, however, certain ways in which the teacher may help. Those things which are presented in such a way that the impression is vivid are best remembered. It is for this reason that practical procedures are much better remembered if demonstrated and that laboratory work, in anatomy, physiology, bacteriology, etc., has proved itself such a great aid to teaching.

Reason is also a strong aid to memory. We can all remember best those things which we understand. In these days of scientific educational methods, that teaching is considered very poor which does not lead the pupils to see the underlying principle of the fact being taught. Facts are, by themselves, easily forgotten but if one understands why the thing is done, the probability is that the fact will be much longer remembered.

The habit of forming right associations is a valuable aid to memory. I can well remember studying history in the elementary school purely as a memory lesson. We began at the top of the page and learned it by rote to the bottom and so on to the next, never once having our attention directed to what it meant nor why that particular bit of history came to be made, nor what sort of connection there was between it and the present. You can easily imagine how much value that kind of work was to us. Because of the failure on the part of the teacher to make associations, it was soon lost.

Now that is just what happens to nurses throughout their hospital training if they are not led to make the proper connections in their theoretical work. It is for this reason that the teacher should know what is going on in the hospital so she can direct the pupils to make the right associations.

The kind of memory the pupils use depends in a large measure on the kind of questions the teacher asks. If she asks questions that can be answered by mere repetition of the test, the pupils will study the text with that end in view. They will use practically rote memory instead of giving careful thought to the subject.

If in the study of the circulation, for example, the teacher asks, "Why is it necessary that the blood should circulate?" "How simple a system could we have and still have a circulation?" and "How do the circulatory and respiratory systems coöperate?" the pupils must think for themselves and if they are led to think in class and to expect a large share of questions that call for thought, they will put more real thinking into their study period, and as some one has said, good memory is really good thinking.

After the nurse has learned the theory in the classroom she has ample opportunity to apply it. In fact much of it should be turned over into habit by repeated application on the wards. Those in charge of her work in the wards should coöperate with the teacher that they may know how the pupil has been taught, to do things, for in habit formation the pupil must make a good start and allow no exceptions from the right way till the habit is well rooted.

Some one has said, "The student should continually carry in mind that facility in the use of knowledge is the end of study." This seems especially true with nurses for no nurse can have achieved her aim in study till she is able to apply the knowledge she has gained. Her success will depend on the amount of adaptation accomplished.

The teacher should frequently ask herself, "Are these pupils better able to work independently than they were at the beginning of the year? Do they know how to concentrate their attention? Can they organize material? Do they think? Are they able to memorize with greatest economy of time and effort? Have they established the habit of verification? Do they apply their knowledge?" If she can answer these questions to her satisfaction she may well feel that she has accomplished the most important things in teaching.

(Gillette, 1915, pp. 115–122)

The Training School's Responsibility in Public Health Nursing Education

By Katharine Tucker, R.N.

Superintendent of the Visiting Nurse Society of Philadelphia

After all, the basis of suggestions for changes in the curriculum of training schools must rest in the last analysis upon our conception of the purpose of training schools. And so I wish to begin with a definition. To my mind, the training school should be the place where women are given, by means of theory and practice, the foundations for the most skilled and intelligent care of the sick. We are almost past the day of the so-called common-sense nurse who meets situations simply as her inherited instincts or acquired habits teach her with only the background of her own limited experience and the folk-lore of her people as basis for judgment. Now intelligent care of the sick must involve some knowledge of the modern scientific approach to disease—something as to causes and prevention as well as a knowledge of particular symptoms and special treatment. For disease no longer is looked upon as an isolated manifestation coming from nowhere and leading to nothing. Neither in diagnosis or treatment can the disease be separated from its causes and effect if thorough methods are being used. Today throughout the medical world we are seeing a revolt against treating hearts and lungs and an insistence on treating the diseased organs only in relation to the whole individual—his mental and social as well as physical self. It was in order that hospitals might meet this new conception and might themselves express this most adequate treatment that social service departments were created to render the work of the hospitals effective and far-reaching by adjusting the environment to the medical situation.

In how far have the training schools kept up with this view of disease and enlarged method of treatment? Many have introduced field work

43

either in the social service department or in visiting-nurse societies for one or two months. Only a few have included in their theoretical work lectures touching upon the social interpretation of sickness. I think it safe to say that the majority of such training schools have felt in doing this rather virtuous, as though they were exceeding what could really be required of them. And well they might, for certainly such a departure has not been required as yet and the schools which have acted on their own initiative in taking the first steps do deserve much credit. But it seems to me that what they have done is only what we should have a right to expect of them, and even more: in looking upon the introduction of such field work as rather an extra flourish, they have stopped short of making the training schools fully meet and express this new attitude toward disease. Training schools have not felt it their responsibility to incorporate in their courses, in proper proportion to the whole, practical and theoretical work on the social side as they have on the physical side of disease. But how is it possible for them to neglect that most important question, the relation of disease to the environment, if they believe the trained care of the sick involves some comprehension of the illness itself? Othewise the training schools must be looked upon simply as a place where women learn the technic of doing certain definite things in a hospital. To be sure, that almost was the old idea from which we are gradually getting away. Not only in hospitals but in factories, department stores and other commercial extablishments it is realized that the best results are obtained and the highest output reached from those who see their task in proper relation to the whole, which implies an intelligent understanding of the whole.

Therefore the question resolves itself into a consideration of what is now omitted from the curriculum that should be and, practically, could be included as to these larger aspects of the problem of sickness. The keynote of our health work today is the cause and prevention of disease. This at once implies a consideration of social problems because of their close interdependent relation to disease. This is the emphasis that seems to be overlooked by our training schools. For all nurses to learn something of present-day knowledge as to preventable causes of illness is essential, for whether she be institutional, private or public health nurse, no nurse can escape the calling of educator. The public thrust it upon her and expect it of her. How many of us when first out of training or even while in training were asked to give advice in a hundred situations about which we knew practically nothing. It is no small responsibility to assume the title of nurse as it invariably means to the public that we have all knowledge in regard to all ills. While this is terrifying at times and a serious responsibility always, it is an opportunity most inspiring and one which as a profession and as individuals we cannot afford to lose. So that our position of educator may be assumed consciously and not accidentally, thoughtfully and intelligently rather than carelessly, it seems to me the duty of the training schools to give the pupils the foundations of knowledge as to prevention which may serve at least to let them catch sight of this constructive approach to sickness and give them an incentive to know more through seeing how much there is to know.

In the suggestions that the Committee on Public Health Nursing Education of the National Organization of Public Health Nursing make, it had been their endeavor to always keep in mind a sense of proper proportion. As far as public health nursing itself is concerned, the suggestions are obviously inadequate, so little detail and so little time is asked, but for general instruction it seems very worth while. In the first year only a point of view could be given, only an attitude of mind could be expected, from a few days spent in the Social Service Department of the Visiting Nurse Society and five most generalized lectures on sickness as a social problem. And yet such a point of view may be sufficient to change entirely the emphasis and interest of the nurse throughout her course. To be able at the very start to visualize the homes from which the patients come, something of the forces at work that brought the patient to the hospital should, and does where tried, vivify and humanize all that otherwise might be impersonal and detached technic. The second year when tuberculosis, venereal diseases, mental diseases and the like are presented from the standpoint of their ravages upon the individual, at the same time to know that there is a group of experts studying the very foundation of these diseases, that is, their social causes; to learn something of these causes, that many are known and can be eliminated; to hear that for the most part these campaigns of prevention depend for their ultimate success upon the work of the nurse, certainly such knowledge will give the student a new eagerness and increased devotion to each daily routine task. And after all is it not the only logical method, to teach about these diseases from the broadest point of view? The lectures should be illustrated by material that the nurses themselves have been both in the hospital and if possible in the homes where the social emphasis may be made real by visits with the Social Service workers. In the third year just as training schools endeavor to give the pupils an idea of the openings in other lines of work, so the committee suggests that five lectures be given on the main types of public health nursing, with some development of the peculiar problems and methods of each. Further, in order that these women who are going out into the world as trained nurses may know something of those larger social problems so closely related to all health questions, the committee has asked for ten lectures on modern social problems such as immigration, labor conditions, prostitution, housing, etc. For the training school so organized that it can offer electives at least to a few well chosen and particularly adapted students, an elective course of three or four months in public health nursing to be given in affiliation with the local public health nursing activities seems desirable. The whole question of introducing electives into the curriculum would of course have to be discussed in relation to the other specialized types of nursing as well. The practicability of such an arrangement would rest on the equipment of the individual training school and the local opportunities.

You will see it is not a public health nursing course for which we ask. We realize this is not the responsibility of the hospitals nor are they equipped to give it, except in so far as they may affiliate for the elective work. It is not even as public health nurses that we ask for this rounding out of the course, though doubtless it is public health nursing work that has emphasized the great need and importance. As nurses and for all nurses we want the training schools to include in their courses such subjects and practical demonstrations as will give the pupils a thorough ground work in all that is implied when we say skilled and intelligent care for the sick, i.e., attention to the social as well as purely medical aspects of disease. The private and institutional nurse need this view and knowledge of the special problems met by the public health nurse as much as the public health nurse needs some knowledge of operating room technic. In this way the training schools would offer an all-round basis for further specialization in any line.

Sometimes I think the growth of Public Health Nursing has been so rapid it is felt by those outside that we wish to swallow up everything: training schools, public interest, even conventions! A pioneer field does bring a kind of leaping, thrilling interest that possibly leads to over emphasis of its own importance. Public health nurses probably have been and are not yet entirely free from this kind of absorption in their own work. However, in these suggestions to the training schools we have most consciously endeavored to put ourselves in their place and to ask only what we felt all nurses need and the training school of high standard could give.

(Tucker, 1916, pp. 113–117)

Teaching and Learning Through Experience

By Bertha Harmer, R.N.

*Assistant Professor, Yale University School of Nursing,
New Haven, Connecticut*

Before discussing our methods which I have been asked to talk with you about, I should like to make this explanation.

The Yale University School of Nursing is fortunate in having received from the Rockefeller Foundation a sum of money which gives it the necessary means and freedom to make a scientific study of the content of nursing knowledge and the methods of teaching best adapted to meet the needs of nursing education. The subsidy granted, while generous, does not in any sense exceed the demand of a school giving a sound, basic education in nursing. The study, also, is not being conducted under ideal conditions, namely, a modern building or with the most modern, up-to-date equipment.

Perhaps it is best that our methods should be evolved under difficulties common to most schools, because such methods should then be more applicable and helpful to other schools.

As the Yale School is now only about one year old it is too early to speak of any of our methods as perfected. They are still under trial and are being tested out in the experimental way that such a study demands. We feel, however, that the methods presented this morning, though not perfected, are educationally sound, and we are glad to share anything we have which may be of use or interest to you or, at any rate, many serve as a basis for discussion.

The subject which I was asked to present was our methods of keeping case studies. But the keeping of case studies is merely one of our methods and is so intimately bound up with our whole educational

47

system of trying to develop in our students character, understanding, knowledge and skill in the care of patients through practical experience, that I have taken the liberty of presenting the more general subject of teaching and learning through practical experience.

This subject was selected because there is a general feeling that, in the effort to break away from the apprenticeship system and to strengthen and improve the theoretical content of nursing education, we have tended to neglect the rich opportunities for teaching in the wards and out-patient department. We have not consciously applied the principles and methods of teaching used in the classroom instruction to developing that part of the student's education which can be obtained only in her practical experience. Principles and methods imply that a course has a definite content or subject matter and definite methods by which this content may be taught and learned. The practical field, that is, any ward or clinic, has a definite content or subject matter and we must use methods which will organize it and get it across to our students. This will undoubtedly result in better, more intelligent care of our patients.

The methods selected for discussion were those relating to the assignment of patients for nursing care and study, the keeping of case studies, records of the student's daily experience, and practice cards which show the student's opportunity for acquiring skill in the various procedures.

The case study method has already been ably presented by Miss Taylor in an article published February, 1925, in the *Public Health Nurse* so I shall endeavor to avoid repetition, and discuss it from a different point of view.

Before discussing our methods or records may I be permitted to present some of our ideas relating to the practical experience which help to determine what methods we shall use and how we shall use them. For to have a point of view, a firm belief that a method has value, that it is worth striving for in spite of difficulties and in spite of the fact that it may be a long time before one can succeed in putting it into effect, is, I feel, even more important than the method itself, and infinitely more important than the form on which the results are recorded. Having a conviction and having accepted a point of view, it is easy enough to prepare a form or record.

As we are concerned with methods of teaching and learning by experience, let us first consider the wise old proverb which says that experience is the best teacher.

All education is said to be a process of growth and development which is brought about by the constant adjustments we are obliged to make. For the students, the practical experience demands constant adjustments in order to work in harmony and efficiently with others in carrying out the many, varied duties required by her patients. With this definition of education, the question for us is how and why *is* experience the best teacher? What are the necessary factors in experience which teach us, that is, which enable us to adjust and which add to our knowledge or skill and develop character? If this proverb is true why is it also said that experience is a very costly teacher, a hard taskmaster, and that we learn by *bitter* experience?

When we analyze our experience we find that what we learn from any one experience depends upon the amount of thought involved in it; that is, what we learn depends upon the keenness with which we observe what goes on about us upon the degree of thought such observations arouse, upon the degree in which our actions are controlled by such thoughts, and upon our ability to see the connections and relationships—that is, the how and the why—between what we and others do and what happens as a result of our doing.

Failure to see and appreciate the connection and relationship of one step with that which precedes and that which follows, to see that the one is the cause and the other the natural result or effect, means that we gain nothing from such an experience which enables us to foresee or to plan what will happen next and no added ability either to adjust ourselves to our environment or to what is coming next, or in any way to direct or control the course of our experience in such a way as to gain the results we desire. We are thus at the mercy of circumstance. It cannot be said that we have learned by experience.

It is this failure to think, then, this unquestioned acceptance of facts and routine methods established by custom—because it has always been done that way—with no conscious effort to establish a richer, sounder body of knowledge and better aims and methods, which makes experience a slow, painful process—a *bitter* experience.

To learn or profit by experience, therefore, a student must learn to observe keenly, to think before she acts, and to learn from the results of her actions how to adjust, direct and control her future experience.

As all education is a process of adjustment the greater the student's power to adjust the greater will be her opportunity for learning and development. If the students are to learn by making adjustments they must know what adjustments are necessary. We, therefore, discuss such problems, our aims and our methods of work with them. They must understand that *our* problems are really *their* problems and that they must share in solving them. In this way, by association with us, they will learn to recognize and solve problems for themselves.

The following quotation expresses this same feeling admirably: "We wish that the pupil be treated as one who intends, and who is expected, to learn for himself, rather than as one who is to be supplied with knowledge by us out of the stores of our information," and that, "If he knew what he was trying to do we believe he could and would do it."

To carry out the above idea, the curriculum, as outlined in the catalogue, is explained—our ideals and standards of work, the sequence of experience from service to service, and the relation and correlation of theory with the practical experience. Then the students are told that our problem and theirs is how to make this experience of greatest value to them and through them to the patients. It is stated that, embodied in this practical experience, and to be found in no other place, there is a definite body of knowledge relating to nursing. But, that this knowledge is scattered, confused, and merged with medical knowledge, varying from place to place, from time to time, under different conditions, and with different doctors and nurses. Many illustrations might be given here. For instance, in small hospitals students often have the opportunity to give treatments not permitted in large hospitals with a larger staff. In hospitals connected with a medical school there is often a tendency to assign to medical students treatments assigned in other hospitals to nurses.

Again, our knowledge of nursing care is too vague and general, that is, not developed and outlined for the individual case. For instance, the treatment prescribed by doctors varies greatly according to the diagnosis, symptoms and individual differences, etc. Not only is the treatment for cardiac patients different from that for, let us say, Hyperthyroidism, but it differs for different cardiac patients and also for different stages of the disease. So far this careful study and differentiation is our present knowledge and practice in nursing, that a student can, and sometimes does, give nursing care to the patients on one whole side of a ward, without even knowing the diagnoses or, knowing this, is conscious of little more. *We* are held responsible for the nursing care—should *we* not prescribe nursing care for each patient as the doctors prescribe medical care? Let me tell you an incident to illustrate this need.

One morning when approaching a room to visit a student nurse who had been ill with diphtheria for about a week, I was met outside by her nurse, a graduate. When I inquired about the patient's condition, she said, "Oh! she is much better; she is taking her own bath." This meant, of course, that neither the nurse nor the patient (a student nurse) knew the danger of exertion or the proper nursing care of a patient with diphtheria. The head nurse knew and was responsible, but instructions regarding the nursing care were not prescribed or written anywhere.

Now through our methods of assigning patients, and through our case studies and experience records, in which emphasis is placed on a program of nursing care based on the needs of the individual patient, we hope to accomplish, at least, three things which will insure sympathetic, intelligent, skilled nursing care for patients and a sound education for student nurses, believing, as we do, that the one insures, and is inseparable from, the other.

First, we with the help of our staff and students, hope to formulate, organize and develop this content of nursing knowledge through a systematic study and analysis of the records kept of the students' experience.

Second, we hope to build up a program of nursing care for each patient, as required, based on a study of the needs of the individual case. This will be done through the case studies.

Third, we hope to have the students understand and practice, even before they go into the wards as well as throughout their practical experience, a method of study which may be used in any scientific piece of work in a science laboratory, the hospital wards or out-patient department, or a community health or social agency, or in any field of industry. To have the students understand and apply this method we feel to be very important because it develops the student mind and makes them independent, responsible workers, able to recognize and solve problems and to learn by themselves.

To get this method, and its application to our study of the practical experience in nursing, across, we take an illustration from a science laboratory which they, themselves, have either done or seen demonstrated. Before doing so, however, we compare the field of practical experience (often spoken of as our laboratory) with a science laboratory. The contrasting features mentioned are as follows:

In a science laboratory we deal mostly with inanimate or lifeless things while in a nursing laboratory we deal with human beings.

In a science laboratory each thing we do is frankly an experiment to find out or to prove something—the result may or may not be—

beneficial—while in a nursing laboratory we do nothing that we are not reasonably sure will be of benefit to the patient.

In a science laboratory the produce of each experiment is thrown away because of no value—what the student learns, only, is of value; while in a nursing laboratory each feeling, thought or action of the nurse is of more or less vital importance because it plays a constructive part in the curative or preventive health program. The nurse here, also, learns by doing.

In a science laboratory, skill, although necessary, is not one of our objectives, so experiments are not repeated until perfected, while in a nursing laboratory skill is one of our primary objectives, so practice is necessary.

In a science laboratory accuracy and scientific precision in carrying out direction or procedures, keenness in observation, accurate recording of procedures and observations, the careful analysis, comparison and selection of data and the statement of conclusions, and, finally, the application or use of such conclusions are all important factors in a science laboratory. In nursing, because of the above mentioned conditions, they are of much greater importance. They are all essential.

As an illustration of an experiment in a laboratory and its application to nursing, we may take the examination of tissues or blood cells with a microscope. As you know, it is advisable, for many reasons, to examine *your* field first with the low power. We see spread out before us a large field in which there are many, many cells. We see that there are two main kinds of cells, red and white, and again that there are different types of white cells. We gain some idea of the relative size and number of these cells in the various groups and their relations to each other, and if we perform certain tests we can actually estimate the total number in the blood and many other facts about them.

Now the study of the student's practical experience recorded on these experience records, which we will examine later, seems to me, analogous to this—it is, so to speak, examining our field of experience with the low power of the microscope. We see, and the student sees, her whole experience spread out before us in proper perspective. We see the number and variety of patients or cases cared for, the number in each group, all the treatments given in their proper relation and all the symptoms observed in their proper relation to the disease or treatment, social problem or nursing care, etc. The records tell us what we have no other way of finding out.

To get back to the use of the microscope. When a student looks through a microscope we have no way of knowing what she sees, understands or learns—she may not be looking at the right field at all; she may have the lens focussed badly; she may be looking at a bubble of air or dust on the slide or lens. What she sees may mean little or nothing to her. To help her, *we* must look through the microscope, help her focus it, direct her observations, have her draw, describe, compare with reference book and record what she sees.

It is the same with the practical experience. When a student is caring for patients, carrying out procedures, charting, etc., we have no assurance that she is learning anything beyond the mere mechanical adjustments required by the procedure unrelated to the individual patient or anything else. Many illustrations might be given of this failure to observe or to relate cause and effect, etc. Just to give one illustration! The other day a student assisting with dressings had no observations recorded on her experience record. When questioned she said, "Oh! I am 'on the dressing carriage.' I have no patients assigned."

Now, as we all know, when that student was assigned to the dressing carriage it was to give her, not only the practice in aseptic technique, but the opportunity to observe dressings, wounds and their treatment in relation to the diagnosis or operation and the patient's general condition.

These records are thus showing us how meagre a student's observations and education may be if we do not have some way of checking up as a means to helping and guiding her in focussing attention on what she is supposed to see and learn. They make it possible for not only one person but the whole faculty, or a special committee appointed, to look through the microscope, as it were, at any student's experience, if desired. This means that the minds of several people, instead of one, can reflect on this experience, evaluate it, and reshape it.

In relation to the recording of practical experience. Dr. Dewey gives us the following food for thought:

> Man differs from the lower animals because he preserves his past experiences. What happened in the past is lived again in memory. And all this which makes the difference between beastiality and humanity, between culture and merely physical nature, is because man remembers, preserving and recording his experiences.
>
> At the time, however, attention is taken up with the practical details and with the strain of uncertainty. Only later, do the details compose into a story and fuse into a whole of meaning. At the time of practical experience man exists from moment to moment, preoccupied with the task of the moment.

So much for the recording of the student's experience and the student's experience record. They should not only be of incalculable value to the students but to us as a means of teaching, of regulating their experience and developing a system of credits based on the actual teaching and educational value of their experience.

Now, let us go back to our study of the blood cells, this time with the high power lens. We see a greatly restricted field in which, perhaps, only one type of blood cells is represented. We are enabled, however, to make an intensive study of this one type noting all its characteristics in detail. The knowledge gained is most illuminating and valuable, but any conclusions we might draw about blood cells and any applications we might make would be very misleading if we did not enlarge our field, compare these cells with others of the same type and of different types, and with the low power picture in the background.

This "high power" examination is analogous to our case study—an intensive study of one selected patient, the emphasis being on the observation of symptoms, the social and medical aspects, and the program of nursing care. Placing patients in a long row of beds, the beds all more or less alike, the patients all bathed, dressed alike, fed more or less alike, all subject to the same conditions, tends to rob them of their individuality, and reduce all more or less to the same level as the uniform does in an army. The case study is an effective way of restoring to the patient his individuality and of meeting his needs as an individual, a member of a family and of the community.

ASSIGNMENT OF PATIENTS

Before turning to the forms or outlines we are using, as a guide to the students in making their studies and records, it is necessary to mention that to each student nurse a selected group of patients is assigned for nursing care for whom she is responsible for varying lengths of time. The patients assigned are selected by the head nurse in conference with the supervisor. The selection depends upon the patients' needs, the student's needs, her experience and ability to care for the patients. Any group of patients may represent a variety of diseases or of problems in treatment, medical, social or nursing; or a group may represent a variety of nursing problems and aspects of the same disease.

The selection of cases, the length of time allowed for observation and nursing care all involve important fundamental educational principles upon which the whole value of the system depends, and should receive the careful thought and study of the faculty.

ASSIGNMENT OF STUDY

To stimulate thoughtful consideration and study, and a sense of responsibility on the part of the student for the individual needs of the patient, the assignment for study is made on the day preceding the actual nursing care. The student is expected to review whatever studies may be helpful in understanding the case, and to think through a program of nursing care to be presented to the head nurse for approval or correction.

To avoid any misunderstanding of treatment, to each chart a card is attached, on which the medical and nursing care prescribed are outlined. These will be saved and filed according to the diagnosis and used for future study, comparison and guidance, and to build up our content of nursing knowledge.

Two courses in the curriculum have a direct bearing on the keeping of case studies, the Social and Economic Aspects of Disease and the Principles and Methods of Case Study. The general plan is to have the students write a case study every two weeks up to a maximum of six in each service. These are handed to the head nurse who, together with the supervisor, corrects and grades them and returns them to the student in conference. The best case studies are copied and passed to the "Case Study Committee," a committee formed to determine what constitutes a good case study, and to select the best studies made in each service during the year. Our plan is to have these printed and used to build up a reference library of case studies for future study and for use in teaching.

The Experience Record is a monthly record but is handed in each week to the head nurse for correction and further guidance as indicated. The experience is summarized at the end of the month by the student, and the completed record handed in to the head nurse or supervisor. The daily record is graded and returned to the student in conference. The summary is filed as a permanent record. In grading the practical experience twenty-five per cent is allowed for the case studies, twenty-five per cent for experience records, and fifty per cent for skill in practical work.

PROCEDURE CARDS AND INSTRUCTOR'S RECORD

To provide that every opportunity will be taken to insure skill through practice in the various procedures, a card is given each student on which she checks those procedures taught in the classroom and ward, and carried out by her in the various services, to the satisfaction of the head nurse or instructor. These cards follow the student from ward to ward or clinic to clinic so that the head nurse may be guided in her teaching and assignment of duties. To insure that, as far as possible, all members of a class will have equal opportunity and uniform instruction, the teaching supervisor in each service keeps a record which gives a picture of the procedures taught and practiced by the whole class or group assigned to that service. This represents, as it were, the *outline of her course* in practical work.

HEAD NURSE INSTRUCTOR'S REPORT

A report of each student in the service is submitted by the head nurse to the Superintendent. The statements made regarding personality, knowledge, skill, etc., are first discussed with the student. In this way, together with the conferences on case studies and experience records, the students are constantly guided and directed and every opportunity taken for teaching and learning by practical experience.

(Harmer, 1925, pp. 124–132)

Preparation for Administrative Positions in Schools of Nursing

By Effie J. Taylor, R.N.

Professor, School of Nursing, Yale University, and Director of Nursing, New Haven Hospital, New Haven, Connecticut

We are attempting in this paper to present to you some viewpoints growing out of an analysis of certain positions in the school of nursing and in the hospital nursing service which carry with them administrative responsibilities, and we are desirous after discussing the activities of these positions to discover how the various officers are to be more adequately prepared for their responsibilities. If we were attempting merely to set up a program of education for a particular objective which excluded immediate needs and for which an entirely new group of workers were under consideration, the problem would be different. It seems desirable, therefore, to consider what should be done to assist those who already occupy administrative positions and what should be done to build up a sounder preparation for the personnel who will occupy these positions in the future.

The conception that specific training out of service is essential for the preparation of the administrative and executive staff to function in the school of nursing and in the nursing service of the hospital, is of fairly recent origin and is not often demanded as a prerequisite. The preparation for these important offices has usually in the past been obtained in service, largely through experience, and more often than otherwise, wholly undirected. Learning solely through experience, while probably of some value to the learner, is a costly, time-consuming, and dangerous procedure, but supported by well-planned courses of instruction in principles underlying the relationships which are associated with executive and administrative responsibilities, it becomes a most effective means of preparation for any type of work.

In order that the subject under discussion may be more clearly presented, let us define in simple terms the positions we have under analysis, and for which we are indicating the need for a well-defined educational program. The definitions are those which have been used throughout the study by the Chairman of the Education Committee and accompanied the master check list, with which many of you here today are already familiar, compiled from diaries kept by nurses holding various positions throughout the country.

The dean or principal of a nursing school is one who gives the major part of her time to the organization and administration of the educational program of the school as a whole. The director or superintendent of the nursing service is one who gives the major part of her time to the organization and administration of the nursing service of the hospital as a whole. The assistant principal or educational director or supervisor of instruction is one who shares the duties and responsibilities of the position of principal of the school with particular attention to the making and carrying out of the teaching program. The assistant director or superintendent of the nursing service (day) is one who shares the duties and responsibilities of the director of the nursing service, with particular attention to the program of carrying out the nursing care, and the assistant director or superintendent of the nursing service (night) is one who gives the major part of her time to the organization and administration of the night nursing service of the whole hospital and to carrying out of the educational program with students and staff on night duty.

For the purpose of setting up an educational program for the preparation of the personnel for each type of administrative position to which we have referred, the various activities carried out by these groups were studied in some detail and it was found that the degree of overlapping of duties was so tremendous that entire differentiation of training on the basis of each individual position was out of the question, as at any time, as you all well know, due to the necessity of relieving those holding other positions and of providing for critical emergencies which arise in any hospital, many or all of the duties may have to be performed by each of the administrative officers. For this reason it seemed very necessary to consider this group as one and think in terms of a general program which would cover the basic requirements for preparation for each of these higher administrative posts. It is obvious that this conclusion does not necessarily indicate that every thus prepared assistant will be thoroughly equipped to become the head of a school or the head of a nursing service. Many desirable requirements are not measured in terms of courses, nor in terms of an accumulation of knowledge. Experience and personal assets must be weighed in the scales of requirement before an intelligent judgment can be made. Qualities of mind and personal attainments, questions of health, social and community understanding and interest, all enter into the appraising of an individual for any position. There are also certain abilities which indicate potential leadership, but these are not necessarily acquired through a course of study.

In seeking to obtain information as to duties and functions, the study was limited to positions usually found in the better type of nursing schools, in those connected with hospitals of average size or above, where the positions are well defined, where the duties in each position are not too widely differentiated for efficient service, and where the working load in each position is reasonable, and the educational side of the program of school and hospital is recognized and carefully provided for.

The master check list was divided into four main divisions and subdivided into many others. Under these divisions the various activities as practiced by members of the school of nursing staff were tabulated. This list of activities covers thirty-one typewritten pages of material, and contains over five hundred and fifty items. It seems to be a fairly comprehensive list, but no doubt there are innumerable activities carried on by the executive nursing groups which are not included in the compilation. It would seem, however, to be sufficiently comprehensive to base some reasonable conclusions upon it.

The four main divisions of the check list are: activities involved in the organization and administration of the nursing school and nursing service; activities concerned with planning and carrying out the program of instruction; activities concerned with the personnel of the school, hospital, and graduates of the school; and the activities concerned with professional and personal improvement, and with community relations. As these divisions are broad and general it may make the discussion considerably clearer and also assist you in grasping the ideas in a more practical way if we enumerate the subdivisions of these main headings as they are carried out in the check list.

Under the first division, "Activities involved in the organization and administration of the nursing school and nursing service," the activities are subdivided into nine groups: activities concerned with the determination of aims, standards and policies of the nursing school and nursing service; activities concerned with the organization of the nursing school and nursing service; activities concerned with the general government of the school and nursing service; activities concerned with housing and living conditions of students and employed personnel; activities concerned with the health of students and employed personnel; activities concerned with the nursing care of the patients; activities concerned with the hospital and school plant and with supplies; activities concerned with the financial and business management of the school and with the nursing service; and activities concerned with correspondence, publications and publicity.

Under the second main or general heading, "Activities concerned with planning and carrying out the programs of instruction," there are twelve subdivisions: studying the needs, abilities and educational foundation of those who are to be taught; preparing the curriculum as a whole; mastering the subject matter to be taught; planning subject matter to be taught in individual courses or units; selecting and organizing subject matter (including content of practical experience); teaching subject matter; making assignments and providing facilities for study and practice; teaching students to study and practice; investigating and evaluating students' needs, abilities and achievements in relation to instruction and study; activities involving contacts with students in relation to instruction; activities involved in providing adequate sources and materials for study and practice; activities involved in records and reports concerning students (not including records of admission and office records).

We now come to the third division with the main heading, "Activities concerned with the personnel of school and hospital and graduates of the school," under which six subdivisions are listed: principal individuals and groups with whom coöperative relationships are established and maintained; typical activities involved in interdepartmental relationships; activities involved in the selection, employment and supervision of graduate nursing staff and other employed personnel; activities involved in admitting, classifying and graduating students; activities involved in extra-curricular activities of the school; activities in relation to graduates of school.

The fourth and last division, "Activities concerned with professional and personal improvement and community relations," is subdivided into ten classes of duties, viz.: making professional contacts; seeking for improvement in professional preparation; seeking to improve professional status; helping to establish cordial relations with members of community; coöperating in community activities; contributing information and assistance to community groups; helping to secure coöperation and assistance from community and from influential citizens in supporting the work of the hospital; in supporting the work of the school, etc.; helping to improve the standards and service of the nursing profession; providing for personal welfare, and in developing and exercising desirable traits.

Under each of these major divisions with the many subheadings are tabulated the chief activities which are carried on in the hospital and nursing school by one or all of its official groups from the head nurse to the director of the school. Considering the fact that the executive group has at some time or other to do or to be responsible for someone else who does one or all of these procedures, it seems reasonable to assume that this group should have learned either through experience or through special training how to carry out or be able to participate in all the activities listed, having passed through the various stages or levels of training by a direct, or in some instances an indirect, route from the head nurse or assistant instructor to the supervisor or instructor level, then to the third level for which we are aiming to construct a suggestive training program. If the activities on the first and second level have not been formerly learned sufficiently at least to understand and interpret them, they must be learned while proceeding with the additional broadening professional content and cultural courses which will advance the administrator to the level on which she can satisfactorily meet the requirements of her more comprehensive responsibilities.

Looking at an objective with a long-range vision is somewhat different from working towards that objective through the process of developing from their base, simple ideas, into more complex systems till the aim is attained. When the subcommittee to study the duties, qualifications and functions of the administrative staff of the school of nursing and hospital nursing service began its work some years ago, with the object of building up a course of study in preparation for the various functions which these officers were required to perform, it seemed a more simple task than the experience of the past three years has proved it to be. One reason for the difficulty is that a voluntary committee, separated by long distances, cannot get together sufficiently often to do group thinking on consecutive parts of its program, and usually not at a time when the material is fresh at hand. The analysis, therefore, has to be made individually, in piecemeal, by correspondence. Thus through lack of the stimulus which is always present when mind meets mind in discussion, rapid and concrete results are difficult to attain. History has repeated itself in this effort, and the work of this subcommittee is still in the state of synthesis on the one hand, and analysis on the other, as we build up only to break down every time a questionnaire, a letter, or a report goes out to each of the members of the committee. There is, however, a considerable unanimity of opinion on certain fundamental factors, which will enable us to present some suggestive principles upon which to develop a program of study to meet the general needs.

In analyzing the master check list to which we have previously referred, it was a unanimous opinion that the majority of the activities carried on in the school and nursing service of the hospital must be learned either in service through experience, or by direct teaching, while in service, or in organized courses of study, and that it was essential for the executive and administrative groups (dean or principal of school, superintendent of nurses, educational director, or assistant principal and assistants, day and night), to have experienced the activities and mastered the subject matter on the lower levels before proceeding to be responsible for the activities on the highest level. In other words, the background and training of these officers should have included the essential knowledge required to function on the head nurse and assistant instructor level, and also on the supervisor and instructor level. It must be noted that we have suggested the prerequisite to be the essential knowledge, and we have not arbitrarily indicated that each step in sequence must have been taken by each individual before advancing to the positions of highest responsibility in administration and teaching. It is conceivable that certain other experiences in life might have provided a part of the prerequisite knowledge, and be accepted in substitution for more arbitrary sequences within the school and hospital.

In preparing a program of study which this committee has under consideration, several points must be kept in mind, such as the individual differences in background, in theory and practice, the personality, the special abilities and major interests of the student. In addition to these points it also must be kept in mind that the courses of study will be given in many different colleges and universities, by a great variety of instructors, where the grouping of subject matter into courses will depend on the facilities, the resources, and the organization of the institution in which the courses are given. It is therefore obvious that any program which may be outlined should at best be suggestive and capable of great flexibility and modification.

In studying the vocational histories of 151 principals of schools, who were members of the National League of Nursing Education, and whose blanks were accurately and correctly filled in, Miss Urch, a member of the subcommittee, found that 55% had attended college, 13% of which held either a Master's or Bachelor's degree; 8.5% had either one or two years of normal school, 15% were high school graduates and 21.5% had less than four years of high school. About 33% of the number before entering the school of nursing had attended college at intervals after completing the nurse's training.

It is very interesting to note that 51% of the total number of histories studied stated no previous professional experience before entering the school of nursing; 30% stated previous experience as teachers; 14.5% stated business experience, and 4% stated experience in various other pursuits.

Another interesting item of information gleaned from this study was that 45% of the total number had felt it essential to take some type of postgraduate work in preparation for the position of director of a school of nursing.

Still another finding of importance was the number of different paths by which these various persons proceeded to the post of director and superintendent. Fifty per cent had been head nurses, 45% assistants, 30% instructors, 23% private duty nurses, 18% night supervisors, and others had held positions in the army, in the public health field, and as office nurses, inspectors, anæsthetists, and as registrars. The analysis does not specifically state the sequence followed from one post to the other, but undoubtedly many of the head nurses were later instructors, night supervisors, and assistants, before becoming directors of schools.

Another vocational study of fifty applicants for matriculation to Teachers College, made by Miss Pfefferkorn, to secure information as to the professional route taken to the position of superintendent of nurses and principal of the nursing school, shows that the position is reached usually by ascending from one level to another. Forty-three of the 50 directors of schools had either been head nurses or supervisors; 23 had been assistant directors; and 30 instructors or educational directors; while others had proceeded to the position directly or after holding minor miscellaneous positions in the nursing field. In the majority of matriculation blanks studied, an average of 4.8 years was spent in other positions before holding the office of superintendent of nurses or principal of the school.

The data studied are probably too limited and too specifically selected upon which to base authoritative conclusions, but the studies carried on by other subcommittees have strengthened the findings sufficiently to form the opinion that it is desirable to proceed to the position of superintendent of nurses and principal of the school through the various steps in sequence, in order that the different experiences will come in logical order in relation to their difficulty and importance.

We may also assume with reasonable assurance that since the study of the duties of the assistants, as compiled in the master check list, indicates that an appreciable number of the activities and responsibilities carried by the superintendent of nurses and principal of the school are shared by and sometimes relegated to the assistants, including the educational director and night supervisor, a similar educational program should be required for this entire group, providing electives and major subjects in sufficient numbers to develop further individual abilities and capacities, and to provide for the different individual specialties and interests.

To return to the matter of the master check list of activities, and to substantiate the opinions we have just expressed, we find a great number of activities which are carried on by every member of the school of nursing staff. The activity described as studying modern standards and trends in nursing and in nursing education is an activity which should be participated in by every staff member from the head nurse to the head of the school. While on the other hand—"studying the individual institution to determine present conditions and needs in relation to nursing service and nursing education"—may more properly be an activity of the administrative group. Another activity in which the entire group may, and should, participate, either individually, or through some form of committee organization is "planning for progressive future developments of the school and nursing service,"—while "arranging for the registration of the school,"—is the responsibility of the executive head.

To consider the activity "studying the needs, abilities and educational foundations of those who are to be taught, in relation to patients, and patients' friends"—the head nurse is the member of the staff who stands in closest relation to these groups. For that reason she needs to know the fundamentals upon which to establish satisfactory relations. She should have had somewhere in her preparation courses or experience which will enable her to teach the principles of health, and how to deal with problems of personality. Such courses are basic for every member of the staff who is responsible for teaching, or for the supervision of the work of others. In analyzing the activities relating to the curriculum as a whole, such an activity as "planning for the coördination of theoretical and practical work" is also a common activity to be participated in by all, while "planning the placement and general sequence of units in the educational program" is the direct responsibility of the higher executive members of the staff. "Studying desirable traits and attitudes to be developed in nursing students, and planning how to provide for such training" is a joint activity, but "selecting, evaluating and defining curriculum objectives" requires a wealth of broad experience, knowledge and great ability. Such an activity as "explaining new orders, treatments and unusual cases" is again the responsibility of the head nurse, supervisors or instructor, while "conducting a course in professional reading and study for the staff" requires the acumen and experience of the educational director or the head of the school.

To continue with the analysis of the check list further would be to accumulate additional examples signifying that there are certain fundamental things to be learned connected with each type of position, and that some items of information are common to all positions. In studying the list in detail, it is evident that some of the activities must be learned as individual procedures in the actual setting. Some may be learned apart from the actual field, and some may be learned only through the application of general principles based on a broad knowledge of many subjects and after several years of experience.

It may be taken for granted that every appointment to a faculty presupposes teaching responsibilities. It is also traditional in schools of nursing that certain positions presuppose the subjects to be taught. For example, in the majority of schools it is taken for granted that the superintendent of nurses and principal of the school will teach the subject of ethics, and quite often the history of nursing. It is quite possible that the major interest of some principals of schools may not be the history of nursing, and that they may not be at all well versed in philosophy and ethics. It is also quite possible that some other faculty member may have spent years in studying either one or both of the subjects, and would be prepared to teach them through her rich knowledge and her special ability in a way the superintendent of nurses could not hope to do were she to devote her utmost energies to the work. And were she to persist in following traditional lines, she would no doubt deprive the students of a rare opportunity, and perhaps place herself in great embarrassment. It would seem reasonable to suppose that in preparing individuals for these advanced positions the ability, the special interest, and the rich experience of each should be further developed and capitalized, instead of diverting the attention of all to new and different fields of thought and study. It will doubtless be conceded that a mastery of certain specific knowledge is essential and basic to all administrative positions, but in no case does it seem desirable that the particular interests of the individual should be set aside and all courses developed upon stereotyped lines.

In aiming to construct an advanced theoretical program for the future for the preparation of the groups under consideration it may be accepted that it should be built upon the premise that the courses essential to a baccalaureate degree have already been covered, and that in addition to the courses usually included in the work for such a degree the professional background content subjects have been credited in former courses. It may also be presupposed that a certain content of pedagogy has been included in former courses permitting the student to enter the essential educational and special subject matter courses upon an advanced level. Should there be an omission in the basic requirements, it would seem necessary that such deficiencies be made up, either previous to or parallel with the subject matter essential for the more advanced standing.

May I say that it is the opinion of several members of the subcommittee that basic to all nursing positions there should be certain broad cultural subjects not concerned with administration or pedagogy included in the general background of education, and that some of these subjects might, to the great advantage of every teacher and administrator, and to the profit of the students, be continued according to the bent of the individual throughout the various years of additional preparation for the higher posts in nursing administration and education. The qualities of leadership, inspiration, and stimulation, are more dependent on personality than upon a knowledge of method and rule, but a desirable personality is developed through the acquiring of knowledge and culture, and through experiencing and reacting happily to a great variety of relationships. For this reason subjects of pedagogical or administrative content will not replace either native ability or general culture and will not suffice to develop successful leaders in either administration or teaching, unless they are built upon a sound and broad individual foundation.

It might be well to keep in mind a conception that the so-called administrative and executive staff is not a superstaff under which all groups must function, and thus be limited in their output, but the group through whom coöperative activities may be carried on and coördinated. The superintendent of nurses who is also the principal of the school of nursing might appropriately be called the "Operative Executive," and she and the other immediate staff should learn to distinguish between responsibility for doing, and the responsibility for seeing that what is necessary gets done.

In an article by Elliott Dunlap Smith, Professor of Industrial Engineering, Sheffied Scientific School, Yale University, entitled, "The Operating Executive: His Relations to the Specialized Departments," these fine points of relationship are clearly described, and the principles underlying these relationships in industry are not markedly different in an organization (the hospital) which is a composite of education and production, or education and service. Professor Smith says, "Such sharing of responsibility is by no means easy to accomplish. Like many other advances in management it makes management better, but more difficult." As management in industry is becoming more difficult, management in any or all of its various phases is also becoming increasingly complicated, and can be directed only through consideration of all the factors involved, and by applying controlled, directed and coöperative methods to procedure.

In the organization of the nursing departments in hospitals there are two main divisions which relate to the two clear-cut, yet interrelated, functions–teaching and service. At the present time no satisfactory system has been evolved which separates specifically these two functions. Ever since the organization of schools of nursing in hospitals, nurse educators have endeavored to solve the problem, in order that the schools might be free to fulfill their primary function and at the same time maintain the integrity within the institution through which the student is directly related to the active field in which nursing can best be taught.

Another conception which is gradually changing is that education and administration are distinct and separate fields. With the building up of service units within the hospital and unit teaching in schools of nursing, we are coming to regard the function of the supervisor and the instructor as so closely related that we are inclined to think of one person carrying both functions with one or many assistants in charge of each departmental unit, medical, surgical, pediatric, obstetrical, etc. Formerly our conception was somewhat different. We had instructors in the theory and practice of nursing, and supervisors in relation to general administration, each group functioning separately in the same ward units and quite often without the least coöperation or knowledge of the aim of the other. You are all familiar with the complex problems which seemed inevitably to arise under this organization, and the handicaps which each group felt through the inhibitions placed sometimes unconsciously on each by the other. The young head nurse in the ward suffered most acutely, for she owed allegiance to each, and was often the recipient of conflicting directions due to different ideals on the part of the highly specialized and presumably authoritative groups, and she had difficulty in determining by which road to proceed.

The new psychology tends to consider the environment of the individual in relation to his well-being and to his whole development. Therefore it is obvious that an organization which deliberately divided the ward unit into such separate and distinct categories, and placed commanding officers over each, would suffer through lack of coördinated ideas. Under the conception that education and administration should be separated, conflicts of prestige, between the two groups ranking on a similar level, frequently blocked the progress of each in developing an ideal ward service and teaching environment.

Perhaps the greatest reason for connecting the educator and the administrator in function is that they must inevitably within a given area perform a great number of the same duties, and we cannot now pigeon-hole these activities as completely as we formerly thought possible, and at the same time develop the whole organization to a high point of efficiency in which all groups may work with comparative ease and comfort. The general checking of functions and pursuits has without doubt established our acceptance of a new point of view.

Administration, therefore, cannot be conceived as an isolated subject. When one thinks of administration it is in relation to something. We think of administration in business, in industry, in education in all its various ramifications, and in government. Successful administration depends upon a thorough knowledge of the rules of the game; an understanding of how to coöperate and make others coöperate; how to coördinate the efforts of the group; how to delegate responsibility and detail and yet keep in touch with fundamental and salient situations, and know where to go for minutiæ; how to look ahead and plan for future developments; how to see something in the future when the signs are in embryo; how to direct and make use of group thinking; in reality administration is leadership, and good leadership is dependent upon capacity and education. It is apparent that in hospitals and schools

of nursing these two great functions—administration and education—
are inseparable, and if we are to attain perfection on the highest level
we may assume that we must begin very early to shape a program of
staff education, either in service or out of service, to define clearly and
to correlate these relationships by theory, and by practical application.

The ward is the hospital in miniature. In it are all the factors concerned with administration and teaching. It is a complete unit, and is
the first and best field in which to study the problems involving coöperative relationships. The importance of the teaching in this diminutive
field is of great significance, and one can early evaluate ability which
will determine the potentialities for the higher posts of administration
and for future leadership.

Significant and far-reaching developments in the field of medicine,
public health, and general education, have had a direct influence on
shaping nursing education, and have demanded a corresponding modification in its educational content. The development of a new system
in an old setting presented many complications, and the conflicts
between the various groups engaged in the administration of the hospital nursing service with its former ideas, and the groups engaged in
attempting to implant new ideals in teaching nursing, resulted in
bringing the various groups more closely together in seeking to solve
what undoubtedly were not separate, but mutual, problems.

For a number of years we have felt the urgent need, and have rather
generally accepted the idea that special preparation in methods of
teaching and related subjects was prerequisite for the theoretical teaching in schools of nursing. This idea has not so generally been accepted
in preparation for administrative positions.

Nursing requires a separate educational content from medicine, yet
because medicine is always building up a new body of knowledge based
on scientific facts, it is constantly releasing to nursing new responsibilities of a highly technical nature, the application of which demands a
more thorough knowledge of the basic physical and social sciences.
The releasing of new responsibilities to nursing changes the activities
of executives, and calls for new knowledge on the part of those directing
the policies of administration, as well as those connected more directly
with the teaching of students.

For certain obvious reasons the organization of the hospital units is
highly specialized, and developed under departments which may or
may not be self-contained.

The modern tendency within these departments is to center all
activities around the individual patient as an individual, and this view-

point tends to a centralization of responsibilities beginning with the head nurse, who is usually the junior member of the teaching and administrative staff, through the supervisor who may also be the instructor, to the assistant and educational director, and to the principal of the school, who may also be the superintendent of nurses. For the reasons we have enumerated, it will no doubt be evident that the preparation of each of the various officers in the administration of the hospital and school of nursing must be developed upon similar lines, and that the content must be differentiated in degree rather than in types of subject matter. In other words, in building up an educational program for the training of the teaching and executive staff, the principles of supervision and administration must both be taught to the young head nurse and continued through to the highest and most responsible officer, the principal of the school of nursing, for each must carry her share of the load in both fields to develop the resources to their highest efficiency.

Under our existing hospital organization it would seem somewhat premature to assume that in presenting a program for the use of the greatest number for whom it will have value, the positions of the principal of the school of nursing and the superintendent of nurses should be separated and a different preparation for each be outlined. If we are to proceed with the idea that certain fundamental preparation in administration and teaching is needed for each executive officer, we will still assume that whether the positions are separated or the authority vested in one individual, the academic preparation will differ only in its emphasis. Much interest has been manifested in discussing the wisdom of the separation of these two main functions by the appointment of two individuals rather than one, as is the prevailing custom. No doubt we have not yet sufficient information upon which to express a worth-while opinion, but we are inclined to think that where experiments have been made, the results have justified the experiment. It is obviously apparent that much will depend on personalities, and the carefulness and accuracy with which the organization and the functions of each position are described and carried out. The principle of separating the school as an educational institution from the hospital as a nursing service is pedagogically sound, but the separation of the director of the school from the actual field in which the practice of nursing is carried on may be subject to a difference of opinion. The nursing service of the hospital primarily functions for the care of the patients, and carries inherent in it a community responsibility, and should not be unduly handicapped in its efficiency by problems which are wholly concerned with nursing education. Where the school and hospital are separated, it is most essential that the executive positions be filled by two individuals who have a similar background of education, resulting in a common understanding of what is owing to the student nurse for a sound and adequate education, and what is owing to the community for the most effective and satisfactory care of its patients. Academic and administrative responsibilities are bound together in each of the positions, and only the closest working relation and impersonal understanding will result in developing each unit on its most efficient level. Connected with such an organization questions of authority arise relating to such items as salaries, housing, and staff appointments, while innumerable ethical subjects constantly present themselves for discussion. "A miniature world court" in the form of a policy making committee on which both sides of the organization are represented, will provide a bridge of connection and will assist in promoting harmony while it will safeguard the integrity of each division. Such an organization can be developed only where the responsibilities of the positions are held in trust as more sacred, and of greater value, than the prestige of the individual who holds the position, and where each has the ability to differentiate between that which is of lasting, or only of immediate importance, or between an opinion and a principle. With such safeguards as have been described thrown around these positions, it seems reasonable to assume that unquestionably the ideal organization would be the separation of these two important positions by the appointment of women thoroughly prepared by experience and education to cope with the immediate problems concerned with the development of a school on the one hand, and on the other, the daily and perplexing problems concerned with the administration of a nursing service for the care of patients. Perhaps no factor can be more inhibiting to long range vision and clear thinking in the promotion of ideals and plans for the future than the daily, harassing, distressing needs which are thrust at every turn upon the superintendent of nurses, and it is well for the school when someone else, less constantly burdened, has its interest in her keeping, and has the vision to think and plan beyond the immediate, and outside the walls of the hospital.

Through the several studies made by the Education Committee it is evident that special preparation is desirable for each official position on the nursing school and nursing service staffs. Whether it is taken during service by means of special courses and institutes, or previous to service in blocks of study for long stretches of time, cannot be determined by arbitrary means. Circumstances such as previous education and background, professional advantages, available resources, must be taken into consideration in individual cases, but it must be borne in mind that no student can make the best of her opportunities for study who is overwhelmed and burdened, both physically and mentally, with the daily and immediate responsibilities of a taxing school and hospital position.

(Taylor, 1931, pp. 154–168)

Through Improvements in the Educational Process

By Myrtle P. Hodgkins, R.N.

Instructor and Supervisor, University of Minnesota School of Nursing, Minneapolis, Minnesota

To express in a little different way the question of what we are doing to improve nursing practice through improvements in the educational process, we might ask what is being done to give the student a keener awareness and deeper understanding of the science and art of nursing. This applies to every phase of her work: observing symptoms, executing procedures, treating mental attitudes, and educating the patient. During the past ten years we have been trying to replace the "training school" with the "school of nursing." To many this has meant merely a change of name; and I sometimes wonder if this change of name should be so promiscuously encouraged. The difference is, after all, fundamental, and unless the policies of the school are such that it can offer a truly educational program, it must still be a training school. Its students through repetition learn to carry out procedures perhaps skillfully but nevertheless automatically, to execute mechanically the orders given by the doctor, but if asked by a patient what would happen if she should ignore the treatment outlined for her, the student's answer would very likely be, "The doctor would be extremely angry." The students in the school of nursing, on the other hand, are taught the basic sciences before beginning their work with patients, and before they are allowed to apply the knowledge so gained they must fully understand the significance of each step in the work which they are about to do.

During this brief discussion we shall not speak of the training school—whether it still be known as such or masquerading under the misleading name "school of nursing." We shall confine our thoughts to the questions of what improvements are being made in those schools which have always formed the vanguard of nursing education. What are they doing in order to assure to the student a clear conception of the underlying principles of her work, thus enabling her to do the health teaching that becomes her responsibility as a nurse?

For a number of years greatest emphasis has been given to classroom instruction. More and more hours of the curriculum are being spent in acquiring the scientific knowledge which is essential to intelligent nursing, until now we find in the better schools a minimum of eight hundred and, in some schools, over fifteen hundred hours being spent in the classroom. In the practice of nursing classes the underlying principles of each procedure are discussed, and the procedure demonstrated by the instructor and by the student. On the ward, when the procedure is done for the first time, and thereafter as many times as is deemed necessary, the instructor is at the bedside to give any necessary assistance.

I use the word assistance with deliberation. The student has, during her classroom hours, learned isolated facts. For her at the time they have little significance as bearing directly upon her work as a nurse. The power of transfer of the average student nurse is no greater than that of a student of any other branch of learning. It is very limited. It is difficult for her to appreciate that she is gaining knowledge for later practical application; she is motivated far more strongly by a desire for a good grade in that one individual course. Not until she is actually caring for her patients does she organize that knowledge and use it to give meaning to her nursing. Not even then does she make a successful transfer unless she is given assistance and direction by an instructor on the ward. We are apt very glibly to say that the ward is the laboratory where the student nurse applies the theory which she has been taught in the classroom. But into what scientific laboratory would a school send its students with no other direction and assistance than the knowledge gained in the lecture hall and reference library? And yet how much more important it is for student nurses to have competent and constant instruction in their clinical experience where their laboratory material is human life! It seems to me that our attention must swing once more from the classroom to the ward. We have taken it for granted that the student will absorb every detail of knowledge poured into her ears by six to a dozen instructors—knowledge entirely new to her at a time when she is perhaps making an adjustment to a completely

different environment and new way of living. Not only this, but more—
we have expected her to make a successful transfer of this knowledge,
thus enabling her to make the best possible practical application of it
in the care of her patients. The ward has been a laboratory without an
instructor; the student has been left to experiment by trial and error
or success, until finally after three years she has if intelligent been able
to learn something perhaps of the skill of nursing.

The weakest link in the chain of educational facilities in the leading
schools of nursing today is ward instruction. The head nurse on the
ward is extremely busy with the duties of administration. She has no
time to assist the students on the floor, no opportunity to give the
valuable suggestions which would help the student so much, no time
for planned personal conferences nor the correcting of written material,
and no time for the study and reading which are necessary to the
teaching of a science so rapidly developing and constantly changing.
A ward instructor freed of all administrative responsibility is essential to
the educational program of each teaching department. Miss Goodrich
expresses this thought in her book, "The Social and Ethical Significance
of Nursing," when she states in speaking of the educational program
on the ward, "such a program as I have suggested obviously demands
instructors with a comprehensive general and professional preparation
and highly specialized in their subject. It entails supervision, bedside
instruction, and case conferences—again time-consuming and costly
program—but of vital importance to the student and to her present
and future patients."

In this new program of ward instruction the effort for improvement
should be made in two phases of the work. First, the concept of
supervision must be modified from that of inspection and criticism to
that of direction and assistance. Is there one among us who does as
good work under a critical eye as when she can be assured of a friendly
spirit of coöperation between herself and the instructor? In the past we
have nurtured in our students from the first the fear and awe of their
supervisors. There are few students who feel that they can take their
personal problems—daily joys and sorrows, questions and difficulties—
to those people to whom in reality they should feel closest. Much
opportunity for inspiring the student nurse with the challenge and
spirit of glorious adventure in the field of nursing education is lost
because of this fearful barrier between student and instructor. Supervisors and instructors should carefully analyze their jobs. What should
be their aim, and how should they set about to attain it? In what way

can they do the very most for the student? In the first place they must cease to think of their work as that of detecting flaws in the work of the students, of merely checking, inspecting, reminding, and reprimanding. As soon as they themselves conceive of their duties in a different light, the student will detect the change in relationship and will be able to help them by giving them the opportunity to help her. If the student can feel assured that she will not be considered inefficient and stupid if she asks for suggestions, she will feel free to make her problem known and receive the assistance to which as a student she is entitled. She will no longer be working under the constant tension and fear which, in the opinion of one physician who has made considerable study of tuberculosis among student nurses and young graduates, are important factors in breaking down her resistance to the disease. The supervisor should inspire in her students the feeling that she has confidence and faith in their high aspirations and is anxious to help them realize their highest hopes and aims. Professor John Dewey, in speaking of the relation between teacher and pupil, says: "The philosophy of the pedagogue is eloquent about the duty of the teacher in instructing pupils; it is almost silent regarding his privilege of learning. It emphasizes the influence of intellectual environment upon the mind; it slurs over the fact that the environment involves a personal sharing in common experiences. It exaggerates beyond reason the possibilities of consciously formulated and used methods, and underestimates the rôle of vital, unconscious, attitudes. It insists upon the old, the past, and passes lightly over the operations of the genuinely novel and unforeseeable. It takes, in brief, everything educational into account save its essence—vital energy seeking opportunity for effective exercise." Again, another time, he states, "It is that no thought, no idea, can possibly be conveyed as an idea from one person to another. . . . Only by wrestling with the conditions of the problem at first hand, seeking and finding his own way out, does he think. When the parent or teacher has provided the conditions which stimulate thinking and has taken a sympathetic attitude toward the activities of the learner by entering into a common or conjoint experience, all has been done which a second party can do to instigate learning. The rest lies with the one directly concerned. . . . We can and do supply ready-made 'ideas' by the thousand; we do not usually take much pains to see that the one learning engages in significant situations where his own activities generate, support, and clinch ideas. This does not mean that the teacher is to stand off and look on; the alternative to furnishing ready-made subject matter and listening to the accuracy with which it is reproduced is not quiescence, but participation, sharing, in an activity. In such shared activity, the teacher is a learner, and the learner is, without knowing it, a teacher—and upon the whole, the less consciousness there is, on either side, of either giving or receiving instruction, the better." When the student feels that instructor and student are both working together for a common end—the prevention and treatment of disease—at that time will the first step have been taken in making the ward experience the valuable adjunct to classroom teaching which it should be but at present falls far short of being.

With this attitude established, the ward instructor can carry on a program which will be truly educational. This instruction will emphasize the correlation of the knowledge already learned and its application at the bedside. I should like to say in passing that the program of study discussed in the remainder of this paper is based upon actual experience which I have had first in the Army School of Nursing, where such a program was developed and successfully carried out in each of the hospital departments, and at the present time in the University of Minnesota School of Nursing, where I am finding it of practical value on the medical service at the Minneapolis General Hospital.

A few years ago our leading educators in nursing were urging a new method of assignment of duties for the student nurse on a given ward. The advantages of the case form of assignment are no longer a theory. Those who have seen the functionings of both methods have had an opportunity to appreciate the increased interest and knowledge of the student working under the new system—none of us would for a moment consider returning to the methods of ten years ago.

The very fact, however, that in giving to the student the full responsibility of the patient we have kindled for her a keener interest in her work, requires that that interest be rewarded with new opportunity for deeper understanding through directed and correlated study. Some hospitals, in a few of their departments, have been able to make a very successful correlation between classroom lectures and ward experience. The doctor's lectures and nursing classes have been given for only those students assigned to the service, and have been repeated as often as there has been a change of the student group. This means, of course, that some students perhaps have been caring for patients for a period before they have had the class material in those particular diseases, but this is far better than the situation existing in most schools, in which there are many instances where the student has her organized study many months after she has completed her assignment to the department where she has had her clinical experience in that subject. By planning the program of clinical experience in such a way as to study first those diseases entailing the most scientific understanding and the most detailed nursing care, the care of the patients will be safeguarded and at the same time the student will have the advantage of caring for patients suffering from the diseases concerning which she is studying. Is there any question but that knowledge acquired at the time when the need for it is felt most keenly and when it can be immediately applied, is most easily learned and longest remembered? The fact that classes held on the individual services are conducted for only a small group of students increases their value considerably. In a small group the instructor can understand the individual differences of her students and so give more valuable assistance to each, and the students always feel much more free to take part in the discussions of the cases. This method of teaching, were it possible throughout the education of the student nurse, would place nursing education in the lead of other forms of learning. The obstacles presented to such a program are many and serious. Can they be overcome? There is the problem of the time involved in repeating the theory so frequently. If the physician who gives the lecture is paid only a nominal sum, the question is also one of money; if his services are volunteered, there is even less chance that he will be willing to take more time from his patients, no matter how interested he may be in nursing education. The answer to this problem will vary with each hospital. With thought and effort an improvement can surely be made over the existing policy. Surely some arrangement can be made whereby the classroom work will always precede or be concurrent with the clinical experience—never follow.

The question of classes in nursing should be a more simple one. Granted that on each service there is an instructor, her program should include classes in nursing for the group assigned to her, and repeated as frequently as the group changes. Whether all the students in a department should change at the same time is a debatable question and depends to a considerable degree upon the number of graduate nurses in the department who can stabilize the nursing service at such a time. In schools where the time on a service is divided into two assignments, one group of ward classes might be given for juniors and one for seniors, making their assignment of patients correspond to the class work given, the date of assignment of the two groups varying slightly in order to make an easier situation in the department. Care must be taken, however, that the assignments to services, including those in medicine and surgery, are not so short and correspondingly numerous that an organized program is made impossible.

Another problem is that of night duty. A program of classes cannot very easily be maintained for the student who spends on night duty perhaps half of her assignment to a department. There are, however, other factors which are tending to decrease the length of time spent by students on night duty. The question of lack of constant supervision during this time is one which is making the value of night duty seriously questioned. Again the need of graduate nurses in the hospital is emphasized.

Still another obstacle which presents a serious problem is that of the number of duty hours for the student. If she is to gain most from these ward classes she must give considerable time to their preparation. These classes should not be conducted in the form of lectures—information showered upon the students by the instructor—but rather should they be a pooling and crystallizing of the ideas and observations of the entire group—those gained from clinical experience and from the reference material assigned by the instructor. They should correspond more closely to the seminars of advanced work in any phase of education, conducted by the students under the direction of the instructor. Only in this way can they be of lasting value to the student. The present heavy schedule of the student nurse, however, allows no time for such study. Her eight hours of duty should include not only the time spent in class but also some time for the study of clinical material on the ward and in the preparation of class and written assignments. This again means the employment of an increased number of graduate nurses— a very excellent way of using the profits which Dean Lyon has told us are brought by the school of nursing to the hospital. There are some who will argue that the first duty of the nurse—graduate or student— is to the patient. For this reason she should not be taken from a busy ward for a period of ward classes. But it is necessary to keep in mind that we are preparing the student for the future. If she can by spending a number of hours (an average perhaps of four hours a week) in specifically learning how to care for her patients most intelligently, is there any question but that time so spent is more valuable to patients as a group—present and future—than would be the same length of time spent in questionable care for the patients then on the service? The greatest good for the largest number must be our motivating thought.

The material for ward classes should include enough of a review in the anatomy, physiology, and pathology of the part involved to form a basis for discussion of symptoms, including any physical and laboratory findings of significance to the nurse; symptoms indicative of complications; special treatments; diet; and, most important of all, the nursing art as particularly applied to each individual disease and the preventative aspects of that disease. Wall charts, laboratory specimens, X-ray plates, and pamphlets should be used to increase the effectiveness of the material presented. Case studies and bedside clinics should always be used to make the correlation and application complete. Where the classes should be held is a matter of some importance. Psychologically the correlation is much more strongly felt if they can be held somewhere on the ward—preferably in light airy room supplied with conference table, shelves of reference books, blackboard, and bed for demonstration purposes. It should be insisted that the students not be interrupted during class hour for ward responsibilities.

The program would necessarily vary somewhat with each department. In addition to ward classes there might well be included short topics given by instructor or student at morning circle. The value to the student giving such a topic can be considerable, but in order to be sure that the subject will be adequately covered and that the information given will be accurate it is very essential that the instructor previously confer with the student about it. Bedside clinics by the medical staff should form an important part of the program, as should also post-mortem study of cases from the department. Planned personal conferences between student and instructor should have an important place in this program. In this way the student can learn before it is time for her to leave the service of any phase of her work which needs improvement or development, and suggestions made to give her assistance in effecting the desired change. Difficulties and problems of the students may be discussed and help given to overcome them. A clear understanding of each student by the instructor is necessary for her greatest possible growth.

And so in review we see a student assigned for a definite period of time—that period to be of sufficient length to allow an organized program of class work—to a department where the atmosphere is one of cöoperation between doctor and nurse, both graduate and student, all working for the ultimate welfare of the patient, the prevention and treatment of disease. There will be an instructor in the department freed of administrative responsibilities who can spend most of her time with the students giving them assistance and direction. A program of classes, clinics, and planned personal conferences, with correlated reference and written work, allows the student to appreciate the opportunity to integrate and apply the knowledge gained as isolated facts in the classroom to the intelligent care of her patients. There are many phases of the educational process which have not been even touched in this discussion. The one which has been considered is, I believe, the one least thought of in the past but one to which we must give our sincere attention if the clinical phase of the course in nursing is to be of real value to the student.

(*Hodgkins, 1932, pp. 198–206*)

Section II
Control of Practice

Introduction to Control of Practice

A major goal for the newly formed Superintendents' Society focused on nursing education reforms as a means for achieving competent practice. Disparities in the quality of available educational models created similar disparities in the quality of nursing service. Nurses who graduated from inferior programs practiced under the same title as, and in direct competition with, those from the more prestigious schools. Yet the public remained unaware that differences existed.

During its formative years, the Superintendents' Society sought to establish educational requirements acceptable to the schools it represented. Those criteria constituted the first steps toward more scientific and systematic practice, and formed the basis for legal credentialing in nursing. Through unified effort and the implementation of sound educational standards, nursing took responsibility for and control of its practice.

Over time, issues surfaced that required deliberate attention. For example, most graduate nurses engaged in private duty work frequently obtained their assignments through directories or registries. Issues related to private duty centered on the establishment of fees, how the fees should be determined and by whom, pay equity with male counterparts, and who should control the registries. Other control issues of the period focused on the attainment of registration laws, implementation of an eight-hour work day, and the recognition of public health nursing as a distinct practice field.

When the Superintendents' Society became the NLNE in 1912, initiatives and strategies begun earlier continued with the same degree of commitment. The papers that follow address many of the significant practice issues faced by the superintendents during the late 19th and early 20th centuries. Although the effects of World War I and the devastating influenza epidemic of 1918 are interwoven in later presentations, of overriding significance is the dedication and self-determination of nurses to control and improve their practice for the benefit of society.

Directories for Nurses

By Miss L. L. Dock

In undertaking to present a paper on "Directories for Nurses," it is with no assumption of special knowledge on the subject, or wish to figure as one having claim to authoritative views, but rather with the hope simply of starting discussion and having light thrown on this practical and important branch of work by the contribution of experience that you will be able to make.

Of actual practical work in the management of nurses' registries I have had none, and of direct observation but little. I do not, therefore, intend to go into technical details, but will ask for a brief consideration of two or three general principles, which seem to me to underlie the work, and which, though as yet perhaps dormant in some minds, will, I believe finally dominate the situation and receive general acceptance. The first is this:

It should be for nurses themselves to fix the rates of payment charged in private duty, and to state these rates to the registry—not the registry to the nurses. This principle is already acknowledged to some extent, and the fact that it is so, marks the last one of an interesting series of modifications, traceable from the beginning of trained nursing to the present time.

The trained nurse of to-day is an evolution from the sister of orders of the church, and the organization and methods of community life, where all needful is done for the individual who, during her life, gives her work, but has no individual liberty allowed her; these were, naturally enough, the models from which the first systems of secular nursing took pattern. Notice, for instance, how closely copied from the sisterhood plan are some of the more conservative German training schools of to-day. The nurses belong to them during lifetime under one arrangement or another, and for the time when no longer able to work, an elaborate pension system is planned with the precision of paternal government. The English training schools present further modifications, though still holding strongly to the idea that at no time must the nurse be a really independent being, but after graduation should rather remain in some more or less protected and dependent relation. When nursing was established in this country, a still further departure from the community idea was taken. The graduate nurse stood free and independent, unbound by promises or obligations to any institution. Her earnings were her own, and she might live where she pleased. One trace only of the early idea now remained, and it is this: The training school undertook to provide her with cases (for which privilege she paid yearly a trifling sum), but as to the rate at which she should be paid, she had nothing to say. This was fixed for her, and from year to year has been handed down until it has acquired the character of an unwritten law, which it would be almost impossible to break.

A distinct shock at first accompanies the thought of a nurse charging more than the regulation twenty or twenty-five dollars a week, yet undoubtedly this last survival of a former condition is beginning to be felt an anachronism, and will soon be discarded, for, when one comes to candid consideration of the question, it is, of course, clear that no one person, or set of persons, can be found to possess an inherent right to say what any other person, or set of persons, shall work for.

I would not seem to fail in appreciation of what has been done for nursing and nurses by these primary methods. The utmost gratitude and recognition are due to those who did so much, not only to train the nurse, but afterward to secure her a just remuneration, yet while believing that their views and plans were the best possible at that time, the natural course of events and daily progress convince one that there will be further changes. Teachers on economics tell us that while the minimum rate in wages and salaries should be fixed, the maximum should remain open and subject to variation.

One takes for granted that no fully trained nurse will undersell another below a fixed point. It is also understood that to a certain extent the law of supply and demand will always tend to equalize nurses' rates. May it not also be freely granted that a nurse has a perfect right to charge a higher rate than usual—if her opportunities or ability can command it?

The second principle I would advocate grows out of the first, and it is this: The woman who nurses ought to be paid equally with the man who nurses. We all know that men—even untrained ones—who nurse, command higher rates than women, while those who are trained charge from five to seven dollars a day. Now, without intending to express any unfriendliness to men nurses (for they are useful in their place, and many patients need them), I yet believe that nurses should strongly disapprove and resent this state of things. The old argument that women must be content to be underpaid, because they take men's work away from them, will not hold here, for it has always been undisputed that nursing is peculiarly a woman's work. Nor can it be maintained that a man must be paid more because he supports a family, for the young men in training schools have no families, but usually make nursing a stepping-stone to medicine, while on the other hand, how many nurses do we not all now who help to keep the home for a father or mother, or educate a younger sister, or give a young brother his start in life? No. This inequality exists, but neither of these reasons explain why it exists, and not until nurses themselves learn to take control of their affairs will it be different.

The principle of self-government lies at the bottom of all we do, but how far we are from carrying out this principle in practice! Our fault in this regard, it is needless to say, arises from the lack of organization, and with the advance of organization it will gradually disappear. To education along this line we must look for that strengthening of our professional spirit which will impel graduates to unify and guard and discipline themselves as carefully as we do our under-graduates, and which will make of private duty nurses a highly organized branch of the service, governed by its own codes, pruned of unworthy members by its own votes, and managed as to its business affairs by its own representatives. The need of strict discipline among private duty nurses is great, and just because it is so, it is difficult for any unprofessional element to enforce it. It seems probable that in time, and from loyalty to a standard, nurses will voluntarily place themselves under a more rigid set of rules in regard to private duty than they will submit to when some other governing body imposes them. They have much to learn in this regard. Some of the comments lately made in "The Trained Nurse" upon my first article on Directories show plainly the one-sided short-sighted views held by many nurses, and their need of enlightenment.

For the standard by which to measure the proper regulations of directories may be taken (with modification as suggested, which time will bring) the dignified and exclusive methods of some of our training school directories. All minor methods, and heterogeneous systems, such as those in vogue in various towns, the directory run by unprofessionals, the directory at the drug store, the directory under the control of the medical society, are to be condemned. They break down professional pride and tend to disintegration, and what we need is to *unite,* and, in uniting, to avoid all appearance of similarity to the intelligence office. Where one good school directory covers the ground, nothing more will be necessary, and in large cities where convenience to the public is an important consideration, would it not be practicable to establish one central directory in which the different schools would unite, and which might stand to them all in the relation of the central post-office to the sub-stations?

It might be so managed that convenience to the public would reach a high state of perfection, and also that the needs of the nursing profession would receive due attention. This seems to be the only way in which graduate nurses can hope to own themselves, as it were, and to avoid scattering, and the appropriation of themselves by various non-professional organizations.

I do not attempt to enter into details, but leave these suggestions to what fate they deserve.

(*Dock, 1897, pp. 57–60*)

Nursing in the Smaller Hospitals and in Those Devoted to the Care of Special Forms of Disease

By Mrs. Hunter Robb

Formerly Superintendent of Johns Hopkins Hospital Training School

If I have to begin with an apology, and ask you not to criticize too sharply the crudeness of the paper which I shall present to you to-day, I cannot nevertheless accept the entire responsibility, for I feel that the fault lies also partly with circumstances and partly with our esteemed chairman. The subject was first assigned to Miss Palmer, but she found her time so occupied on assuming the duties of superintendent of the Rochester City Hospital that she wrote that it was impossible for her to prepare the paper. Our chairman in casting about for a substitute and knowing my good nature of old, has taken an unfair advantage of that knowledge. While I feel that she has conferred an honor by putting this task upon me, I am convinced that I have assumed a burden which is too heavy for me. The subject is one upon which I would speak gladly only after months of careful study. But it is too important and far-reaching to be touched upon lightly and in the short time at my disposal I have not been able to grapple with it with any great satisfaction to myself.

The question of providing nursing in the smaller hospitals and in those devoted to the care of special forms of disease is not a new one. I am sure that many of us in days gone by, as well as at the present time, have turned and are still turning the problem over and over in our minds. We have pondered it in the night season, and have had it with us as a continuous underlying current of thought through our busy working hours. For there is no doubt that this class of nursing goes far towards the making or undoing of our present system of caring for the sick both inside and outside of hospitals; its influence is far-reaching, and largely by the results obtained in these institutions will the profession of nursing rise or fall. It is, therefore, a problem that demands our most careful consideration and deliberation; it is not to be taken up lightly or passed over hastily, but discussed carefully and kept before us until, as a convention, we are satisfied that the system of nursing in other than our large general hospitals has been made as perfect as possible.

We will first take a brief survey of this class of institutions and then consider their work and influence upon the nursing profession and their relation to the large hospitals.

In making up our list of hospitals we find that we have, indeed, a varied selection. There is the small general hospital, hospitals for children, for the general diseases of women, for women and children, for obstetrical cases, for gynaecological cases, and private hospitals for the insane. Again we have hydrotherapeutic establishments, special hospitals for the carrying out of the rest cure and for the treatment of nervous disorders, private hospitals and sanitariums, hospitals in connection with large industrial enterprises, factories, railroads and mines, emergency hospitals, hospitals for infectious and contagious diseases and those devoted to diseases of the eye, ear and throat. But, besides these hospitals, we have another large class of institutions which provides homes for the poor and feeble and which necessarily have wards connected with them. These are called by various names, such as homes and infirmaries, but inasmuch as part at least of their work is connected with the nursing of the sick, they are to be considered in this respect as hospitals.

Hospitals of one kind or another would then appear to be almost numerous enough. They form a network which reaches from ocean to ocean and from the north to the extreme south of the land. But it may be said that while the number of large hospitals hardly exceeds one hundred, the smaller are many times as numerous.

The existence of these small and special hospitals are the outcome of various factors. Some have been founded from pure philanthropy or as memorials of departed friends; others are the monuments of wealthy people, who wish to perpetuate their names, and in a country where fortunes are made as rapidly as in America this form of bequest is not unusual. Others, again, are integral parts of medical schools or universities, and their existence is demanded by the medical professors as necessary adjuncts to medical instruction. But, perhaps, a larger class still is the result of specialization among physicians, who open private hospitals, or so-called sanitariums, in which their own particular class of patients is cared for.

A study of the past and present history of hospitals, and more especially those of the last class, goes to show that the possibility of establishing and carrying on so many various hospitals and the continuous increase in their numbers is in a large measure due to the present system of nursing. Previous to the organization of Training Schools for Nurses, and for some years after, we find comparatively few hospitals in existence; but with the advent and success of the trained nurse the question of providing for the proper care of the sick in hospitals was solved, and forthwith we find both physicians and laymen rushing into hospital construction, with the result that we have numbers of hospitals in operation to-day, with much to be grateful for in connection with them and not a few things to deplore.

Of those with which we are dealing at present, the small general hospital probably ranks first in point of usefulness, as it opens its doors at one time or another to all of the diseases for which the special hospitals are designed. Certainly, last in rank comes the private hospital or sanitarium, opened by the specialist for his own particular patients and for his own personal profit.

That any kind of a hospital which does its duty by its patients has a perfect right to exist would seem to be beyond question. Nevertheless it must be insisted that each owes a duty to the public as well and must be open to commendation or censure, according to the system employed in providing proper nursing for its sick. Upon investigation we find several methods employed. Some have organized training schools or offer a post-graduate course to nurses from the smaller schools. Others, again, employ graduate trained nurses. In a few co-operative nursing is established, one school undertaking the care of two or more hospitals. Still others are under the care of religious orders, and a few employ a corps of paid attendants who have never attended any regular school.

These various hospitals we may divide into three groups:

(1) The small general hospital or cottage hospital, containing from fifty to seventy-five or one hundred beds. Hospitals for children, for women and children, lying-in hospitals, hospitals for gynae-cological diseases, for nervous disorders and for rest cure cases.

(2) The very small general hospital, providing from six to forty beds. Sanitariums, hydrotherapeutic establishments, hospitals for

infectious and contagious diseases, emergency hospitals, institutions for the insane, railroad and similar hospitals, and eye, ear and throat infirmaries.

(3) Infirmaries and homes. Hospitals for incurables.

With but few exceptions it will be found that the nursing in the first and second groups is done by training schools established in connection with each hospital. With many of the institutions in the third group we also find training schools; others, again, are cared for by paid attendants by the post-graduate system and by paid trained nurses.

But, unfortunately, in all of the groups, dozens or even hundreds of hospitals are met with containing only from six to ten or twenty beds, and yet maintaining training schools for nurses. The well-known circular of information is sent out offering apparently the same advantages as the larger schools. The course of instruction covers two years; the pupils must be of a certain age, though frequently they are taken as young as eighteen; they have certain hours on duty, time for rest and recreation. It would appear also they have the same classes and lectures, for, according to the prospectus, they are instructed "in the general care of the sick, making beds, changing bed and body linen, giving baths, dressing bed sores, making bandages, in the application of fomentations and of poultices, in cupping, leeching" and other accomplishments. We meet again and again the same old list, but whether it means much or little, or less than nothing, it is often impossible to say. Certainly for the uninitiated and ignorant woman who knows nothing of hospitals it is a fine bait. But as an addition we have the statement that after the probation month the pupil will receive each month for the first year a certain number of dollars and an increased number of dollars monthly for the second year, and this ostensibly to cover the cost of uniform and text books. Finally examinations are held and certificates of qualification are presented. But when one reads in the "Trained Nurse" such statements as this, "Two nurses graduated from the ———— hospital with all honors," one certainly is justified in inferring that honors were easy in such cases.

Now why is it that all these small and special hospitals adopt this method of nursing, and offer such inducements, and why is it that the demand is supplied by so many women? In the first place competition is so great in these days that the public demands, and rightly so, to be well taken care of. Again, physicians know that with trained nursing their results will be better and will not lend their names or allow themselves to be connected with any institution that is apparently lacking in this respect. A third and most potent reason is the fact that training schools are cheaper and the pupils are easier to manage than graduate nurses. In fact, in many instances the pupils are a source of distinct profit, for in some of these schools they are required not only to do the hospital nursing, but are also sent out to private duty, sometimes for weeks at a time, during their two years' service, while the $10 or $15 per week which they earn goes towards the support of the hospital and school, and in some instances forms quite a large item. This is perfectly well known, despite the fact that one never reads of the nurses as financial benefactors, all the glory and honor of that kind going to the managing body of the institution.

Perhaps the best excuse which could be urged in defense of the system is that more and better work and a stricter discipline are possible in a training school than can be obtained where graduate trained nurses or attendants are employed.

Again, the apparently liberal offer of an education and compensation at the same time attracts women, good, bad and indifferent, in sufficiently large numbers to keep the vacancies filled, if one is not over particular as to requirements. And perhaps it is too much to expect that a woman who has never seen the inside of a hospital should be competent to differentiate between the different grades of schools and their advantages. The compensation is also an added inducement, and she may not realize that for a present small gain she is sacrificing future higher professional standing and better opportunities. I must add also that people have not yet quite got over the habits of thinking that if a woman is a failure at everything else she is at least fit to go into a hospital and become a nurse, and unfortunately it happens that, although such an incompetent has no possible chance for entrance into the general hospital school, she is still received with open arms into the private and special hospitals.

The small general hospital, with fifty beds or more, is generally justified in having attached to it an organized training school. The so-called cottage hospitals found in the smaller cities or in thickly populated country districts have a comparatively wide scope. They meet a need which can be supplied in no other way, and their usefulness is at once apparent. One occasionally reads, in the nursing magazines, short articles in favor of the training afforded by these cottage hospitals as compared with that obtainable in a large general hospital in the city. It is argued that the nurse is better equipped for her work in that she comes into more direct contact with her superintendent and the physicians, and also because from the very smallness of the field she is able to study and become well acquainted with any case that is of peculiar importance. But certainly it would appear that if a large general training school is properly systematized and managed, it must naturally follow that the pupil gets all and a great deal more than she can in a small hospital. Where this is not the case there is something wrong with the management of the larger school. As a proof that pupils from the smaller hospitals do not always find their training sufficient, superintendents of the larger general schools could tell how often application is made to them by graduates from these, as well as from schools belonging to special hospitals, stating that they wish for a larger and more varied experience. We know, however, that many of our small general training schools do excellent work and turn out competent graduates. Where they are offered by graduates from larger general training schools, who are good managers and disciplinarians, and are enthusiastic in their work, every opportunity is seized and utilized for the advantage of the pupils, who can thus secure a thorough and fairly wide training. Again, when the nurse has graduated she often finds her field of work right in the town or surrounding country where she is among friends.

The amount of good accomplished by these cottage hospitals, both within and without their walls, is inestimable. They fill a long filled want and rob illness in town and country of half its terrors, and are of unspeakable comfort to the physicians, who are usually their promoters and warm supporters.

In some instances, particularly in hospitals connected with churches, we find the nursing done by members of religious orders, sisters or deaconesses. For some reasons it seems to me to be regretted that in some church hospitals the sisters are giving up this branch of their work in favor of nurses and are establishing training schools in connection with these institutions. Might it not possibly be better that a certain per cent. of the sisters should be regularly instructed in nursing, so that from their number a permanent staff of skilled workers would always be obtainable?

Turning to the remainder of the first group, which are all established for the care of some particular class of patients, we find, alas, that training schools again abound, and the same attractive circulars are being issued for the enlightenment of applicants. With few exceptions, these hospitals are established in cities and therefore cannot plead isolation. No doubt women who enter these schools become well grounded in the care of one particular class of patients and their diseases, but it is absurd to claim that she graduates from there with a thorough, all-round training in both the practice and theory of her work, which would justify her in assuming the title of trained nurse. It is true that she may make the care of that particular disease her specialty and attempt nothing else, but even then, everything else being equal, she cannot long be as efficient even in this limited sphere as the graduate from the general hospital, who, aided by an intelligent and varied knowledge, supplemented by wide experience and practice, can speedily adapt herself to any particular class of cases. If we think of the future of the women who enter these hospitals, it would seem that but little can be said in justification of the managers of such hospitals in their position as organizers of training schools. We are compelled to think that the welfare of their pupil nurses with them is a matter of no importance. To have the patients well cared for with as little expense and friction and with as much ease as possible is their first consideration. Experience may have shown that this end can be most easily attained by establishing a training school, but we may well ask whether the means are justifiable. It is puerile to argue that the pupil nurse is a free agent and need not enter such a school or stay after she is there. But can we reasonably expect that a woman who is ignorant of hospitals and their methods can be in a position to differentiate between what is advisable or inadvisable, more especially when the institution has the support of many good names?

I do not mean that these special hospitals do not turn out some excellent nurses. I believe quite to the contrary, for there are always some women bright and clever enough to profit by their work no matter where they are placed; the greater the pity that their privileges are not broader and more complete. Many of these special hospitals undoubtedly fill distinct needs and it may be to the interest of both patients and science to have them in our midst. Children's hospitals, private hospitals for the carrying out of the rest cure and the treatment of nervous patients and separate hospitals for the insane are necessities. It does not, however, follow that they should each organize a training school, and that hospitals and sanitariums opened by individuals for their own private gain should have in connection with them training schools for nurses, is a condition worthy of the severest condemnation.

One especially glaring instance has just come under my notice. I have recently been told of a private special hospital owned by one man which accommodates thirty patients; his training school for nurses numbers twenty pupils. The promoter's sole plea is that he tried graduate nurses but they did so badly that he was obliged to open a school. These same graduates were no doubt products of institutions equally as bad as his own.

Such examples are repeated over and over again and yet graduates from such schools receive the same title and claim from the public and their fellows the same recognition awarded to trained nurses, who have given of their best time and strength to qualify themselves in well equipped schools to do their work thoroughly and be an honor to their profession. Every year these hospitals and graduates are on the increase until they threaten to take entire possession of the land. Right-minded, deep-thinking men and women among the laity who interest themselves in hospital work are averse to this system of multiplying small half-equipped training schools, and the question has been put to me, and I am sure to other superintendents many times, What other way is there? What else can be suggested which would seem to promote better results than those obtained by the methods now generally in vogue?

Exclusive of training schools we have five courses left open to us. The nursing could be undertaken (1) by the graduates of smaller schools willing to give their services in return for a post-graduate course under competent instructors, (2) by paid competent graduate nurses, (3) by attendants under the supervision of trained nurses, (4) by adopting the system of co-operative nursing, or (5) by members of religious orders, previously trained for these duties.

Of these various methods I would here, as in my paper on "Educational Standards for Nurses," make my special plea for co-operative nursing whenever such a scheme is feasible. This method I am happy to say has already been put into practice in some few schools. For nine years the Illinois Training School, of Chicago, has successfully provided for the nursing of two large institutions with its pupils, thereby adding largely to the experience and competency of the pupils and at the same time helping to elevate the standard of nursing work. It has also been for some years in operation in Milwaukee, and in 1894 we read that "a new system has been introduced into the Utica, N.Y., Hospital, whereby pupils from the Faxton Hospital Training School do the nursing." The writer adds, "The cost to the city is less than formerly even should twice the number of nurses be on duty there." The Emergency Hospital, of San Francisco, is provided for by pupils of the

Children's Hospital; of the Sloan Maternity, New York, by pupils from the New York Training School. In Washington the Columbia and Children's Hospital arranged to interchange pupils, and at one time there was a suggestion that the Garfield should unite with them. Certainly if such special hospitals, as those for children, women and children, lying-in hospitals, and hospitals for gynaecological and for nervous cases are so situated in the cities that they could operate with a general hospital or other institutions, they owe it to the women they take into their schools to do so. The first move must naturally come from the trustees or boards of management, but the actual success demands wholly upon the superintendents of the various schools, and now that we are getting on a more common plane as to teaching and requirements for entrance and graduation, the plan seems more feasible than before. But its accomplishment will require much patience and self-sacrifice on the part of some of our number and the only certain reward which I can offer to them is the feeling that they will have rendered possible the attainment of the greater good to the greater number.

Some special hospitals offer a post-graduate course to graduates from other schools who wish for further training. The weak point in this system lies in the fact that they cannot offer an all-round experience, and if a graduate from one special hospital enters another of a similar kind offering her a post-graduate course, she only adds to her experience the knowledge of one other special disease. Only when a woman has already a general training and then enters a post-graduate school for the sake of perfecting herself in the cure of one particular class of cases is the post-graduate course made use of in the right way; unless, as already suggested by Miss Davis in her paper on "A Post-Graduate Course," we can find some general hospital whose managers will be willing to organize its school on the post-graduate basis and thus offer opportunities for further development to all kinds of graduates.

Training schools in connection with hospitals for the insane are as yet few in number, but the tendency to increase them is growing and undoubtedly in the care of this class of patients there is room for much improvement. But can these hospitals any more than any special hospitals offer sufficient variety in nursing to produce all-round trained nurses? Experience shows that their graduates also try for admittance into general training schools and are willing to give two more years of their time without pay in order to gain more experience in their work. It would seem that the plan adopted by the superintendent of one hospital for the insane might be a good one, that is to appoint a certain number of trained nurses as supervisors and let their staff of assistants be paid permanent attendants. Such also might be the system in emergency hospitals, infirmaries and homes and hydrotherapeutic establishments. Hospitals for infectious diseases, the eye, ear and throat infirmaries should certainly be under the care of graduate trained nurses or else under the co-operative system.

Such plans as I have outlined are given to you in the way of suggestions. Some of them have been tried successfully. No doubt there remain others, still better, to be discovered. In any case it is a duty incumbent upon each trained nurse to use her efforts against the establishment of any more small half equipped schools and to use her efforts towards improving, where it is possible, those already in existence, and the strong distinction between thoroughly equipped schools and the half-equipped ones should be to put the best schools on a purely educational basis, withdraw the monthly allowance, increase the time of training, and in return offer a broad and liberal education to women who would become trained nurses.

The writer would beg in conclusion that any one who may read this paper will remember that it has been written entirely without prejudice or without any feeling of "looking down" upon the small or special schools. It is simply a plea for the broader and more liberal education of all who call themselves trained nurses. It is only meant as an effort to draw us as a profession nearer together, to place nursing the continent over on a distinct and sure basis beyond all questioning. It has been said that "the country is swarming with ill-paid stenographers who cannot spell or punctuate, with starving sewing-women who sew badly, with cooks who do not know how to cook, and in many cases with so-called trained nurses who are lacking in tact, good manners, and education." Some women are given the popular term "born nurses" when they are especially remarkable for good sense and adaptability; but we know that nurses are *made* not born, and the rule has but few exceptions, that it is the woman whose general education is the best who is able to do one particular thing best. If this be true in the simplest things, how much more is training required for work as complicated as nursing. Dr. Weir Mitchell says that a woman to be a nurse requires education, tact, good sense, good manners, and good health. Given all these requirements, and nothing less should be the standard, we owe it to such a woman in preparing her to be a trained nurse to give her the best that the work of nursing affords. By making this our standard, by lengthening the term of service and lessening the daily practical work, so that her brain may be in a good condition to understand the theory of nursing, and she may do her practical work with more understanding, and by bringing these small and special hospitals into line and touch with our large general schools we shall all be the gainers.

(*Robb, 1897b, pp. 59–68*)

What Has Been Accomplished in the Way of Legislation for Nurses

By Miss Mary W. McKechnie

Superintendent of the New York Infirmary for Women and Children

Within the past year, through the efforts of the State Nurses' Associations, bills for the regulation of professional nursing have been framed and introduced in the Legislatures of five States.

When we consider that it is only two years since concerted action toward this end really started, and at the time of the Congress of Nurses in Buffalo in 1901, the New York State Nurses' Association had barely taken shape, we have reason to be proud of the measure of success that has crowned these efforts, and of the results that have been attained.

Of the bills presented, only one, that of Illinois, has met with defeat; still the effort in this State cannot be said to have been entirely unsuccessful, for although the bill has failed to receive the Governor's signature, a brave fight has been made, and we hear that the good results of organization among nurses in Illinois, has alone been worth working for.

In these four bills the fundamental basis has been the same. Each has contained the following provisions arranged to conform with the existing laws governing other professional schools in these States; viz.—

1. Registration for Nurses and license to practice only on presentation of a certificate from a State board of examiners, and the right to use the distinguishing title of "Registered" or "Graduate" nurse.

2. A State board of examiners composed of nurses, selected from nominees from the State Nurses' Association, to be appointed by

the Governor of the State, with power to determine the standard of education and qualifications necessary in an applicant before entering upon the practice of professional nursing.

3. Penalties for infringement of these provisions and for false representation.

The States now having laws governing professional nursing are: New York, North Carolina and New Jersey.

The laws in force in these States enable any resident, 21 years of age, of good moral character, holding a diploma from a recognized training school for nurses, who shall receive from the State board of examiners a certificate of his or her qualifications to practice as a registered nurse to be known and called a registered nurse, and to use the letters R.N. after his or her name to indicate that he or she is a registered nurse, provided he or she shall first cause such certificate to be recorded in the County Clerk's office with affidavit of his or her identity and place of residence.

Examination waived. Nurses who have graduated before the passage of these laws, will upon recommendation of the board of examiners receive a certificate without examination.

Nurses in training at the time of the passage of these laws and who shall graduate afterwards, will upon recommendation of the board of examiners receive a certificate without examination.

Nurses that have had at least one year's experience in a general hospital and were practising nursing on the date of the passage of these laws, will upon recommendation of the State board of examiners receive a certificate without examination.

Practical examination. Those nurses who have been engaged in the actual practice of nursing before the passing of these laws, and who shall, within a specified time, satisfactorily pass an examination in practical nursing conducted by the State board of examiners, will receive a certificate.

In New York State full examination goes into effect January, 1906, and all those wishing to engage in the practice of nursing as registered nurses after this date will first require to pass an examination by the State board of examiners. In Virginia and North Carolina the law takes effect January 1st, 1904.

In the progress of these Bills through the intricacies of State Legislation much pruning and reconstructing has been necessary and many modifications have been made, but enough of the original remains to make us feel that some steps have been gained in the right direction.

Opposition encountered. In New York State the opposition came from the Buffalo Nurses' Association, a body of nurses opposed to the New York State Nurses' Association.

The objections raised were "that the medical profession was not recognized on the board of examiners" and "that the State Nurses' Association was not a representative body and should not have the exclusive right to nominate for appointments on the board of examiners."

The first objection was covered by the fact, that three physicians were to be found on the Board of Regents of the University of New York, and the second by the fine array of figures presented by the Nurses' Committee on Legislation showing that the State Nurses' Association represented one-half of all nurses practising in the State.

Objection to a minimum course of two years' training in connection with a general hospital, came from those persons interested in the large sanitariums in the State.

The Bill was amended to include "training schools connected with hospitals and sanitariums maintaining proper standards in this and other respects" acceptable to the Regents.

In New York State the Regents make the rules and regulations governing the examination of candidates and grant certificates.

The board of examiners advises the Regents in the making of rules and regulations and recommends candidates for licensing certificates.

Opposition in the other three States was mainly directed against the two years' course of training, and came from those having commercial interests in special and private hospitals, and from the "bogus nurse" schools giving a "short time" course of instruction.

In the North Carolina Bill the bad effect of this opposition is seen, in that no course of training in a hospital is required, and any applicant passing a satisfactory examination in the subjects given, is entitled to a certificate and license to practice. North Carolina has two physicians on the board of examiners.

New Jersey has gained nothing in the way of an educational standard, has no State board of examiners, and does not recognize the State Nurses' Association. New Jersey suffered from the influence of "short time" schools for nurses, received no support from the public press and little from the medical profession.

Although it is now a recognized fact in these States that special preparatory education and personal qualifications are necessary to fit a nurse for the practice of her profession, no standard of education has yet been defined. This is a question that will confront those whose duty it is to make rules and regulations for the examination of candidates.

It would seem fitting that this Society, which from the time of its organization has stood for better and higher standards of education for nurses, should take some definite action on this important subject before it adjourns, and I would suggest that a committee be appointed to outline what the Society considers the minimum requirements for registration in:—

1. Entrance examinations to schools of nursing, with definite requirements in education and personal qualifications.

2. A definite course of study, with minimum of subjects to be studied practically, and minimum length of course of training.

(McKechnie, 1904, pp. 62–65)

A General Presentation of the Statutory Requirements of the Different States

By Annie W. Goodrich, R.N.

Miss Goodrich. I think it is wonderful that we have come together in this great hall to-night at the end of only eleven years to discuss the question of legislation concerning the practice of nursing. I know of no feature in our progress that is more encouraging or more inspiring than our legislation. Are our laws, you say at once, so satisfactory? No, certainly not. They are conspicuously weak and inefficient in almost every state, but what does legislation evidence? It evidences organization, unity of purpose, strength, professional progress, and, above all, the establishment, to the satisfaction of the community, that this profession has a definite service to render to the race. As it is written on the statute books of one of our states—"An act to amend the public health law relative to the practice of nursing."

To go into all the details this evening of these statutory differences would take far too much time that could be more profitably devoted to discussion. Nor is it necessary that we should, for we can now refer to those who desire to make a study of these matters to various publications: The bulletin issued this year by the Board of Education in Washington; the Annual Report of the New York State Education Department, together with their pamphlets, such as the syllabus and the handbook containing a summary of the laws, etc.; Miss Louie Croft Boyd's "State Registration for Nurses," published by Saunders & Company and now under revision; and, for immediate study, to the comprehensive and interesting exhibit prepared for the convention by Miss Giles.

But in order that those who are not immediately in touch with our legislation may have a clear understanding of the papers to be presented, I beg to submit certain statistics, together with a brief outline of the statutory requirements and results already obtained.

We had some difficulty in getting information. A questionnaire was sent out. Possibly some of the copies did not go to the right authorities, but I am very grateful to the many who did reply and I naturally feel that I am, perhaps, greatly at fault myself, because in the many phases of work that came up this last winter unexpectedly I was unable to give it the attention of which it was worthy.

There are now laws regulating the practice of nursing on the statute books of thirty-three states, seven of which are compulsory; that is to say, they forbid the practice of any person as a graduate, trained, or registered nurse without a license. The others are permissive only "who may practice as a registered nurse." They were obtained in the following order: in 1903, four—North Carolina, New Jersey, New York, and Virginia; in 1904, one—Maryland; 1905, four—Indiana, California, Colorado, and Connecticut; in 1907, seven—New Hampshire, District of Columbia, Iowa, West Virginia, Minnesota, Illinois, and Georgia; in 1909, nine—Wyoming, Washington, Texas, Oklahoma, Nebraska, Delaware, Pennsylvania, Missouri, and Michigan; in 1910, one—Massachusetts; in 1911, five—Tennessee, Idaho, Oregon, Wisconsin, and Vermont.

The information concerning the total number of schools registered as maintaining standards meeting the requirements of the law, is too incomplete to be of value. In a number of states the schools have not as yet been standardized. The total number reported as registered in the different states is 508, representing 14 states. The total number of nurses reported as registered, 32,972, representing 20 states. This is unquestionably an underestimate of the number. The largest number registered in any state is in New York, 8,960 having registered with 128 registered schools.

The population of New York was reported as 9,113,614 in 1910. The daily average of patients reported last year in registered hospitals was 31,424, making the proportion of hospital beds to inhabitants approximately 1 to 290. (This includes the nine registered state hospitals for the insane, whose total number of beds is something over 18,000.)

That report applies to hospitals for the insane, though this is an item that will interest you. Nearly 50 per cent. of the beds that we report in the registered hospitals are in the nine state hospitals for the insane. That statistic is appalling to me.

The second state is Massachusetts, which reports 6,000 registered; their total number of beds, 6,505, exclusive of beds in hospitals for the insane, the latter numbering 10,764. The population of Massachusetts in 1910 was 3,366,416—one hospital bed to about 515 patients, exclusive of beds in hospitals for the insane.

I remember, a few years ago, reading an article in an architectural magazine calling attention to the need of architects conversant with hospital construction and saying that the proportion of beds in the hospitals of Massachusetts at that time to the inhabitants was one to one thousand, and at the present rate of increase it would soon be about one to one hundred.

There appear to be four distinct lines of legal requirements—preliminary education, professional training, licensing tests, and registry.

Preliminary Education.—In nineteen states there is no regulation concerning the educational qualification required; six require high school training or its equivalent; four one year of high, or its equivalent; three require completion of the grammar school.

Evidence of Educational Qualifications.—Where institutions are registered, the diploma is a certification that the requirements of educational qualifications are met. In some states a statement of the educational qualification is required on the educational blank. In one state, only, evidence of the educational qualification is required to be filed and approved by the Registering Board before the admission of the pupil to the school of nursing. This is a recently made requirement and has caused much agitation in the state where it was issued.

Professional Education.—Twenty-one states require a two-year course; nine require three years; two make no requirement, and the requirement of two is not known. Twenty require the experience to be obtained in a general hospital, six in a hospital or sanitarium, two do not specify where the experience shall be obtained, two specify that the experience shall be in medical, surgical, and obstetrical nursing in a public or private hospital, one requires medical and surgical nursing.

Licensing Test.—All the laws require an examination, but provide waivers, generally to include all those practising nursing at the time of the passage of the act. Seventeen laws have a reciprocity clause providing for the registration without examination of nurses registered in other states whose laws have equal requirements. All laws require a fee from applicants for registration. In five states the fee is $10; in the remainder, $5.

All those items are rather important. About the question of the fee I do not dare talk very much, because I feel that I shall take somebody else's time. But if a fee of ten dollars can possibly be required that, of course, gives a fund in the treasury for the carrying on of the inspections and other expenses, which will be of infinite value in standardizing the schools. The fee of five dollars in a small state brings in so little money that it is impossible to do very much work.

Boards of Examiners.—The Board of Examiners in twenty-nine states, including New Jersey, whose law has just been amended, is composed wholly of nurses. Nine boards have nurses and physicians, two states have no board of examiners, in one state the board is composed entirely of physicians. I am sorry to have to say so, but I am going to say it, that it is much easier to get information where boards are composed of nurses than otherwise, because we are interested in our own profession and members of other professions have something else to do. In eleven states the nomination of the members of the board is made by the State Nurses' Association, in twelve by the Governor, in four by the Board of Health. In seventeen states the board is appointed by the Governor, in six by the Medical State Board, in one by regents.

Regulations are made covering the salary of the secretary, the amount appropriated ranging from $50 to $500. The amount paid to the examiners is $4, $5, and $10 daily, when occupied. There are also regulations governing meetings, dates of examination, etc.

Inspection.—There appear to be two definitely appointed inspectors, one in Illinois, and one in New York. The law in one state, Idaho, provides that the president of the board shall inspect the schools; in Iowa, that a member of the board shall do so. Three states report inspection of a somewhat similar character—Virginia, New Hampshire, and Washington. A not inconsiderable number report informal inspections.

At least ten states have issued a syllabus, prepared generally by the Board of Examiners for the state by the State Nurses' Association. In one, Virginia, the syllabus issued by the National Hospital Conference has been adopted.

I will quote from two of many letters I received:

The direct results of our registration requirements have been in the change from a two-year to a three-year course in all schools, and the discontinuance of the former universal practice of sending out pupils for private work. Indirectly, we are getting results through the enlightenment the Act has brought to pupils themselves as to what should be

required of them and by them, and through the supervision all schools
are being made to feel they are under, by both the State Association
Executive Board and the State Board.

Conditions are still deplorable in even our best schools—both
through indifference and lack of funds—but we know them to be
appreciably better than they were five years ago, when our legislation
was secured.

Registration in our state has made improvement in most of the
training schools, one poor school has gone out of existence. I don't
feel there is one school that we could call indifferent. One member of
the board visits the schools in the state as it seems necessary. We visited
each school the first year the law was in effect, and many the second.
The schools seem anxious and willing to do what is expected of them
and are friendly to the board.

In almost every communication we have received, while the ineffi-
ciency of the law has been deplored, it has been asserted that, nevertheless, such laws have had beneficial result in raising the standard of the
schools and leading to greater uniformity in curricula. I would like to
make one recommendation concerning the work which could be done
and should be done, I think, by state associations. We believe that very
valuable knowledge could be obtained, and far-reaching work be done,
if, in every state, reports could be made to the State Nurses' Association
of the institutions in that state, their number, their nature, and other
important details—in the states where inspection obtains, by the
inspectors, in others, by the Board of Examiners, who could so divide
the state as to minimize the work of each member. In states without
legislation some method of obtaining this information could be determined by the State Association. These reports to be submitted by the
State Associations to the American Nurses' Association, who could
then prepare a report for the Board of Education in Washington.

A comparison of the statistical report of the Bulletin of Education
with the reports received from the Board of Examiners shows great
discrepancies in statistics. These reports come directly from the institution to the Department. Undoubtedly many hospitals do not report,
nor has there ever been any attempt to classify properly the institutions;
and it seems to me that the above suggestion might aid such a classification.

I beg to state here that while this statistical report is included with
Miss Nutting's monograph, she was in no wise responsible for the
preparation of the statistics.

My study of the various laws, which has been extremely superficial, I must admit, together with the knowledge I have gained during the past eighteen months, lead me to believe that in the New York State law we have more nearly approached the ideal than in any other. Our strength is threefold. We come under the Public Health Law and are, therefore, admitted to have a definite part in the health of the community. By the placing of the schools under the Regents, we have become part of a world-renowned and almost unique educational system. The regulations governing the education of the nurse are, therefore, in the hands of educational experts, and such regulations must accord with the regulations governing all the other professions. We have the assistance, and this is no small item, of machinery already well established, as the divisions of the Department exemplify. We do not have there a department of law, of medicine, of public schools, etc., but we have the statistical division, the examinations division, the inspections division. And our third and greatest strength lies in our law's requirement of co-operation on the part of the Department of Education with our State Nurses' Association. Our Board of Nurse Examiners is, it is true, appointed by the Department, but the nominations of the members are made by the State Association. I only wish that our Advisory Council and the Inspector were nominated by the Association also.

The New York state law has, however, a great weakness—a weakness that retards our progress and handicaps the Education Department beyond words. Our law is permissive only, though in the face of the splendid and ever-increasing response on the part of the graduates of our registered schools—the number coming up for examination increasing every year—we cannot fear for the future; and the history of our state is but the history in a greater or lesser degree of every other. Nevertheless, I want to make one earnest plea for compulsory legislation—not who may practise as a registered nurse, or who shall practise as a graduate, trained, or registered nurse, but who shall practise as a *nurse*. Surely, if we can call ourselves the American Nurses' Association we can go on the statute books in the same way. I make a plea for such registration, not for the protection of the nurse, but of the community. We are, in truth, public servants, and the knowledge that we should bring to our service is too great, and our responsibility too wide, for us longer to allow the individual institution for the sick to determine what our professional preparation shall be. Such legislation would necessitate a compliance with the educational requirements on the part of every school of nursing. The short-course school, a greater menace to the public safety than is generally realized, would be obliged to change its name, and such legislation would turn back into the attendant class many young women who, while personally qualified, are not educationally equipped for the scientific preparation so evidently needed for the wider fields of nursing activities of today.

I have said our laws are weak and inefficient, and so they are. That our educational system is defective none can dispute; but as we listened to that superb report of our Interstate Secretary yesterday, it seemed, despite the shadow of patient, lonely struggle in the waste places, an extraordinary picture of organized progress, and the more extraordinary because of the demanding nature of our work. Whatever her field, I think we must unanimously admit that the nurse is more entirely excluded from outside interests—social, civic, educational—than the members of almost any other profession, and we can not but ask wherein lies her power, to what is due this ability to organize so forcefully, progressively, and harmoniously.

The nature of our calling developing, as it does, all the highest attributes in human nature, unquestionably plays the greatest part; but I am inclined to think that two very potent factors in this development have been certain features of our institutional preparation, features that we are at present striving to modify, if not abolish—the militarism, that splendid drilling in the subordination of self to the machine, and the overdemand in work and responsibility which is so wonderful a developer of resourcefulness, executive ability, and indomitable courage.

Do not understand me as deprecating the modification of either of these features. I am the ardent advocate of such modification; but a building whose foundation-walls project beyond a certain elevation would not be structurally correct, and we have gone beyond our foundation-wall. I am only paying a passing tribute to a system to which I believe we are deeply indebted.

We have been in existence as a profession not more than fifty years, and our first society was organized here barely twenty years ago, but we are meeting this week in this metropolis of the Middle West, a great organization, representing over twenty thousand members and thirty-eight state associations, together with two national bodies representing special activities—one of an equal number of years' standing, and the other in formation.

Can we not boastfully say we have our patriots, our educators, and our statesmen—with what a record of professional work! Consider the remarkable development in the Red Cross nursing service in two years only, for which we are indebted to the great organizing ability of one of our members.

We read with pride the letter of transmittal accompanying a monograph on the educational status of nursing, the work of another, a letter which, I believe, has a sufficiently important bearing upon the subject we are presenting tonight to permit of my reading:

DEPARTMENT OF THE INTERIOR
BUREAU OF EDUCATION

Washington, D.C., February 23, 1912.

Sir: Within comparatively recent years the trained nurse has become an important and constant helper of the physician, not only in public and private hospitals, but also in the home, taking the place of untrained watchers who, however willing, can render only an ineffective service. This work of nursing has rapidly advanced to the position of a profession requiring careful preparation for admission. Thirty states of the Union have enacted laws for its regulation, and all the other states will probably do the same within the next few years. In several of the larger cities, nurses are employed by the boards of education to visit the public schools, to look after the minor ailments of the pupils, and to assist in caring for their health. For the education and training of nurses, schools have been established and are maintained in most of the states. There are at present more than 1,100 such schools, with an attendance of approximately 30,000 students. For this reason the education of nurses and the educational status of nursing have become questions of general importance and public interest on which the Bureau of Education, in pursuance of the purpose for which it was established, should give information. I recommend that the manuscript be published as a bulletin of the Bureau of Education.

Respectfully submitted,
P.P. Claxton, Commissioner

The Secretary of the Interior.

Could we ask for more definite approval, or by a higher authority, of the work of one of our educators?

And to obtain legislation in not thirty, as the commissioner said, but in thirty-three states, must we not in each state have had some leading spirits following the footsteps of the women who played so important a part in our first legislation only ten years ago, one of whom is to give the history of legislation tomorrow, one whose part has been great indeed, not only in her work in the state, but in the legislation of all the states through the pages of our *American Journal of Nursing*? Have we not here evidence of statesmanship? Despite our defects, unsolved problems, even failures, as the steady tread of this triumphing army sounds in our ears, we dare to say they have, indeed, builded better than they knew.

(*Goodrich, 1912, pp. 212–222*)

The Eight Hour Law for Pupil Nurses in California After One and One-half Years Practical Demonstration in a General Hospital of One Hundred Beds

Mrs. Pahl

Superintendent, Angelus Hospital, Los Angeles, California

When the eight hour law for women in California was amended to include pupil nurses in training schools, the problem which confronted the hospital authorities throughout the state seemed a very difficult one to solve in a manner which would mete out justice to the patient, to the nurse in training and to the hospital, but being law-abiding citizens we immediately set to work to adjust our training schools to the provisions of this new mandate.

The hospitals of California are not unlike those of any other state, embodying many kinds and conditions. Consequently I speak only of the type of which I have most intimate knowledge, a general hospital of approximately one hundred beds, owned by a corporation of citizens of the town in which it is located.

In the larger cities the hospitals have resolved themselves into hotels for sick people, and like hotels for well people they have developed into elegant hostelries for those who demand luxurious surroundings and institutions of simple appointment for those who desire less expensive accommodations, but the problems for all are the same. First to give the best possible care to the sick, second to give the best possible instruction to the pupil nurses in the training school and third to come up to the standard of efficiency and success which the sponsors of the institution expect.

Consequently the first thing we did under the eight hour law was to increase the number of pupil nurses by one-third, that the patients might receive plenty of care. The next thing was to add one-third more instructors and supervisors to the training school staff that the sixteen hours off duty of the pupil in each twenty-four might be wisely and profitably divided between recreation, study and rest.

The next thing made necessary by the foregoing, was to raise the hospital rates to cover the increased expense. A prudent person regrets the necessity of adding materially to the always heavy burden of illness, but this is one of the inevitable contingencies of the operation of the eight-hour law. Another trying detail of its development, from the patient's standpoint, is that patients who do not have a private or special nurse, but depend upon the general or floor nurse for their care must needs have at least five different nurses enter their room in twenty-four hours. Hence it is incumbent upon the training school management to so instruct and perfect the work of the pupils that the care given to the patient may be so systematic and uniform that these numerous changes may be accompanied by no break in the continuity or acceptability of the service rendered.

In the training school in which I am especially interested we had established the eight-hour schedule for pupils on day duty long before the coming of the eight-hour law and the change from a fifty-six to a forty-eight hour week was not as radical as in many schools, but the apportionment of the time is necessarily quite different, and in order that there might be no question of exactitude, and that the burden of the detail of keeping each nurse's time might not devolve upon the busy head nurse but upon the pupils themselves, a time clock was installed. The instructor makes out a daily schedule of hours, which is posted in a conspicuous place and each pupil checks off every minute she is on duty. These time cards are subsequently inspected and the system works out most satisfactorily.

With the extra hours now to be profitably accounted for, a thorough course of study, class and lecture work, is outlined which fills all of the spare time day by day. We employ an expert instructor who develops the course in theory which is followed up by an instructor in practice. With the excellent facilities available for educating our young women, we find that we are developing a school of nurses whose active brains are guiding their busy fingers with an applied skill and intelligence beyond the possibilities of the tired nurse who was on duty ten or twelve hours a day, day after day.

We also have a law for State Registration, under the control of the State Board of Health, and by the provisions of this law we have a State

Director of Training Schools. This office is at present being filled by a most able woman, who working under the jurisdiction and in conjunction with this honorable body, has practically established a uniform curriculum throughout the state. With a uniform curriculum of high standard, time to study and time to play, we feel that the young women who take up the vocation of nursing with the true spirit of service and the desire to excel under these most favorable conditions which obtain in California, can not fail to be especially well fitted for their profession.

A detail of the arrangement of the nurses' time which keeps them fresh and fit, is that each nurse works eight hours a day for six days and rests upon the seventh, but that seventh day is not always, or yet often, on Sunday.

If a pupil nurse is on duty and her eight hours of service are completed either at seven p.m. or ten-thirty p.m. as the case may be, she has that night off duty, all the next day and night and reports for duty the following morning, which gives her at least thirty-two consecutive hours of freedom from hospital work. If her day off duty falls upon a day in which she has class or lecture she must report for these, otherwise she has the time to herself unbroken. The nurses on night duty have the same amount of time each week, which they are allowed to spend with their relatives or friends. We find that this arrangement keeps the pupils in good health, content and happy and fit for hard work and study.

It has been suggested that this method must be detrimental to the school discipline but we maintain that a school for young women whose ages average twenty-two years is no kindergarten and if they cannot deport themselves in a manner becoming young women who are soon to take their places in a profession which is the very essence of poise and dignity and womanliness, they have no place in that profession and the sooner this is discovered and the sooner they are eliminated from the ranks the better. I may say here that we long for the time when the parents and the public schools will earnestly work with us in giving the necessary fundamental training to these young women, when the parents will instruct them in good morals and character building and at least teach them the proper use of the knife and fork, and to hang up their own clothes and when the graduates from the public and high schools can solve the simplest problems in percentage, divide fractions or spell beefsteak; then the training school instructors can give their undivided attention to developing a profession instead of teaching morals and arithmetic.

The hospitals, which all thinking people know full well are important and necessary institutions of the commonwealth, have received scant justice at the hands of the public, probably either through ignorance or because of politics. There may be hospitals whose management may be justly criticised—that is true of many schools and churches and institutions of municipality and state—but as a whole the hospitals deserve great credit and praise for the enormous amount of good work they conscientiously do, and they should be encouraged and upheld instead of being picked to pieces, as is often thoughtlessly done.

The fallacy seems to obtain that hospitals owned by citizens are large dividend paying institutions, but any business man would laugh in scorn at investing his money in a business which would fetch him so meager a return for his investment as the average hospital. The average hospital in California that is doing splendid work in caring for the lives and health of the citizens of the community in which it is located has no endowment, and must needs be self supporting, and while it is an old sentiment that a man cares more for his property than he does for his life, there is no good reason why a hospital maintained for the care of the reasonably well-to-do citizens should be a public mendicant.

We have demonstrated that it is quite possible to operate this eight-hour law successfully from the pupil nurses standpoint, and from the standpoint of the hospital, but we cannot lose sight of the fact that the burden falls heaviest upon the public, for the increased cost of operation under this new law must be met and it is the public that pays, and where the people, from whom the hospitals drew their patronage, are unable to pay, the training schools have closed.

According to the provisions of the law as it now stands if a nurse's eight hours of time has expired, she must go off duty, no matter what she may be doing or how critical or important the work she may be conducting.

Every effort is made to so plan a nurse's work that she may not be engaged in important duties when her time comes to leave the floor, but it is impossible to always be able to accurately gauge the duration of a case. It does not infrequently happen that the nurse must be changed at a critical part of an accouchement, or in the middle of an operation, for ten minutes past ten does not mean ten o'clock, and the iron hand of the law is over us, and again the public pays, perhaps by the loss of the life of a much longed for infant, or an infection caused by a break in the continuity of the surgical technique. The remedy for these exigencies is with the people as neither the hospitals nor the nurses asked for this law and if it does not please the public it is within their privilege and power to change it.

We think if the law provided that during the third or senior year the pupils might be permitted to care for private patients in hospitals, for a period not to exceed four months in the aggregate, during which period of special work the provisions of the eight-hour law relating to the hours of pupil nurses in training schools did not apply, it would add much to its efficiency, but the degree of success with which the present law is demonstrated depends largely upon the mental calibre of the hospital superintendent and the woman at the head of the training school.

In closing I would say that if this amendment to the eight-hour law for women was made to include pupil nurses in training schools with the sincere purpose of securing for the nurses more favorable conditions under which to work and more thorough and advanced instruction in the theory of their profession, this purpose has been accomplished, and while the law as it now stands, has its defects, it is a long step in the right direction.

(Pahl, 1915, pp. 178–183)

The Relation of the Private Duty Nurse to the Public as an Educator

By Carolyn Gray

City Hospital, New York

Last winter when the date of this meeting seemed far distant, I foolishly agreed to write a paper on "The Relation of the Private Duty Nurse to the Public as an Educator." It was a cold stormy day and May seemed a long way off. It is a failing of mine to have unlimited confidence in my ability to do almost anything six months hence! Now that I stand here before you, my many years of hospital work point with accusing fingers at the few months of private duty experience which I have to my credit. Yet those few months have done valiant service in helping me to understand some of the problems of the private duty nurse, and have filled me with respect for the women who are able to do this exacting work successfully year after year. It is, therefore, with a feeling of admiration and a very keen appreciation of the difficulties which beset the pathway of a private nurse that I attempt to speak of her opportunities as an educator.

One is reluctantly forced to admit that many nurses are not in any true sense of the word educators. This is a lamentable fact; and the responsibility for it must be put on the schools that have attempted to train them, but have failed to make them realize how numerous and diversified their opportunities are. Private nursing is a most important field, and needs many of the best recruits we can give to it. Granted that it has many disadvantages, it also has many compensations, not the least of which is the heart-felt appreciation shown by the majority of those served. No one can deny that the private duty nurse is at the present time a public benefactor, but no one has ever yet dreamed of the good she might do if she were better equipped for her work.

Because I want to stimulate your imagination, I am going to ask you to visualize as clearly as possible your ideal nurse. Endow her with all the physical qualities you think she should possess. Dress her in the uniform that appeals most strongly to you. Add any touches that will make her more satisfying and more clearly perfect in your opinion. Then presuppose that she has the scientific knowledge of hygiene, psychology, sociology and all the other "ologies" that she will need. It is just here that I always experience difficulty in filling in the picture of my ideal nurse, because almost every day I hear of some branch of human knowledge that it is absolutely my nurse should have.

Let us follow our nurse as she goes about her work, sometimes in the homes of the poor, other times in the homes of the rich, for need of her services opens every door to her and makes the circle of her influence almost limitless. In almost every type of home there are many problems other than the care of the patient which the nurse, if she be a keen observer, cannot fail to appreciate. Our ideas regarding the proper care of children have been modified to a great extent in recent years, and the opportunities for suggesting wiser care, more rational feeding, a more sympathetic recognition of childish limitations, particularly where there is any abnormal mental or physical condition, present themselves in endless variety. In the homes of the poor it might be possible for her to suggest a wiser outlay of the small income showing possible economies, especially in buying food with high nutritive value for a limited expenditure of money. She could also serve as a connecting link between the families of the poor and the many agencies for relief, advising them to whom to apply for the specific help needed.

Much has been done to increase interest in the maintenance of health and disseminate a knowledge of hygiene, but even after such knowledge has become common property, it often fails to function in the lives of men and women until *some one* has applied it and shown how to adapt it to the special needs of the individual and his environment. Not infrequently an attack of illness puts the patient in an apperceptive frame of mind which makes him or her a very apt pupil. This represents a valuable opportunity for a most useful form of education and it is to the credit of our ideal nurse that she is well enough equipped to make good use of all such opportunities.

In addition, think how often it is possible for her to interpret the rich to the poor and vice versa, as well as to show how the right solution of social problems affects not one special group but *all* the members of a community. We are daily coming to recognize more fully the interrelationship of different classes. We have learned from sad experience that the unhealthful condition of our slums affects not only the slum dwellers but even the residents of our most exclusive sections. Tuberculosis is no respecter of persons and though it often originates in the slums, it may easily be carried far from them. I am reminded of the experience of a woman serving as a factory inspector who found among the packers of sanitary drinking cups a girl in an advanced stage of tuberculosis. The health of all who use drinking cups was endangered by the conditions that make this possible, and it is the duty of the nurse to bring home such knowledge to those who can use it as a weapon for prevention.

For three years we have stood aloof and watched the gigantic struggle going on in Europe. Despite the warning voice of prophets we, as people, have felt it the part of wisdom to keep out of the struggle, and have quieted our conscience by sending such alms as we could spare. Latterly, our attitude has entirely changed and I interpret all our war preparations as an evidence of our realization that the solution of the European problem affects *not* only Europeans but the whole civilized world. If our nurse has a broad enough social viewpoint to recognize the value of the diversity of national characteristics, and also has the common needs of all peoples, she can, as she goes from one home to another, be a potent factor in instilling an idea of internationalism that will help to make those with whom she comes in contact humane as well as *patriotic*.

Always and everywhere our ideal nurse should serve as a recruiting officer to the ranks of pupil nurses. She knows full well that the demands the training makes are more than offset by the fascination nursing has for the woman who really finds it her vocation. With so many recruiting officers our ranks should be well filled. The fact that they are not makes one wonder why? I have often wished it were possible to have all the graduates of our schools answer this question. From a wide variety of answers, I suspect we would find that *long* hours are a determining factor in keeping many young women out of our profession. Perhaps it is only honest for us to admit that the governing boards of training schools have made many of the conditions such that our private duty nurses who know these conditions have educated the public to believe that the life of a nurse is undesirable. Possibly, if our schools and their graduates, through their alumnae associations, could coöperate with the governing boards of training schools, to improve these conditions it would be possible to make the advantages so apparent that those who had been kept away by the long hours and other limitations would gladly join our ranks.

Moreover an honest interpretation of the history of nursing schools and their relative position in many hospitals forces one to realize that they will never attain their maximum of usefulness until they are endowed. It is the private duty nurse who comes in contact with those who have the means and would have the desire to endow our schools if they knew the benefits that would result from such endowments. This opportunity is indeed a privilege and one that many private duty nurses are not cognizant of.

Last of all our ideal nurse has a wonderful opportunity to educate the public regarding the necessity for nursing legislation. Every bill introduced by nurses in every one of the states that has nursing laws has had for its purpose:

1. Improvement of the care of the sick.

2. Better education for the nurse so as to fit her to give this care.

3. Protection of the public by making it possible for them to differentiate between the nurses who have qualified themselves and those who have not.

Not until public opinion has been educated to realize that the legislation for which we are working will really benefit the public, even more than the nurse, will the opposition be overcome. We are convinced that public opinion in regard to nursing problems depends more on the private nurse than upon any other representative of our profession. Perhaps when each and every private nurse makes it her special business to know all about proposed nursing legislation and is able to meet the arguments for and against it intelligently, so that each one does her share to educate public opinion, we shall find we have more friends than we need.

In conclusion I would summarize the opportunities of the private duty nurse as an educator as follows:

1. Application of scientific knowledge to various problems of the home. (a) Training and feeding of children. (b) Wise expenditure of limited income. (c) Application of hygienic principles to individual needs.

2. Applications of social science to social problems.

3. Serve as an ideal to young women seeking their vocation.

4. Help to improve the quality of public opinion regarding the scope and importance of nursing, and the need for endowment of nursing schools.

5. Enlighten the public regarding the purpose of and necessity for so-called "Nursing Bills."

If the ideal nurse whom we have in mind is to act as an educator along these various lines, she must of necessity keep herself informed of the scientific discoveries that affect her work and she must know enough about the different problems with which the members of her profession are struggling to discuss them intelligently. I anticipate that some of you are questioning how she, with her long hours of arduous work, can possibly do this. My answer would be: Let her.

First. Take advantage of all the literature published by the boards of health of our cities and states, of the various pamphlets published by insurance companies, as well as the popular books on health subjects which are available in most of our public libraries.

Second. Join the alumnae association of her school and take an active part in all that her alumnae attempts to do.

Third. Subscribe to *The American Journal of Nursing* and *The Modern Hospital*.

Fourth. Attend as many of the meetings of the state and national associations as possible. This will be a good beginning as it will suggest new possibilities and additional means for improvement.

If our ideal nurse is to be able to meet all these opportunities intelligently, can nature endow her too generously or nursing schools over-educate her? Rather is it not necessary that such an important connecting link between our schools and the public should be in a very true sense an *ideal nurse*?

(*Gray, 1917, pp. 267–272*)

The Present Conditions of Supply and Demand

By Mrs. Bessie A. Haasis

Educational Secretary, National Organization for Public Health Nursing

It would certainly seem that the subject of the present conditions of supply and demand should be approached by the questionnaire method, but as I had no desire to precipitate an avalanche in our office I did not try this method, but have instead drawn some deductions from the requests that have come into our office for nurses and from information received from other centers from which nurses are sent out.

If it were simply a question of quantity I could sum it up in a few words: the demand is overwhelming and the supply inadequate but improving. But since it is not only a question of quantity but of quality as well, I would like to draw your attention to a few facts that are decidedly interesting and decidedly up-to-date.

During the past year there has been an unprecedented increase in the demand for public health nurses, both of the specialized type and the kind who can carry on generalized work. The conditions which have led to requests for special nurses have been somewhat as follows.

The findings of the draft have stimulated a great interest in child hygiene, in the correction of defects during the school period, and we find states such as North Dakota, for instance, passing laws enabling each county to spend money from the public funds for school nurses.

The demand for school nurses comes from all over the country, and even in places where the nurse asked for is supposed to do a generalized piece of work, it is almost always taken for granted that she will at least start her work, make her initial approach, through the families she reaches through the school children.

During the past year the various organizations engaged in tuberculosis work were relieved of the necessity, under which they formerly labored, of spending a great deal of time in the raising of funds. This has given them the funds that they previously had and sometimes an increase and the opportunity to spend their energies in the actual work of fighting tuberculosis. In addition to that we have had beside the tuberculosis soldier problem, the problem of what to do with his family, and this has increased our demand for nurses who are specially qualified to do tuberculosis work alone, or to approach community work from the angle of tuberculosis.

The Children's Year program, which succeeded in getting measured and weighed over six million children, has greatly stimulated the demand for nurses to carry on child welfare work alone, or to approach community nursing through child welfare work.

Just recently we have heard that there is an increasing demand for mental hygiene nurses, nurses who have had experience with the care of mental cases, and who have also had social case work and who understand family and home problems, who can take their part in the adjustment of the returned soldier who is suffering from some mental disease, to his family and to his community.

It is generally supposed that there has been a great increase in the demand for industrial nurses. This has not been the experience in our office. As Miss Strong put it, in Massachusetts, although there is a law which requires every industrial concern employing over one hundred employees to also employ some one who can take care of the injuries adequately, the nurse sought is much more likely to be the friend of the manager's wife than the nurse that has had special training.

There is also a great misunderstanding among nurses themselves about what industrial nursing consists in, and we have had a great many nurses come into our office, who have done first aid work inside factories, without any social, or family, or home, or community work, who considered themselves industrial nurses. That is not the generally accepted sense of the term "industrial nursing" as used by public health nursing organizations. I cannot see that there is any great demand today for industrial nurses, although more than half the nurses that come in and ask for positions express a preference for this kind of work. The same is true among social workers. Mrs. King of the National Social Workers' Exchange recently told me that they were having exactly the same experience that large numbers of people who have had experience in factories in some capacity or other during the war, perhaps only two or three months, on the shutting down of the factories, come out feeling that they have had good training and experience in industrial social work, and that they also were being flooded with a large number of workers for whom there were no positions.

For the special activities in the nursing field we are having requests, not only for staff workers, nurses who will work on a staff of say five or ten in a city of considerable size, but for nurses who can organize such a service for cities of all sizes.

Besides these demands for specialized nursing, we are feeling, very acutely, the demand which has been the direct result of the Red Cross splendid peace time program of developing public health work in every community which is not already provided with it. This also calls for nurses who can take care of a small area by themselves, or for others who can coördinate the work in areas that are insufficiently, or inadequately, covered at the present time by two or three nurses under independent organizations.

It is needless to repeat the fact that the influenza epidemic taught the United States the great value of having some organized nursing service in each community which should be capable of expansion during an emergency to cover the homes of the entire population of a given area. This has also brought a demand, and, of course, for this work the emphasis is laid on the fact that the nurse must have organizing ability, and be able to adapt herself to unusual conditions, if they arise.

The program of the United States Public Health Service during the war, which built up as nearly as possible the model health administration around each cantonment, also has done considerable to stimulate the demand. Some of these extra cantonment zone units have gone on after the military organization disbanded through the support of the civilian population of the city, or the county. A number shrank in size considerably when outside subsidy was withdrawn, and some few have disappeared entirely. They have left their mark, however, and, sooner or later public health nursing will be revived in those communities.

The propaganda, which has been carried on by various organizations interested in public health nursing work, has also had this effect: we have all worked together. The publicity has merged so that it is hard to tell, when you read an article in the newspapers, whether it was stimulated by one organization or another. There is a remarkable unity of purpose about these various organizations to establish at least one nurse to every county in the United States and as many more as are needed for centers of population where there is congestion.

It is hard to consider the present demand for public health nurses without a look into the future. It is difficult to go to meetings of social workers these days without hearing a good deal about the future care of the sick. At the recent conference of social workers in Atlantic City social insurance was on everybody's lips. As Mr. Lapp said, every risk that is measurable can be insured against. The risk of illness *is* definitely measurable and there is no reason at all why it shall not be insured against.

The labor organizations, which formerly have been somewhat hostile to social insurance, including insurance against sickness, have some of them now come out and favor it, notably in the case of New York State. When that comes—and I cannot believe that it will be five years before *some* state in the Union will pass some such laws—there will be a demand for a vast number of nurses to care for the sick in their homes. To my mind, the discussion of the attendant ties right up to this. If people are to be insured against the sickness that they may have and insured that they may have the health that they need, this will be paid for out of taxation and the nurses and the attendants, if they are needed, the household helpers if they are needed, will be paid for and organized into a single service for the entire population.

In addition to these requests for workers, we also have many requests for teachers. This is one of the calls which has been most difficult to meet. The National Organization has a scholarship fund of $10,000 which it is hoping to spend during the coming year for the education of women for such positions. Normal school or college graduates if they have been engaged in public health nursing will be eligible. Familiarity with the technique of teaching and a wide acquaintance with the methods in public health nursing are necessary to equip them to direct public health nursing courses.

So much for the demand. The supply has been seriously interfered with during the war. But during the war also there has been a distinct change in the character of the students that have been taken care of in various schools of public health nursing. At the present time there are nine recognized post-graduate courses, four months in length; and four summer courses not less than six weeks in length. There are in addition to these a number of courses which have not yet been recognized by the National Organization through lack of teaching personnel or of adequate field work.

Of these various courses twelve are taking undergraduates. New post-graduate courses are being projected in four states.

During the past year, as you heard yesterday, the Red Cross has set aside a large scholarship fund to prepare nurses, primarily those returning from military service, for public health nursing. The indications are that the courses this summer and fall will be filled to capacity.

During the past year the capacity of courses for graduates has hardly been taxed. Some courses have had one and some have had two students. Only one that I know of had as many as twelve in an eight months' course. The scholarships of the Red Cross are designed, for the most part, to increase the number of public health nurses rather than to raise the quality of the public health nurses already in the field. In past years about half the students, who have taken post-graduate courses in public health nursing, have had experience in public health nursing, and from that realized their need for instruction and entered the course. The other half have been nurses who have not had experience in public health work, getting their first introduction through the course. Because of this decision of the Red Cross to award these scholarships largely to those who have not done public health nursing before there will be a preponderance, no doubt, of workers new to the field in the courses this year.

One of the most interesting things in the development which I hope Miss Stewart will tell about is of the course for teachers in the Department of Nursing and Health, at Columbia this fall.

In addition to these courses preparing post-graduates, there are a large number of hospitals (I have a list of over one hundred), which have given their senior students from two to eight months in public health nursing instruction and experience. This is a practice which the National Organization has been delighted to see initiated in any city, where the public health nursing was carried on in such a way, that to send students into it would enrich their training while not depriving them of any of the education which they needed in their hospital and which would insure them, in the public health organization just as definite teaching as the teaching they would get in any department of the hospital itself.

The stand has definitely been taken that it is an injustice to send a student to a visiting nurse association, to a city board of health, or to any public health nursing agency which depends upon such students for the work which they will accomplish. I feel that no organization is justified in taking students, unless it can guarantee them three hours' classwork a week, unless it will start them in as students with some one else who knows how to do the thing exceedingly well, and will explain to them the different steps in the procedures, and keep a check on them exactly as a check is kept on students going into a new department in the hospital. Where possible we are very anxious to have developed an affiliation with schools where post-graduate courses are being given. However, it is not always profitable to turn under-graduates into a complete post-graduate course, for reasons that I will speak of later.

The National Organization is exceedingly anxious to have a complete list of the hospitals which give their students experience and instruction in public health nursing during their senior year. Every few days we receive a letter from some nurse asking, "What hospitals in my state give public health nursing during the senior year?" I can only go to the list which I have assembled by writing the various State Nurses Associations and State Leagues of Nursing Education. I would take it as a great favor, if any of you here who are connected with hospitals, which have recently made affiliations, would see me at some time during the conference, and give me the name of your hospital and the organization to which your students are sent.

A number of hospitals are giving their students experience and instruction in their social service department, where visiting nurse organizations, or public health nursing organizations are not available. Sometimes this is done even when visiting nurse organizations are available, because it is felt that it fits in better with the hospital routine and makes for unity in the control of the students. I would like to make it clear that while it may not always be true, it is very frequently the case that such experience does not give the nurse the same attitude towards the public health problems that experience in public health nursing organizations, or with a group of school nurses does. Hospital Social Service Departments lay a great deal of emphasis on the social case work side and less on the community aspects of disease. However, it is an excellent affiliation and there is no question that such experience is useful for the nurse in deciding what kind of work she wants to enter after she finishes her training.

The question arises, how far shall this practice of giving under-graduates experience in public health nursing be extended? I would say just as far as we can be assured that it will not rob the course in the hospitals, because we need every bit that the hospital has to teach, just as has been pointed out that in the hospital the nurse needs all the experience she can possibly gain during her training. We would not impoverish the hospital training for the sick with two weeks, or two months, or four months in public health nursing, if it leaves her a poorer nurse than she has been before.

Also we would extend it, as I said before, only where the student can be assured good teaching.

It seems to me that in the very near future things are going to crystallize and we will have a more definite line of demarcation between what the under-graduate and the post-graduate student should have. I think we cannot expect the under-graduate courses, the under-graduate instruction in public health nursing, at the end of the senior year to do the same thing for the nurse and produce the same kind of product as will a post-graduate course given to an older nurse. As in other fields, it is not simply the content of the course which makes the public health worker. We feel the need of women of maturity, of experience, with knowledge of dietetics and the problems of patients in their homes. Undoubtedly the post-graduate will be able to take more advanced instruction if she has had some public health work during her under-graduate days. Of course if the hospitals will demand college graduation for admission, then the college graduate taking her under-graduate course may get, in four months, at the end of the senior year, enough public health nursing to make her able to go out and take the qualified positions we expect of graduates and post-graduates where they will not have the constant aid of the supervisor. Until the standard of nurses going into training schools is raised as to age and education, we cannot expect this to be the case.

During the past year public health nurses have come under very hot fire from various groups. In the first place, we have been called to account for not turning out *enough* public health nurses for staff positions.

We have also been criticised for not turning out public health nurses that were well enough trained, and that we feel is a well-founded criticism. We hope that, through the League of Nursing Education more and more hospitals will give their students training in contagious diseases, in mental diseases and especially in venereal work, also that more nurses will have adequate preparation in the care of children. This is one of the greatest defects in the graduates of ten or fifteen years ago, who try not to enter public health work. They have had more or less casual experience with children but lack the modern methods of caring for infants.

We do not want to do a single thing to hasten any preparation of public health nurses which is going to cut down their present training.

However, if the drudgery could be eliminated, if the teaching could be improved, so that the nurse could learn more in two months than she had before in four months, we believe that the course should be shortened. We look for splendid results from the investigation which Miss Goldmark is to make. We feel that for the supervisory positions a post-graduate course including sociology, preventive medicine, the principles of teaching will still be necessary. Of course our ultimate aim is the endowed school with the college graduate as the student applying for admission. This may be a long time off but there is no reason why we cannot keep our eye fixed upon it.

(Haasis, 1919, pp. 207–215)

Main Issues in Public Health Nursing

By Edna L. Foley

The main issues of the year in the public health nursing field are that it wants more nurses, better equipped nurses, more clearly defined and closely coödinated work between doctors and public health nurses, fewer patients and a better educated public. There is too much preventable illness. Perhaps more legislation might help but our public is not yet educated up to an honest enforcement of such legislation as we have got. The doctor, being a man, may swear at the quacks and cults that are entering his domain; the nurse, being a woman, may only wring her hands when she finds an indifferent health department a smallpox patient attending a public school or when she traces a child's blindness to neglected eye-inspection of the new-born. We have no laws as yet that keep city and state public health nursing out of the politician's spoils basket but such health laws as we have are so indifferently enforced that we have no reason to believe that more laws will give the public better public health nursing. Perhaps the remedy lies within ourselves, who knows? Legislation is sometimes a panacea, more often than not, a soporific, and so, the public health nursing field turns to the training schools for help and to the members of the League for nursing education for the solution of its problems.

In a recent paper discussing the relation between the specialist and the practitioner, an eminent physician, as well known locally for his tireless consideration of his patients as he is for his apparently, intentional lack of consideration for nurses caring for those patients, closed by saying:

> And I trust there has been manifest in this paper the thought that whatever we plan for specialist or practitioner, it must never be forgotten that the interest that is paramount is that of the patient.

And so naturally my theme resolves itself into "Our patients,"—
who are they? What do they ask of us? What are we giving them? As
a public health nurse and a training school graduate, I can only answer
the first question by saying—"Patients are our reason for being." If
Eve had never tasted the apple, if Pandora had not lifted the lid, or if
we were all Christian Scientists, presumably, we should still require
nurses for the two greatest mysteries of human life would still have
occurred, even in the Garden of Eden. I leave to makers of dictionaries
the definition of the word "patient." To the average Public Health
nurse, it has grown to embrace every other human being except herself.
Neither rich nor poor, well not sick, escape her imaginary net. If she
only would—or could—apply her excellent maxims and programs to
herself, we should soon have a race of super-women, husky tolerant,
magnificently sane.

WHAT DO OUR PATIENTS ASK OF US?

Comfort, surcease from pain, gentle, deft handling; helpful instruction of the homely, practical kind; health, a chance to work and live as
Americans should. A simple enough program, seemingly, but how
many hospitals have time to teach nurses to dress, painlessly, extensive,
loathsome, exquisitely painful wounds? In how many medical wards is
the cardiac patient's rest, diet and general care, of prime importance,
especially when there are medical students to be taught the use of
brand new stethoscopes and a rush in the surgery withdraws half the
necessary nursing force.

The atmosphere of many hospitals reminds me of an open-air school
that I once inspected. Nearly all of the children ran afternoon tempera-
tures which the physician could not explain. As I stood watching the
youngsters, the teacher, a woman uncommonly well equipped to teach
six grades at one time, talked very much like this: "Children, let me
see how nicely you can put your papers away. Hurry, hurry, hurry."
"Children, show me how well you can do your number work. Who
will have the first answer for me? Hurry, hurry, hurry." These poor
little tykes, each one with a tuberculosis history or tendency "hurried"
in a state of breathless tension from morn till dewy eve. The teacher
was a good woman. The children loved her, but she was no more fitted
for her particular job than most of us are equipped to run aeroplanes.

And so, when the patient asks "health" of the public health nurse or of the physician either, for that matter, they are not always ready with the charm that produces results.

Dr. Green of the *American Medical Association Journal* said before members of the Woman's City Club of Chicago last week, that there was only one medical school in the country giving its students an opportunity for practical work in public health, although perhaps six of eight were giving theoretical work. We are doing better than that for nurses. At last counting, there were 19 courses in public health nursing endorsed by the National Organization for Public Health Nursing and a larger number of hospitals annually are trying to give their students some theory or practice, or both, in public health nursing. That is the beginning of our incursion into the realms of preventive medicine, our attempt to meet the needs of the patient who asks only for "health." What we are giving our patients, depends largely upon what we ourselves have been given. And here the public health nurse finds herself face to face with what may prove to be the crux of the whole situation. *Public Health* means health for all, not health doled out by municipal departments, nor cures secured by the joint efforts of the hospital, staff and the United States Pharmacopeia. It means also protection from preventable disease in schools, workshops and homes alike; instruction, education, and the foundation of health habits. Good health is the inalienable right of every citizen, man, woman or child, and since this vague, almost unknown quantity is the right of every citizen, should not good public health nursing be the concern of the laity, as well as of the handful of nurses who are struggling with this big problem? The National Organization for Public Health Nursing was founded in this belief. It is not necessary to explain its work and aims to members of this audience. Its phenominal growth during the last eight years came in response to the many and various demands made upon its personnel. But perhaps it is necessary to state that while its policies and programs have been planned and executed almost entirely by public health nurses, its work has been financed largely by non-professional friends. In fact only 7 per cent of a large budget of 1919 came from its active membership.

It would be difficult, if not impossible, to measure the debt of public health nursing to certain generous, far-sighted citizens of Cleveland, Chicago, Boston, Philadelphia, New York and other cities. Their annual individual gifts have ranged from $34,000 to $5, and in time, vision and service they have given almost as generously as the nurses themselves.

Our magazine was given and has been edited by lay-people all these years. Some of our best committee work and published reports have been done by non-professional members. Nor has all of our support come from individuals. The expense of the time, energy, thought and service given their various duties by officers, directors and committee members, has been invariably borne by the organizations employing them.

Consequently, the members of the National Organization for Public Health Nursing know how to value such volunteer service. We know too, that nursing is the ephemeral element in public health—the desire for health is here to stay. The demand for public health nurses grows annually, but it is becoming a trained demand. Just any nurse will not do. She must have had experience, or a post-graduate course, or both. She should have personality, as well as a hospital diploma. When the average community asks for a public health nurse, it wants a young woman with poise, initiative, good manners, resourcefulness, but it wants a nurse. It may get the nurse, the woman whose hands are willing to serve the physical needs of her patients. Does the fault lie with the public health nursing field, or with the hospital that fewer and fewer nurses are willing to nurse? Must we go elsewhere for the people who are neither unwilling nor unprepared to nurse the sick? A few years ago, such a graduate nurse took to school teaching, or got married, now she is saying rather frankly that any person can give nursing care, she herself prefers to teach, to supervise, to inspect, to educate. Does this mean that we shall have to leave the nursing care of the sick and helpless to the graduates of short courses, or shall we readjust both our training school and public health nursing methods so that we may have better nurses who will, at the same time, be sufficiently intelligent to have a social and health education added to their hospital training, using all three eventually for the good of all kinds of patients and the greater glory of their profession.

The average American girl has ideals. She is good potential material. Inarticulate she may be but she is plastic, imitative and desires to be useful. Hard work alone does not phase her, but uncongenial companions, whether superiors or juniors, do. The shortage of the right kind of nurses that most institutions are facing now may be due as much to the lack of leadership as to the aftermath of the war. The directors, the attending staff and the doctors, as well as the day-director and chief-nurse, make the hospital atmosphere.

No matter how much we shorten its hours, or soften its edges, nursing, like motherhood and teaching, will always be hard work. It will require courage, devotion and the missionary, as well as the pioneer spirit. The sick, when they are not afraid of death, are the most notoriously ungrateful people alive. A woman can only nurse them for one of two reasons—economic, or vocational. As a means of livelihood merely, nursing is a trade. It is not first cousin to a profession, but as a means of livelihood, plus a means of rendering service, nursing, wherever done, is an act of mercy, and that is considerably better than a mere profession. We should cease to quibble over these meaningless distinctions of title—private nurse, public health nurse, and what not, "By their fruits shall they be known." We need better, as well as more nurses before the public health nurse field can be sufficiently and adequately developed.

As public health nursing has developed during the past year, it has clearly demonstrated three services that the League for Nursing Education, because of its first hand contact with the laity, the medical profession and the pupil nurse, may render nursing and nurses. It can aid in bringing about a closer, more intimate contact with non-professionals, both individuals and groups. It can effect between physicians and nurses a better understanding of their singleness of ultimate aim—well patients. At last and by no means least, it can recommend, and possibly bring about a readjustment of the hospital training of nurses so that they will be given an opportunity to prepare to specialize and will be taught to appreciate the dignity of their calling and the extent of the service they are being equipped to offer their fellow men. This work rightly belongs to the League.

(*Foley, 1922, pp. 221–226*)

How Can General Duty Be Made More Attractive to Graduate Nurses

By Anna D. Wolf, R.N.

Associate Professor of Nursing, Superintendent of Nurses, University Clinics, University of Chicago, Chicago, Illinois

This title suggests the following assumptions: First, that "General Duty" is necessary. Second, that it apparently has been a service undesirable, perhaps undesired both by the administrator and the appointee and that it has been assigned to others than graduate nurses. Before attempting to answer the question asked, let us for a few moments consider these inherent implications suggested in the subject.

In our present understanding of the term, general duty in a hospital means a service rendered by a graduate nurse who has been appointed at a given salary to assist with the nursing service in any one of the many departments of a hospital. This may involve actual bedside care of patients, service in the operating rooms, or in the out-patient clinic. It is not a particularly new type of service. Our sisters of the profession in England have long since used successfully in their nursing homes graduate nurses to care for the sick. In our own country, from the statistics of the American Medical Association we find that 5,261 hospitals are conducting their service without students and are employing graduate nurses and unprofessional assistants to care for their patients with varying degrees of success. From the Public Health Organizations which have always employed graduate nurses for the required service in the family we can learn much of the successful activities and satisfactions derived by the graduates through such a service.

The administrators of schools of nursing and of nursing services in hospitals with schools of nursing have come to the realization of the fact that for the sake of carrying out a real educational program for their students they must rely upon other than student service for the care of patients; and again that they are responsible for a tremendous exodus of graduate nurses from their schools each year and that many of these nurses are not finding employment. To verify these facts only turn to the recent studies of the Grading Committee and the appalling figures will arrest your attention. The unemployment of many graduates during the past year has been before us constantly. We can be assured that these numbers of unemployed will be increased and not decreased in the years to come with the same output of our schools as at present. Although one might point out other salient reasons for the employment of general duty nurses, these two reasons remain paramount to my thinking: (1) That such employment will stabilize the nursing service of a teaching hospital, enabling a better selection of students and a better teaching program to be carried out as the students will not be depended upon entirely for the nursing care of the patients; and (2) That such employment will offer graduate nurses an excellent service which will prove profitable for both employer and employee.

The second implication of the title indicates that the service of general duty has not proven satisfactory to the graduate. What are the reasons for this? Why should nurses not want to do this type of nursing? For what purpose have they received their nursing education? What is there about general duty nursing that makes it unattractive and undesirable?

Unquestionably there are those nurses in our profession who do not like bedside nursing, the personal contact with the patient and his family. They find such service irksome and tiresome when continued for a long period of time. They feel this type of service is menial and not deserving of ambitious women. They prefer other types of nursing service found in administrative and executive work, in teaching, in public health, where they think an opportunity for their individual development may be greater. Fortunately for the sick in the community, a large group of our graduates are interested in the service to patients. They do want to care for the sick and because of this desire, continue in private nursing. Why should our graduates feel that the very nature of general duty is undignified and not worthy of their attention, time and service? I believe we administrators have a real responsibility for this attitude. We have felt that the service to patients was in a sense a lower level of nursing than, for instance, the service of teaching a nurse how to care for a patient. We say too often "Oh, yes, she is a private duty nurse," or, "She is a general duty nurse, she is capable of much more than that kind of work;" as much as to say that type of worker is below a high standard of service and mentality. That very attitude of nursing executives, head nurses and instructors is, I believe, the most serious unattractive feature to be overcome. Unless we who are executives honor such work, give the worker a high status, and have faith in her work, never can we expect from her a high degree of service, never will she be happy and satisfied. Many of you will say "But the nurses have proven so unsatisfactory in their work; they are not interested and are only a transient group." That may be true, the nurse may be at fault, perhaps she should never have been allowed to graduate. But I wonder how many of us have examined our own attitude regarding this kind of work and have really made the nurse feel her work was of the utmost importance; that it provided a better care of the patient; that her service *was superior* to a *student's service*. That is the sore point with the graduate. She has been made to feel her service is not as valuable as a student's. In my recent experience with graduate nurses representing thirty-eight different schools, I have found an excellent nursing service. As one of my head nurses said to me one day, 'The graduate nurse sees more to be done for a patient than a student, she knows better what to do." This response should not be exceptional but constant. If we are graduating students we should anticipate that their service as graduates will be better. The complaint from superintendents of nurses that graduates are not as buoyant, resilient and enthusiastic as students is often heard. It is true that as age advances these particular attitudes of youthful expression may not be so pronounced. However, maturity and continued interest in nursing, both found in the graduate, are splendid attitudes upon which to depend. Many times enthusiasm breaks through the austere door of this severe maturity and over and again, "that desire to learn something new" is just as keen in the graduate as student.

If we wish to receive the highest degree of service from the graduate, we must first have faith in her and in the service we ask her to render, dignify the position, build up confidence in the work, and make the conditions of her appointment and service satisfying to her.

What do ordinary individuals expect from their jobs to satisfy them?

The nature of the work must maintain their interest; the hours of work must be reasonable, allowing time for recreation and rest; compensation must be fair and adequate for the qualifications of the incumbent; the individual must feel that there is a dependence upon her service and that she is growing intellectually in it and is becoming a better prepaid woman for whatever else she may choose to do.

Should we expect our nurses to be content in their work with less?

Every nurse seems to enjoy one particular type of work more than another. As far as possible consider her choice of service. That choice, I have found, is very apt to be due to many factors. It may be a choice because of a desire for broader professional experience. In some cases a nurse will want to rotate from one department to another after a period of a few months in each in order to enlarge her background of clinical experience. This is apt to be the case with the young graduate who is trying her wings and wants to determine which phase of nursing appeals to her most, or again this appeals to the nurse who has been out in the field a number of years in private nursing or public health and wants to "brush up" on various principles and methods in nursing, or to become more familiar with recent research studies in the care of patients.

Again we find the choice of an individual for one type of service only. She dislikes rotating, she prefers remaining in one department indefinitely. She feels the importance of specialization; the value of knowing one type of work thoroughly; she enjoys particularly contact with a group of patients whose treatment she has followed throughout their stay in the hospital; whose family interests her. In this group is the young woman who is further preparing herself for operating room work who aspires to be a head nurse or supervisor in such a department if her administrative, executive and teaching qualities are developed sufficiently; or the nurse whose opportunity for out-patient service has been limited and who feels the importance of this work and enjoys it so greatly she wishes to remain in it. Often we find nurses who are especially interested in the care of medical patients or surgical patients; who prefer the care of women, to men or to children. Again there are those who do not want executive responsibilities against those who do want such work, or those who do not want night duty opposed to those who enjoy night duty. These choices of nurses seem legion. However, if a nurse is to be satisfied in her work, her choice of service must be considered, difficult as it often is to administer the situation. If her first choice has not been granted, she must be made to realize thought has been given her preference and time should be taken to confer with her about it. For the time and trouble an administrator may take to consider these individual preferences, she is repaid by the more successful work accomplished by the nurse whose interest in her work is retained.

A fair working day and week should be maintained. Would that it were possible to give every nurse a whole day off each week and one day a four hour service! Why should this be considered too much time off for the nurse when, except with hospital employees, practically every other worker in the community receives it. An average forty-four hour week should be our aim. Undoubtedly it will take a long time to become effective but it ought to be our goal. None of us could argue that the general duty nurse's work is so light that she doesn't need so much time off. Her work is strenuous. It results in mental as well as physical fatigue; it is of such an intimate and responsible type that she deserves reasonable periods for rest, recreation and study. Other factors relative to her time which deserve consideration are that her time be regular and that hours on and off duty be known sometime in advance. We have found posting hours for the week on Monday fairly satisfactory to the nurse. At least her day off and her half day are rarely disturbed, though she may be requested to change her time on duty to meet emergencies of one type or another. Generally speaking, nurses meet these requests cooperatively although one finds those who do not respond as cordially as others. It has been helpful to have a corps of nurses for a "P.R.N. service" who may be called upon for relief wherever needed.

To have both day and night services average the same amount of time has proven successful. Evening service, if on an unbroken shift, and night service are popular where otherwise they are irksome and undesirable unless compensation may be greater, thus serving as an attraction.

There is a danger that nurses may be so imbued with the idea of "limited time" that they forget the human service to be rendered and that this service must always be accomplished irrespective of their time on or off duty. We have rarely encountered nurses who are not willing and do frequently work overtime if it is necessary for the care of the patient. Graduate nurses have not lost their sense of service; they gladly and willingly give it if they are not imposed upon.

For continuous service vacation periods should be granted. My conviction is that this is a factor of great importance and will do much in preventing a large turn-over of the staff.

With most hospital appointments compensation includes not only monetary salary but housing, board and laundry. To offer salaries that are adequate for service rendered, that take into account the years of service of the individual and that will allow for certain yearly savings will attract and hold a desirable type of young woman. An increase of salary for satisfactory tenure of service should be given.

If graduate nurses are required to live in quarters assigned by the hospital, much can be done to make their condition of living agreeable. Every effort should be made to provide single rooms which alone can make possible privacy and solitude which everyone needs, especially when the group includes those on day and night service. As few rules and regulations concerning the conduct of the group should be made as is possible to maintain happy and contented group life. If regulations are necessary they should be instituted by the group. If the group is a carefully selected one upon which rests the responsibility of discreet and proper conduct, the problems of discipline are practically nil. The group values the trust and confidence put in it and rarely takes advantage of its responsibility.

However well arranged and administered the living quarters provided by the hospital, I believe provision to live out of residence should be made for those nurses who desire it and that adequate funds be allowed so that a proper standard of living may be maintained. The same financial arrangement should obtain in regard to board. Without doubt greater satisfaction would result for both employer and employee if this were done. It is a much better business arrangement. The nurse would appreciate the cost of living if each month she whould have to pay out of her salary a certain sum for room and board. The likelihood is that she with one or two friends or a member of her family would live together in an apartment, setting up a home for themselves and having more nearly a normal life. A better morale of the group will likely exist because of these adjustments.

With real appreciation of the importance of adequate compensation, I believe the opportunity for study is held by ambitious graduates even more desirable. This advantage can be arranged for in hospitals which have no immediate connection with a university center although it stands to reason it is more easily arranged in those in close proximity or affiliation with a university. Every effort should be made to encourage and arrange for the nurse to have formal class work if she desired. To have a group of graduates interested in their further education should bring to the hospital conducting a school of nursing an alert personnel whose interest in the program of that school may be depended upon. From such a group one should find young women who may be recommended for other types of work necessitating enlarged professional and educational background.

Staff education which may include regular conferences, clinics and demonstrations is an advantage and is enjoyed by the graduate. It is difficult to secure always one hundred per cent participation; however in our experience we have found the majority greatly interested in group meetings where there is opportunity for discussion on clinical subjects.

An informal type of education must be carried on constantly. To the new nurse joining the staff a great deal of personal thought and care must be given in orienting her to her new work. She must have a clear understanding of what the service entails before her appointment. A visit through the hospital; an introduction to various members of the staff and an effort to make her one of the hospital family all tend to bring about a friendly relationship between her and the older members of the staff. Particular attention and help with the hospital's routines and methods must be given her in the early days of her hospital experience. She is often homesick for her own friends and her own hospital unless she is fortunate enough to have one of her school on the staff. She has to give up much that is dear to her and accept new policies, principles and methods of work. Her adjustment to this new service is as difficult as the hospital's adjustment to her. In fact, it is more frequently more difficult as often she has never had this type of service before and she has no similar experience to help her make new adjustments except her initiation in a school of nursing, as many a graduate has said: "I feel just like a probationer all over again." There are a tremendous number of things the new nurse must learn and is eager to learn. Her introduction must be thoughtfully and skillfully made. The process of her adjustment may be sometimes rather painful but in most cases after sincere effort has been made on the part of the administration and the appointee, the nurse will tell very sincerely of the values received, of the stimulation through various types of contact; in meeting nurses from many different hospitals, of learning new methods of work, and so forth.

There are of course nurses who not only find the adjustment difficult but the work exceedingly distasteful. The service in no way appeals. For the sake of the group it is best to urge this young woman to seek elsewhere further opportunities for her endeavor. A consideration of her dissatisfactions proves, however, a real benefit if used for furthering the better administration of the service. It is difficult to secure adverse criticisms from the staff which seems content. Our educational system has not fostered it. We should urge suggestions for improvement and change which may be profitably used. Among distasteful features sometimes mentioned are those relative to relationships existing between head nurses or other executive officers and staff nurses; certain undesirable combinations of hours; certain methods of nursing procedure; rotation of service; lack of opportunity for individual expression and development. Sensitiveness to these undesirable features and a whole-hearted, thoughtful consideration of them with a remedy in mind should be expressed by the administration.

To maintain a satisfying type of general nursing service in a hospital with students may present features less desirable to the graduate nurse than one in a hospital without students. In a recent questionnaire answered by thirty-two graduates doing general duty, reasons that service with students might prove distasteful to the graduate were: "the danger that all interesting work would be given to the students;" that "graduates and students would be put on the same professional level;" that "students may not have the proper advantage if working with graduates;" that "one preferred working with nurses of one's own age;" that "only routine would be given graduates;" that "the student might be dissatisfied if the graduates had more privileges and the graduate dissatisfied if she had to conform to rigid rules of students." On the other hand, reasons for preferring to work in hospitals with students were that "staff nurses would feel more responsibility and be more alert;" that "there would be an incentive to the graduate as she will be closely observed." "She would be an example;" "an assistant in a teaching program;" "there would be an opportunity of learning more when teaching others;" "less danger of falling below standard;" "an opportunity to keep in touch with newer methods of conducting a school and probably re-interest them in class work;" "the enthusiasm and interests of students would prove a stimulas to better work." These answers are indicative of the general feeling that the student is "the worker" in the field of institutional nursing and has not yet been appreciated as a "student" in the full sense of the word. Undoubtedly, to conduct a service with graduates in a hospital conducting a school of nursing will mean a more diligent effort to choose the staff more carefully and make the service of the highest type. Students should be made to appreciate the advantages and opportunities of such work and anticipate that service as a valuable graduate experience. In looking forward to institutional appointments, many students have the idea that immediately upon graduation they should assume the responsibilities of a head nurse or a supervisor or an instructor. Our system of having students or very young graduates in charge of wards and assisting with supervision promotes this impression. We must emphasize the importance of having greater clinical experience before assuming such responsibilities and that this experience can be obtained through well-conducted general nursing service.

Another factor which may bear upon the satisfaction derived from a general duty service is the employment of a supplementary staff to assist with many simple tasks easily carried on by an unprofessional group. To have ward assistants to make up beds, to help with baths and treatments, to take patients to clinics, X-ray and other departments, to care for physical surroundings of patients, to assist with service of diet and many other duties of a similar nature relieves the graduate nurses of necessary services which do not require professional preparation.

To summarize briefly, the following are constructive suggestions which may result in promoting a more attractive general duty service for the graduate nurse.

1. Nursing executives should feel their responsibility in building up a higher status for the general duty nurse. This must entail a deeper appreciation of her activities and out of it must grow an honest spirit of respect and admiration for the service rendered. This attitude should extend to all the various members of the school and hospital staff.

2. The interest of the group should be stimulated and retained. Each individual nurse must feel that she will be given an opportunity to engage in the service she prefers. Choice of service must be considered of great importance as it will undoubtedly mean the retention of the keenest interest of the nurse, all other things being equal, consequently the best service.

3. A forty-four hour working week should be our aim. A weekly schedule should be arranged so that the nurse may know her program in advance and that she may have sufficient time for rest and recreation. Night and day services should average the same number of hours. For continuous service a vacation period should be provided.

4. Adequate compensation with an increase for satisfactory tenure of service should be granted. Effort should be made to secure allowances for room and board which would permit the nurse to live out of residence if preferred.

5. Every opportunity for educational advancement should be given. These opportunities may be offered through formal class work in a nearby college or university or again through a definite staff-educational program which may include personal and group conferences, discussion groups, demonstrations and clinics.

6. The services of the graduate nurse should be limited to those requiring a professional background: By the employment of supplementary staff to assist with many simple but very necessary tasks, the graduate is relieved of much monotonous and less interesting work and feels her professional services are of greater value.

7. Self-expression should be encouraged and individual capacities should be recognized.

Criticisms and suggestions from the staff when utilized stimulate greater cooperation in the service and may promote individual development. Increased salary as a reward will not satisfy the ambitious nurse. Recognition should be made of her abilities which may warrant a promotion in the service.

(Wolf, 1928, pp. 209–217)

Section III
Recruitment

Introduction to Recruitment

A desire to improve health care in America prompted many reform efforts by the early nursing leaders of the Superintendents' Society. Reforms such as a uniform curriculum for all schools, a three-year course, shorter working hours, a graduate nurse staff, and pay equity dominated speeches at the annual conventions. However, leaders knew that without better qualified nurses, their efforts to improve nursing education and practice would not succeed. In light of this, the Superintendents' Society instituted drives to recruit new members into the profession.

Strategies to recruit new students motivated the society to examine conditions at their schools. Too long hours on duty and too few hours in class created overtired and unprepared students. Word of this to potential candidates often dampened their enthusiasm. Unless they obtained shorter hours for students and other reforms, it would be difficult to attract young women into nursing. Advisors at high schools and colleges said that they would not recommend nursing as a career because the working conditions were too hard.

Through the years, a shortage of nurses occurred as the demand for their services grew. New opportunities in specialized areas increased and the number of hospital beds rose steadily creating new jobs for nurses. Competition for new recruits became more difficult as women entered professions previously closed to them. As a result, the superintendents initiated campaigns with pamphlets, fliers, and leaflets designed to attract new recruits. Nurses addressed audiences at high schools, colleges, and women's groups extolling the virtues of the nursing profession. They sought intelligent, willing candidates who fit the model of the ideal nurse.

Over time campaigns responded to subtle differences in requirements and an ever changing supply and demand for nurses. Factors like the woman's movement, specialization in nursing, and the economic climate provided a backdrop for various recruitment campaigns. Attracting women into nursing meant competing with several more lucrative career opportunities opened to women during the early woman's movement. Increased specialization meant that more nurses had more job opportunities in such areas as public health nursing and psychiatric nursing. World War I and the influenza epidemic prompted larger drives for nurses to fill vacant military and civilian positions. The need for nursing teachers at training schools was so great that it became more patriotic for nursing instructors to stay at home than go abroad during the war. During the 1930s, too many private duty nurses for too few jobs prompted an oversupply of nurses. Recruitment efforts refocused to find less but better qualified students. Hospitals began to hire graduate nurses, forever changing the employment pattern of nurses in America.

The following speeches deal with recruitment of nurses. They center on recruitment of pupil nurses because during most of the years covered in this book, students, rather than graduates, provided nursing care in hospitals. Later, in the 1920s and 1930s, when hospitals started hiring graduate nurses, nursing leadership redirected recruitment campaigns to reduce the oversupply of inadequately prepared nurses.

The Supply and Demand of Students in the Nurse Training-Schools

By Anna L. Alline

We have heard not infrequently of late that the number of applicants to the training-schools is decreasing. The facts do not bear out this statement. We find in the statistics that the increase in the number of student nurses is at the rate of several hundred a year. To give it in round numbers: in 1890, there were one thousand five hundred students in the schools; in 1900, eleven thousand; in 1903, the date of the latest available statistics, there were thirteen thousand seven hundred. This goes to show that it is an increase in the demand rather than a decrease in supply. This surely is a matter of encouragement. Nurse training came as a response to a need and has, through the power wrought from intelligence, fidelity and self-sacrifice, become a permanent institution, really essential to the welfare of human kind, and so closely allied to the medical profession that they are inseparable. We may well turn back once more and call to mind that it is woman's work and appeals to all that is highest and best in her. The mother nature always has, and always will, turn to the care of the helpless, whether it is the helplessness of infancy, sickness or old age. It will not change; there will always be that element in it that appeals to woman, and always that nature in woman that responds to the need. We can rest assured of an increasing demand and can be equally sure that there will always be a large proportion of women who prefer this form of occupation to all others.

In preparing to open this discussion, a letter of inquiry was sent to the schools represented in this Society. Many replies were received not only of definite information asked, in the form of statistics, but long letters of explanation and description of conditions, which are of great value. A study of the reports of these schools, together with a personal knowledge of training-schools from Maine to California and visits to nearly a hundred schools in the past six months, has convinced me that our problem is one of conditions in the schools. While we have schools all over the country, in the city and rural districts—large schools and small schools that have, up to date, had no difficulty in filling their classes with desirable students; and this, too, when the course was increased in length from two to three years; some making monthly allowances, and some on the non-payment basis; some requiring a high school diploma for admission, and others one year in the high school or its equivalent, it is equally true that some schools are not receiving enough applicants and are greatly distressed. The uneven distribution thus shown is directly due to the state we have long been struggling to produce. In our early years of organized effort, many a question was left unanswered, except by the phrase "We must educate the people." This has been accomplished to a considerable extent, one result being that a prospective nurse applies to several schools for information and naturally chooses the one that will best fit her for her chosen work and not leave her broken down in health and spirits, a rather wise and not at all unreasonable foresight. Her selection is finally made after a study of many features. Let us consider some of these features.

The reputation of the school is of no small moment: her history and traditions are as far-reaching as doctors, nurses and patients travel. One of the strongest factors working for good is a competent superintendent having a long term of service. When a superintendent severs her connection with a school, there is usually a period of two or more years during which the position is filled by a succession of people, for varying lengths of time, with a senior nurse filling in between, till the course of instruction is a farce; discipline is most lax; and the school in a deplorable condition. This reacts directly on the care of the patients and the public confidence is shaken. It takes years to get the school back to a good standard and there is always a class or two graduated that has not had thorough training. Often the superintendent takes more responsibility than she can handle well: superintendent of hospital and training-school, medical interne, housekeeper, drug clerk and so on, actually attempting to carry out the detail work of each office. What instruction can she give? How can she fulfill her promises to the students to give them a course of training? She cannot and she knows that she cannot. If she is unable to demonstrate this to the Board in such a way as to be afforded sufficient assistance to meet these obligations, the responsibility should be no longer continued. Furthermore, the instruction should not be just what could be given impromptu. Lessons should be prepared and the *method* of instruction given much attention. Under such conditions as our class work is given, it requires even greater ability to teach than under model conditions. College professors read, study and discuss subject matter and method all the time in order to properly instruct their students. From what we know of the teaching in the training-schools, is it any wonder that the nurses fear the state examination? We institute state regulations; it is for us to see that the instruction is provided and that sufficient time is given the student to enable her to profit by it. It is to be hoped that the time has come when we can speak of the relation between superintendent and nurse as that of teacher and student, and that it means friendship rather than the feeling and attitude of superior and subordinate. I have recently found instances of the form of discipline that humiliates. That is always degrading; it cannot be uplifting. It is well for us as those having charge of this important work to have a season of self-examination, see where we stand, find out if we are true, search for the weak points, and aim to strengthen them.

With our prospective applicant let us look at the schools themselves and we may see that remedies can be suggested to improve conditions—sane remedies. The hours, of course, must still come first and we again have our mathematical problem. How else can we present it with such force? Seven days a week instead of six. Fifty weeks in a year, not to mention six legal holidays, recognized in all walks of life except nursing, which takes a working week out of the fifty. Seven working days mean fifty-six hours a week; no other occupation requires even that number. While this is the least that is possible for a student nurse, many are the ways of increasing them. Six to nine months of a course is spent on night duty and the nights are twelve hours long, eighty-four hours a week. This eight to ten-hour day and twelve-hour night is not mental work alone, nor entirely physical. It is both and it is both of them all the time. Over and above this time of physical and mental occupation, which is quite enough to expect of mortal woman, one is supposed to pursue certain studies, and even this is not the end. If nurses on duty all day do not attend class in the evening, they relieve night nurses for class. Night nurses in some schools are called at one o'clock in the afternoon to attend classes. More often than not, nurses assigned to maternity, emergency and operating-room service are "on call" night as well as day for weeks at a time. We all know these things only too well, but they will have to be the burden of our song till these pernicious practices have ceased. Pernicious is not too strong a term, for such demands rob a woman of her health, which is all the capital a nurse has. It is her right to guard it and it should be the care of all hospital authorities to see that her health is maintained throughout the course.

The next essential of proper conditions is a room for each nurse, away from the hospital atmosphere, plain, comfortable and healthful. The question of food needs also to be kept before us. As a rule, good food material is purchased, but it is not properly cooked or served. One point that need never occur is the unvarying menu. To be able to say today what will be served to you the first, second and third day of every week and every month is in itself enough to rob you of an appetite for it. Food poorly cooked or served is an extravagance and this is one instance where hospital economy is seldom practiced, however much it is preached. These points are more or less known to the applicant and considered by her and her friends. She also looks to the requirements for admission. From a careful study of the reports sent in and the schools themselves, I find that it is not the long course that keeps out the nurses. In fact, it has little bearing on the subject. The general feeling of our superintendents—in fact, of all graduate nurses—is that the three years are necessary, unless the students can come to the school much better prepared than are the majority of those in training. More years in school attendance and better home training—otherwise, a preparatory course is the only substitute for the approved term. This leaves the two years' course quite out of the question. The non-payment system and the monthly allowance for years past have been discussed from every point of view. Out of the seventy-nine schools reporting on this, eleven make no allowance of money, only three of these mention non-payment as a cause for a decrease in applications. The length of course in these eleven schools ranges from two and one-half to three and one-half years; two of them ask a fee for the preliminary course; several require high school diplomas for admission; some have the eight-hour system; and all have nurses' homes. With these varying conditions the non-payment system may be said to have practically no effect on the question.

Raising the standards has been suggested as a cause of our difficulty. Can we not honestly say that raising the standard tends to improve conditions and call in a larger number, because it will be better worth while? This has been proven time and again, the world over. We are not so unlike other people. The road we are traveling is new to us, but has been traveled many a time before. One year in the high school, or its equivalent, is not high, it really is as low as can be accepted, if we call it a school at all. It means virtually this: that a girl leaves school at the age of fifteen and for the six years prior to entering the training-school, she has not occupied herself in a profitable way; for six years she has been contented to drift. It will take a year at least to get her into the proper attitude to apply herself or receive instruction. There are two evils resulting from placing these incompetent women in the school. First, we are caring for our sick with an inferior grade of women, which we have no right to do, and second, we are doing a great injustice to the graduates of the school, as well as to the better class of students. Can we shirk such responsibilities? Any school, under such conditions, runs down; the right kind of women will not enter; and its graduates will not recommend it. Patients, too, soon learn to go to the hospital where they may have intelligent care. Any hospital attempting to care for its patients without proper consideration for its nursing force, is accepting patients under false pretences just as much as it would in having quacks instead of doctors or adulterating the drugs. Such things are termed criminal practice. The whole trend of the times is toward better educational advantages. We not only desire but have great need to fall in line, to help and be helped. The very subjects we would outline for a preparatory school are being developed in the high school course. Things are coming our way and we must be alive and alert, when the opportunity offers and not let it pass by. While the high schools and our preparatory schools are uniting on common ground, the betterment of the conditions in our schools should claim our attention. This is really what we are doing, but we must have any amount of patience, courage and perseverance. How are we doing it?

To quote from the nurse practice act of the State of New York after stating the minimum requirements, it reads: "and registered by the University of the State of New York, as maintaining in this and other respects proper standards, all of which shall be determined by said Regents." The minimum requirements are specified, but "other respects" gives a wide scope, not only in the matter of instruction, but number and kind of instructors, hours, housing, food, cleanliness, general appearance, and all things which tend toward the better quali-fied nurse. For the most part criticism of the schools has been received kindly; it is given in a kind spirit with the sole purpose of being helpful. It is directed to the officer immediately responsible, whether it be the superintendent of the school, chairman of the committee or president of the board. In this way it is decidedly educational. It often cuts close to the nerve and gives another point of view; it is having good effect. There are some, of course, who do not wish to conform to the regulations. It is to their advantage, through the medium of the purse, or otherwise, to continue in the old way. This is a simple matter. They go on in their own way. The name is stricken from the list of registered schools and the regents have no further responsibility. Do we fully realize that this method of procedure gives us two classes of nurses? Those of the first class are registered; those of the second are not. The outcome of this must be progress. We will have schools that are schools—not treadmills. We must be reasonable in our demands of students and reasonable in our care of them and their instruction. This can be done where the facilities are limited, by the development of school affiliations. To further this development it is important to have definite contracts in regard to time, number of students and subject, placing these contracts on file in each institution. Schools should make their course of instruction more uniform, that affiliation need not seriously affect the theoretical course. Much can be done by the study of a systematic outline such as the one suggested by the State Board in New York. Complete records should be kept of the standing of each student, the practical and theoretical course covered by each and the full outline of the course in progress. This will preclude the interruption of the course by a change in officers and be especially helpful to the students in training. Superintendents should be registered nurses, have registered assistants and registered permanent head nurses. Registration should be required for eligibility to membership in all our societies.

Honest advertising is perfectly legitimate and commendable. State the case attractively and fairly. Then see to it that you make it good. Advertise in periodicals of widest circulation among the class you desire for the work. A consistent solution of the whole question may be expressed in four words—standards, inspection, registration and examinations. Inspection is a means of keeping the schools up to the standard, making registration effective and examinations practicable. To insist on registration of schools and nurses or attempting to force the matter is futile. Let them decide in what class they wish to be. It is more effectual to lead people than to push them. There is always room at the top and competition is a healthful stimulus. It is the policy of the Education Department of the State of New York to be tolerant of conditions so long as there is evidence of honest effort toward improvement. More than this, the Department is ready to assist in every possible way. It is a matter of education to the recipients whether they be students of the school, officers in charge, or even ladies' boards and trustees. On the other side, the Department is just as ready to sever connections with any institution which cannot for good reasons, or will not for other reasons, meet the requirements. The regents have the necessary power and from my personal experience, though limited as to time, as you know, I am confident that for New York State, at least, our future is secure, if we do our part and work together quietly, rationally and steadily.

(Alline, 1907, pp. 29–36)

How the Training School for Nurses Benefits by Relation to a University

By Louise Powell

1. A University has a distinctive and enviable standing in a community; some of this distinction attaches to the Training School connected with it and gives the school and the nursing profession a desirable social position.

2. It instills the nurses with some of the college spirit, which leads one into the better things of life.

3. It secures space in the University catalogue, for advertisement of the Training School among desirable young women, such advertisement carrying with it the University's endorsement.

4. The affiliation, including participation in Commencement exercises, proves attractive to College young women, increases the number of applicants for entrance to the Training School and raises their standard; this in turn raises the standard of the entire school.

5. It secures for the school recognition with consequent co-operation of the faculty, alumni and undergraduates of the University.

6. It gives a grade of teaching to the nurses not possible in a school not so connected. The Universities call to their faculties, the best obtainable teachers and the nurses profit thereby. Physicians may be very successful in their profession and still be unable to teach; such usually are connected with private hospitals and teach in their Teaching Schools. A school connected with a University, gets for its instructors men who pre-eminently are teachers. The resulting instruction must excel. The same standard of scholarship that obtains in the University likewise will obtain in the Training

School. The pupil becomes a student of nursing and pays her tuition by service in the hospital instead of being practically an employee in the hospital, receiving a little desultory teaching as compensation for her work.

To epitomize: A Training School connected with a University, compared with one that is not, gets more applicants, gets better applicants, gives them better training and enjoys a higher professional and social prestige.

In 1909, two years ago, the Board of Regents of the University of Minnesota authorized the establishment of a school for nurses, with two objects in view—first to furnish a nursing service for the University Hospital, and second, to give a thorough training to nurses.

In March of that year the first class, numbering seven, entered the University for a four months' preliminary course. This course is taken at the student's own expense, and a tuition fee of $25 is charged by the University. A high school diploma is required, preference, however, being given to women of broader education. The applicants must meet the training school committee in person. The work during the course is as follows:

Anatomy, three hours weekly, for 16 weeks; 48 hrs.

Physiology, three hours weekly, for 16 weeks; 48 hrs.

Materia Medica, three hours weekly, for 16 weeks, 48 hrs.

Bacteriology and Hygiene, two hours weekly for 16 weeks; 32 hrs.

Chemistry, two hours weekly, for 16 weeks; 32 hrs.

English, three hours weekly, for 16 weeks; 48 hrs.

Physical Culture, two hours weekly, for 16 weeks; 32 hrs.

Five hours a week is spent with the Superintendent of the Training School in which time she takes up History of Nursing; 14 hours.

Ethics and Etiquette; 12 hrs.

Personal Hygiene; 10 hrs.

Hospital Economy; 15 hrs.

In this course is taken up the construction of a building, heating, lighting, plumbing, general finish of walls, floors, etc., and finally each department is taken up with its use, equipment, management, care and cost.

The last four weeks are spent in familiarizing the students with principles of nursing, terms, etc., as preparation for the course in practical nursing given by demonstration for 6 hours each week, during the two months of preparation.

The classes during the preliminary course are given in the University with the exception of the class with the Superintendent. This is held in the class room at the Hospital.

Examinations being acceptably passed, the students come into residence for two months on probation. Since the school was started there have been 17 applications withdrawn, 7 rejected, 21 accepted, 4 resigned, 1 dismissed, 1 preliminary course only.

There are at present 16 nurses in training. Of this number, 3 in Normal, 2 College, 6 University, 5 High School only.

At the close of her paper Miss Powell spoke as follows:

I know you will all want to know whether our applicants are adequate for our needs. Most certainly not, and I don't expect them to be for several years for several reasons. We have no reputation, no large number of graduates to go out and tell what beautiful training we are giving them. It is the only school, I think, in that part of the country which charges a fee. At a conservative estimate it costs a student not a resident about $125. The doctors got a little panicky during the last spring at the outlook of sixteen nurses to open a rather large hospital, and there was considerable talk, and meetings held, looking toward letting down the bars until the school was large enough. To the credit of Doctor Board I would like to say that he fought very bravely for the preliminary course and we have succeeded in getting an appropriation for the first two years to pay twenty graduate nurses until our school is large enough.

As to the quality of the women in training I cannot speak fully from my short experience. I found eight students in the school when I got there, and eight have been added since. There was only one class a year. I insisted that we take in another class, giving us two classes a year.

The quality of the probationers when they come in is to me strikingly different. They are certainly better prepared to do the work easily and attack their problems more intelligently. And I feel certain the doctors get better service and the patients better care. The reports of the head nurses confirm that.

I have not had time as yet to exercise my supervision, or to know how these subjects are taught in the University. I propose during the next years, if possible, to attend the classes myself. I know that there are great improvements to be made in certain classes. I asked two classes of students who have been in the school from a year and a half to two years to give me their opinion as to whether the work had been valuable. And in both classes the reports begin by saying there is not time enough to get the work properly. One of the students told me that she felt if the women outside knew how valuable the course was there would be no lack of applicants. There are certain subjects that they feel should be more closely related to the nursing work, and that will come as soon as we have classes large enough. The hospital seems perfectly willing to take suggestions from me as the head of the school, and I think will act upon them as soon as the school warrants it.

The attitude of the university to the school, I think, is very fine. They show in every possible way that they regard the students of the training school as students of the university. I encourage this by having the nurses take part in the large gatherings of the students, and having them use a hall which is for the benefit of the women students. The university library is at our disposal, and at my request a number of books of interest to nurses have been put into the library.

I feel very hopeful of the situation. I feel that the university has taken hold of it in a reasonable way. The movement originated with the doctors, and they are all interested. The President of the university has expressed an interest in this department, and I am hoping and working for the granting of diplomas, which are granted by the Board of Regents at the university, with nurses in the caps and gowns. This will be one more way of cementing the union and having our work looked upon as a department of the university.

(Powell, 1911, pp. 150–154)

Report of the Committee for Approaching Women's Colleges

By Isabel M. Stewart, Chairman

Members of the committee appointed August, 1912. Miss VanKirk, Miss Edna Foley, Miss Susan Watson, Miss Charlotte Burgess, Miss Laura Logan, and Miss Isabel Stewart (chairman). Miss VanKirk was unable to act, and Miss Florence Patterson was appointed in her place. Miss Katherine Tucker was appointed later in the year.

After considerable discussion as to the purpose and scope of the committee's work, it was decided that our first object was to interest college women in nursing, and next to induce more of them to take up the work as a profession. The following methods of reaching college students were suggested:

1. Through addresses and talks before groups of college women.
2. Through the publication of articles on nursing in college papers.
3. Through the distribution of literature dealing with the opportunities in nursing as a profession.
4. Through fraternity organizations which have members in the nursing profession.
5. Through vocational bureaus for college women.

To outline any general system of campaign we felt that we must know something of the representatives of the various colleges who are already engaged in nursing. Miss Patterson very kindly took this matter in hand and wrote to all the co-educational and women's colleges in the United States and Canada, asking for the names and addresses of any graduates who had entered nursing schools. She also wrote to a large number of training schools asking for information about students or graduates who were college women. The results were not so satisfactory as we would wish. Many colleges keep no records of their graduates, and a number of the institutions written to failed to answer. Miss Patterson succeeded in securing the names and addresses of seventy-two college graduates who are, or have been, in nursing work. They represent thirty-two different colleges or universities, and are scattered over many schools, eight students having received a degree from Columbia University being included.

The replies came in so late that it was impossible to do much toward organizing our publicity campaign this year, but we feel that there is now something definite for the committee to begin on next college year.

Through our correspondence with these nurses and through discussions among our own members, we find that one of the greatest difficulties we have to face is the lack of enthusiasm among those who should be our spokesmen. When urged to speak or write in the interests of our propaganda, we find a considerable degree of hesitancy and several of our most enthusiastic and most successful workers frankly state that they cannot conscientiously urge their friends to enter nursing schools so long as present conditions exist. They mention particularly the long hours of duty, the needless repetition of much of the purely manual work, the meagreness of the theoretical work offered, and the unintelligent application of the old traditions of discipline and etiquette, which are so contrary to the spirit and practice of the modern college. These nurses are most loyal to nursing itself. They see all kinds of wonderful possibilities in it. They plead for more highly educated workers, and are eager to forward the interests of the profession in every possible way, but they cannot present the advantages of a nursing education with the conviction and enthusiasm that are required, if we would induce intelligent young women to enter our ranks.

Unfortunately, there are too many who have been induced to take up the work—only to find that the picture is not quite as it was painted—often the choice of a school was unfortunate. They drop out, discouraging their friends by stories of their experiences, which we must admit are not all unfounded. Fortunately there are not a few college women who are happy and successful in nursing work, and the great possibilities before the profession will, we are convinced, induce many others to come in, but effort should be directed especially toward educated applicants as to the means of entering the better schools, and arranging for such recognition of college work as other educational institutions offer. In medical schools, colleges, etc., credit is given for all previous work which bears on the professional training, while in nursing schools the student gets no credit at all for even the best courses in Anatomy, Physiology, Bacteriology, etc. Many medical schools reduce the course by a year (or in some cases more) for students presenting a college degree. We offer no special inducements to such students.

The committee feels also that it would be of great advantage if the League of Nursing Education could prepare some definite statement, defining the subjects which a girl might cover in her college course, with a view to entering a nursing school later. If she could there be exempt from these courses even though she put in the full time in her practical work, it would be of advantage to her.

Several of the committee feel also that there should be opportunity for specialization allowed in the third year of the nursing course; otherwise the college graduate who wishes to take up District Nursing or Social Service work must add another year to her period of preparation before she is ready for active service. This makes it very difficult for us to compete with such professions as teaching, social work, secretarial work, etc., where the additional preparation is seldom more than a year, and often not that for a college graduate.

The fact that it is becoming more and more common to link up nursing schools with universities or colleges raises the question of the nature of such affiliations. We have had several protests against a certain type of so-called affiliation, where there is not the slightest pretense of adopting university standards or of improving the real status of the school. It would seem to the committee that some effort should be made to prevent the discrediting of nursing education among college students which must inevitably result from this practice.

Members of this committee have assisted by advice and criticism in the publication of the little pamphlet on "Opportunities in the Field of Nursing." Through the Nursing and Health Branch of the Teachers College Alumnae Association, copies have been sent to all the women's colleges in the country. The replies which have been received from the deans of these colleges show that there is a good deal of interest being awakened among college students and college officials, and that the information we have been able to supply is much appreciated. Copies have also been sent to a number of prominent fraternity members, and it is hoped that by this more personal method, we may reach people more efficiently.

The committee ventures to suggest that the rather cumbersome name which it bears might be simplified into some such title as "The

Collegiate Committee." It has been suggested also that it could strengthen itself considerably by adding to its members a few influential lay members who are closely identified with college interests, and who might help in securing funds by which to carry on the work. The lack of money is a serious handicap, especially where publicity work of any kind is to be undertaken.

It has been further suggested that representatives from the new National Association of Public Health Nursing and possibly from the American Nurses' Association might be asked to serve on this committee, thus making it more fully represent the whole field of nursing.

(Stewart, 1913, pp. 35–38)

The Training School Prospectus and its Educational Possibilities

By Sara E. Parsons

Massachusetts General Hospital

Of course, the prospectus of a school, no matter how attractive, will never take the place of *real educational opportunities*. The success of a school depends upon its graduates. If students are carefully chosen and trained and find in their graduate work that their preparation fits them adequately for the duties that devolve upon them and that they compare favorably with graduates from other schools, these graduates will establish the reputation of the school and secure for it a continuous train of applicants. But a school must not rely wholly upon that advantage. To meet the increasing demands, it must progress and improve its curriculum every year, and be ready for intelligent scrutiny into its organization and educational advantages.

As all candidates cannot visit the school, the school must go to them by proxy in the prospectus. The prospectus may be a most useful instrument and serves not only the school which it represents, but is its legitimate advertisement, and best of all, it may be an *educator* of prospective applicants and of the general public as to the status of nursing schools in general and of opportunities in the nursing field.

We must not forget the value of first impressions when composing our announcements. The size, style, color and type must be considered as well as the subject matter. Much depends upon whether the school is new with its history to make, or old with an established reputation; whether the school is connected with a large or small hospital.

Much also depends upon the class of applicants to which the school makes an appeal. It is absolutely necessary that nothing but the truth be stated in the circular.

If the school is old enough to have established a definite curriculum it should be presented so as to give the inquirer a good idea of the time spent in lecture and class work (in points preferably), and the topics considered in each course.

It is safe to assume that any intelligent applicant will wish to know as much as possible about a place in which she proposes to spend three of the best years of her life.

Illustrations of the hospital, class rooms, nurses' homes, etc., will all be interesting to her. They may either be inserted into the circular or put in as loose leaves. She will be interested in the location of the hospital, its advantages and a brief sketch of the history of the hospital and school, and statistical data will enhance the value of the announcement. Emphasis should, of course, be placed on the educational advantages, but the hours for work and recreation, equipment, expenses, etc., will be matters of vital interest.

If she is wise, she will want to know what her opportunities are to be afterwards and what the alumnae of the school stands for. The prospectus is an opportunity to educate the public as well as applicants to an extent never utilized. The public is pretty well informed as to other educational institutions, but knows little about schools of nursing or of the opportunities in the field of nursing. On the contrary, it is misinformed and has prejudices and delusions that are very detrimental to our profession. These opportunities should be presented with the usual ratio of compensation. Every well known school sends out hundreds of circulars every year.

Probably nearly every applicant sends to three or four schools for information—if each applicant and her friends read in every circular that desirable schools must provide theoretical and practical instruction in surgery, medicine, pediatrics and obstetrics at least; that schools connected with hospitals having less than 50 beds with a daily average of patients less than 30 are not recognized by the National Red Cross Association; by the Army or Navy Nursing Bureaus; such information would do more towards obliterating undesirable schools and in saving young women from wasting three years, than anything else that could be done.

This instruction should form the preface of the announcement. The names of those who control the schools should come next with the names of the officers and instructors. Under the name of each instructor should be given a summary of his or her qualifications for the position he holds. Such information will be considered by a thoughtful candidate.

Following that should come the descriptive or historical sketch of the hospital and school with the general information concerning required qualifications of applicants, expenses, illness, hours of duty and recreation, calendar of classes, details of curriculum during entire course. Scholarships, loan funds, elective courses and post graduate opportunities should be stated.

The living accommodations should be truthfully described and it is legitimate to call attention to special features of the school and locality that are especially desirable or peculiar to that particular school.

The prospectus as an allurement to attract desirable candiates cannot do better than to append a list of names of its students in training and the cities and states they come from. A good deal of useful information can be gleaned from such a list. Names and addresses of old graduates who are living in different parts of the country may be given for reference.

As an advertisement, the prospectus may be sent to vocational bureaus, schools and colleges and distributed liberally among doctors who are interested in the school.

(Parsons, 1916, pp. 171–174)

The Results of Organized Publicity in Interesting the Public in Nursing

By Carolyn E. Gray

Secretary of New York State Board of Nurse Examiners

Organized publicity applied to nursing was a war-time measure and today our main interest is not so much in the results which *were* obtained, but rather in the question of publicity in general and what results we may expect to obtain from it in peace-times. The splendid publicity work carried on by the Nursing Committee of the Council of National Defense plus war-time enthusiasm brought to our schools such large numbers of young women that only a year ago, our main problem was to provide accommodations for larger classes of pupils than had ever before been admitted. This required much careful planning and many adjustments, which were hardly complete, when the epidemic of influenza swept the country. Possibly if we had known what the months of October and November were to bring us, we could not have provided for the emergency better. Hundreds of our nursing schools were filled with probationers and it will always be to the credit of these recruits that they faced the terrible ordeals of the epidemic with courage as great as that displayed by our soldiers in the front line trenches.

When the terrors of influenza had somewhat abated and we were struggling to get our classes started and live up to schedules which had been temporarily abandoned, the armistice was signed. Welcome as this was, it entirely reversed our problem, and some of our students who had stood bravely at their posts all through the awful days of the pandemic, lost interest and enthusiasm to such an extent that they left our ranks. To my thinking, the most remarkable thing was that the fascination of nursing was strong enough to hold so many, rather than the fact that the loss of war-time enthusiasm and returning fiances took a smaller number from our schools. However, I do not belittle this problem, which has been a cause of worry and anxiety from the standpoint of the superintendent of a nursing school who has witnessed her classes grow smaller because of the gradual leave taking of war-time recruits. Added to this there has been a very decided drop in the number of applicants to our schools and from many parts of the country we hear that the nursing schools are facing a serious shortage of pupils, which in hospital terms means a lack of nurses to care for the sick and carry on the multitudinous tasks which by some strange process of reasoning are classed as "nursing."

The lime light of publicity which flooded our schools, perhaps more completely than ever before, showed many weak points in our system for which many members of this League are seeking remedies. I interpret the purpose of this paper to be the question whether publicity will again help us to fill our schools with the pupils we need so badly.

Looked at from the proper standpoint, we offer *education* in return for definite work, and this we must stress and emphasize because any attempt to attract pupils on any other than an educational basis means, to my thinking, complete failure. Education for a profession and for life is, in terms of advertising, the goods we have to sell. Always when we are facing a shortage of pupils there is danger that this may be lost sight of, and we are all familiar with the suggested panaceas of "short courses," "lower standards," "increased allowance," etc.

Fortunately we have a goodly number of schools that never lose sight of their educational function, and these illustrate my point, that the appeal of nursing education is quite as potent to fill our schools as various other forms of education are successful in filling our colleges and universities.

This brings us to the anomalous position which our schools occupy. They are never listed with other schools and cannot be found in catalogues, books or any of the printed records where educational opportunities are usually sought. Moreover the educators of this country are in many instances woefully ignorant of what we offer, and still think of our schools in terms of apprenticeship rather than education. Despite these facts our attitude in regard to advertising is one of shrinking and a feeling that it is not dignified. I believe I do not exaggerate when I state that many of us were "horrified" the first time it was suggested to us that we advertise our beloved school. Yet it is necessary for all schools to advertise. Our universities, colleges, professional and private schools all advertise systematically. They suffer from no false standards and are frankly competing to attract the best young men and women of the country to their respective doors. Our daily papers and magazines devote many pages to advertising the claims of universities and colleges that are already far better known than even our best nursing schools. And the advertising is done by experts who know the psychology of the art and do it effectively. Moreover, college festivities, graduation exercises, and various social functions are always well written up, because they furnish interesting news items, and while primarily this is not advertising, it serves the purpose of advertising in the best sense of the word. In comparison with this, we find not a word about hospital training schools. They are not listed as educational institutions, are not found in the advertising pages of papers, or magazines and are rarely mentioned in the news items. The interesting articles on nursing published in the daily papers during the war were red letter events, and were part of a regularly organized campaign.

Another comparison that is of interest is the relative number of students required by nursing schools. In the United States there are approximately 48,000 to 50,000 pupils in training and from 14,000 to 15,000 pupils enter each year. This total of 15,000 students, which we must enroll each year, is far in excess of the total enrolled in any other group of schools. There are few professions whose annual number of graduates even approaches the number leaving our schools *annually*.

All this is relevant to the existing condition, which is that the nursing schools are today in need of a large number of pupils and are making no systematic efforts to inform the public of the advantages which nursing education offers.

It would seem that we have reached the "parting of the ways" and will have to rid ourselves of the obsession that it is undignified to advertise, and because of our great need and past failure to use this means, make a serious study of how best to make it serve our purpose.

It is true that in a few instances individual schools, whose need has been great, have advertised successfully and perhaps I can best tell of the methods that have been used to increase the number of pupils in a large school.

1. Descriptive booklets were attractively bound and printed, showing a series of pictures of the outside of the hospital, nurses residence, surroundings, etc., also a set of interior views of the interesting things one might show a visitor on a tour of inspection. Each picture was

accompanied by a few lines of description. A detachable printed post-card was inserted at the end, so that if the booklet proved interesting, the reader could use the card to request further information. In response to these cards a circular of information was sent out. This went into detail regarding the theoretical and practical course offered and attempted to answer the usual questions that applicants ask. The picture booklets were printed in February and in March distributed to the reading rooms of the high schools, public libraries, women's clubs, religious societies, and by means of alumnae members over as wide an area of country as possible. These attracted attention and brought results which more than repaid the initial cost of getting up the books which had been considerable. Moreover, the use of these books simplified the office work to a very great extent, and, in one instance, made it possible to dispense with the services of one of the two clerks that had formerly been kept busy.

2. Interesting articles were printed in various religious publications. Several were written by pupil nurses. This is perhaps the cheapest and most effective method of advertising, if one is fortunate enough to have pupils gifted with literary ability. The testimony of pupils in training carries weight with parents and guardians, and the pupil is nearer the view-point of the applicant and knows the things that will make the strongest appeal to a prospective beginner.

3. A few schools have used posters of quite large size, showing a few attractive pictures, with a brief but interesting statement regarding the school. These posters are sent far and wide to high schools and displayed on the bulletin boards. They have proved a successful means of interesting young women, and are cheaper than books.

4. Page advertisements were carried in school publications and such magazines as the *Young Women's Christian Association Monthly* and the *Extension Magazine of the Catholic Church*. The writer of these advertisements must be familiar with the psychology of advertising, should use pictures and make sure the page is too attractively gotten up to be skipped by the reader. It is a good plan to have reprints of these pages and send them to the various Young Women's Christian Association branches, including the summer camps asking that they be posted on the bulletin boards. Considering the initial outlay this proved very profitable advertising. I would like to emphasize the advantage of the full page advertisement over the usual one of six or ten lines,

inserted among many similar ones, because the latter did *not* bring results even when inserted in rural and Canadian papers.

5. It seems probable that our main source of supply must come from the high schools and colleges of the country, consequently our profession must be kept in the foreground so that these pupils in thinking of what they intend to do when school days are over, will at least know about nursing. In many parts of the country representatives of our profession have made addresses in the high schools. As one of these representatives I made some sad mistakes and for a time was quite discourged until I learned the method of approach. Later I came to the conclusion that addresses in the high schools are perhaps the very best way to arouse interest that will later bear fruit but it is not the quickest way to secure immediate returns. The first, second and third years I attempted this I didn't get any pupils but since then each year has brought a number and in several instances they have come from high schools where they heard the address given as long as four years ago. I remember quite distinctly how well prepared I felt as I wended my way to my first high school address. I had listed all the advantages of our school, and felt quite confident I had the right method of approach. Imagine my discomfiture to face what seemed like a sea of blue and pink bows adorning the heads of *mere children*. These children were surfeited with classes and lessons, the educational appeal fell flat. They were far more interested in "doing things" and a few stock stories of hospital happenings were all that saved me from utter failure. I decided never again to attempt such a thing, and never did. Before I made another address I secured a sct of slides illustrating a visit to the hospital and simply attempted to describe what the illustrations pictured. I closed my address with an invitation to visit the hospital and one busy spring entertained ten groups from various high schools. These groups came at stated times and every effort was made to try to show them, as nearly as practicable, what had been shown on the screen. It took time and patience to entertain them and answer their questions, but it resulted in a far better attitude on the part of both the pupils and the teachers who accompanied them, and cleared away many misconceptions and prejudices.

Miss Nutting, Miss Wald and Miss Goodrich who made addresses in colleges could tell you better than I about the success of their efforts. As evidence of their success I submit the large number of college women enrolled last year.

During the time that I was engaged in carrying on this publicity campaign, I began to wonder whether the stereotyped letters I sent out in answer to inquiries were all they might be, and thought I would like to know what other schools were doing. With the help of a friend I sent inquiries to thirty schools and I assure you I learned much from the letters and literature I received. We women who are superintendents of training schools are all too often so busy that office work and letter writing is not as important from our point of view as it is from the point of view of the applicant. Some of us need to learn the value of courteous and cordial letters that will encourage timid writers to persevere. We who know how much nursing has to offer should not hesitate to tempt prospective pupils in every possible way, and I think you will all agree with me that form letters with a rubber stamp signature are not apt to be tempting.

As a result of my personal experiences I am a firm believer in advertising and also a firm believer that a knowledge of nursing does not necessarily make one a successful advertiser. I enjoyed my experiences, and learned much, but am convined that one who knew the art of advertising could have applied that knowledge to my problem with a larger measure of success than I had. The few facts I learned were paid for by costly mistakes, and, even yet, I dislike blue and pink hair ribbons.

The exigencies of the war taught us the value of organized publicity and as this is costly it would seem to be justified only in time of great need. Some of you I know will consider the present a time of great need, and I am inclined to agree with this opinion. If the hospitals all over the country would share the expense, it might not be prohibitive. A publicity expert would map out a campaign and would see to it that interesting articles on nursing subjects were published simultaneously in a large number of papers. By means of pamphlets similar to the splendid ones written by Miss Isabel M. Stewart of Teachers College, the principals of high schools and the deans of colleges could be reached and in many, possibly untried ways, we might be able to arouse and develop an enlightened public opinion regarding our hospitals and schools that would prove a tremendous asset. Many of us who have struggled with problems that should be a matter of community concern and knowledge, and have realized the ignorance of the public regarding these problems, have come to question whether the highest form of loyalty to our beloved schools consists in keeping all knowledge from the public.

In our effort to attract pupils, to improve standards and secure legislation, public opinion of the right sort would prove the greatest help in the world. Are we as a professional group wise in continuing to ignore this asset?

(Gray, 1919, pp. 197–203)

The Recruiting of Student Nurses

By Katherine Olmstead

Executive Secretary, Central Council for Nursing Education

The shortage of workers. It is true that there is a shortage of nurses. There is undoubtedly, as Dr. Parnell has said, a shortage in all the professions, in all the occupations into which women are entering. We know that twenty-five years ago there were exactly two occupations for women, nursing and teaching. At the last census in 1910 we found that there were three hundred occupations in which women were engaged, and since the war that number has been more than tripled.

There is besides a wave of influence going over this country which makes everybody want a quick and large money return for service. We are finding that in vocational conferences this influence has affected not only the business men and women, but the young girls entering a life profession. Young women can, after a six month's course in a business college, with very little experience enter less laborious fields at the same remuneration and shorter hours than can a registered nurse. You will realize that to a certain large group of our young women this makes a very strong appeal.

We are finding another condition that is healthy. The women's colleges, especially throughout the middle west, are crowded. In one small women's college in Illinois fifty-eight young women were turned away last year because there was not room enough to take care of them in the college. So that there is a tendency toward higher education on the part of young women.

With those two things in our minds we can classify our young women into two groups: one group affected with the desire to get money and what money brings—clothes, finery and pleasure; the other group— those who are eager for a higher education, who are eager to know the joys of service. Those of you who were at the Des Moines Student

Volunteer meeting last winter will remember those 5000 young women, eager and anxious to hear about how they could be of the greatest service to humanity whether in China or Africa, or here in America. You will realize that there is still a large group of our young American women who want to do the kind of work that nursing offers.

PURPOSES OF THE CENTRAL COUNCIL

Now what are we going to do as nurses? Do we want the first group in our training schools or do we want the other group? In Chicago and in the surrounding states we have decided that we want the latter group of young women and we are going to get them into the training schools; not into every training school, but into the best schools for nurses in that part of the country. We are trying to mobilize our forces and we have formed what we call a Central Council for Nursing Education. It originally started with the lay boards of some of Chicago's best training schools. These men and women, realizing that they needed more student nurses, held meetings and decided to form a Council. They wanted to disseminate knowledge throughout Illinois and the central west about nursing education, to overcome the newspaper publicity that has been given to short courses. We can do it. We have never yet tried to get the finest and best things about our nursing profession before the public. These spectacular short courses where a thousand women are turned out in a few weeks calling themselves public health nurses, and graduate nurses, have news value and it gets into the newspapers. What we are going to do is to get good facts and also do things which have news value. We are going to try to talk, not alone to students of the high schools and colleges, but to groups of young women who are in business. We want to meet the parents through women's clubs, to meet fathers through business clubs, and try to create a wave of sentiment for the better and higher type of nursing education.

Throughout some of our central states the hospitals are very much interested in the recruiting for their own schools. Some of our states are already beginning to form councils and committees for this work and are recruiting for all the accredited schools in their state. This may be all right if you are absolutely sure that all the accredited schools in your state meet with the best educational requirements, but I doubt if such conditions exist in many states. I do not believe campaigns of this kind can be successful, because I doubt if there is a thinking woman in our profession who will go out and urge keen young high school and college girls to enter the profession under the handicap of a poor inadequate training. If we are going to try to attract the finest type of young women, we must see that they get into good schools. If we have an organization strong enough, and if we can mobilize our own forces effectively, those training schools which are not really educational institutions and are not attempting to be, will either be starved for lack of pupil nurses or else they will raise their standards in order to be able to attract the better group of young women.

TYPES OF PUBLICITY

We know we have been too quiet in the past. We have not carried out our nursing propaganda work with a sufficient amount of publicity. There are several kinds of publicity. Some of our best and biggest and finest pieces of work have had a certain amount of dignified publicity connected with them and it has not hurt them in the least. The publicity that we are going to carry on will take the form of lectures to different groups of people. The postal card which you have seen will be sent to all the young women having had high school or college education (or its equivalent) throughout the central states. When they write in to the Central Council for information on nursing as a profession, leaflets and literature on nursing will be sent to them. At present we are getting a pamphlet printed. Have any of you ever compared the catalogues from nurses training schools and those from clubs and schools and colleges? They are just as different as black from white. In the college and school catalogues you see the most attractive pictures—recreation, parks, playing and fun,—and in ours we show the style of buildings, and what the hospital board is doing. You can't expect young women to enter our training schools if we do not make them attractive and if we do not give them a proper knowledge about the training which they are going to get.

These pamphlets we are going to get out describing the opportunities in our training schools we hope will be very effective. We must portray our profession attractively and in a dignified manner, placing emphasis on the educational value of the training. In order to keep these pamphlets up to date we will have loose leaves for each hospital that enters the Council, prepared with our assistance, with pictures of its training school and a statement of its requirements. These will be put in the pamphlets that will be sent out for general distribution.

We know that we must have some way of bringing before mothers and fathers the real life of the students of our training schools. They have the most exaggerated ideas about what goes on there. Whose fault is it? It is our fault largely. When I was a pupil nurse my pet story when I went visiting was to tell how a D. T. patient chases me all around the ward. Pupil nurses do not realize what harm they are doing to the profession by such stories, but we must make them see that this kind of thing gives an entirely wrong impression about our schools, and that they can do more than anyone else to change this impression if they will only tell the true and fine things about their life and work in the hospital. If every pupil nurse could be inspired to send a postal card or write an encouraging letter to every girl friend of hers who is of proper age to go into training school, it would help a great deal.

I am very much in favor of the moving picture as a means of bringing before the people some visual conception of what is actually being done in nursing. It would make a deeper impression than anything else. A good moving picture of nurses' training schools would have a powerful effect throughout the country. But it must be a real picture, not a fancy one. It must show the real life of the student nurse and do it in an artistic way.

There is one thing that we must get rid of, this bugbear of hard work and drudgery and over-fatigue that has become firmly associated in the public mind with schools for nurses. The only way to change that impression is to change conditions—not in one or two schools, but in all schools for nurses.

FINANCIAL SUPPORT

Now all this publicity work is expensive. We are sending out thousands of leaflets, pictures and post cards into the central states and we expect to get a number of replies. We are hoping to have each state organize its own forces, and to send members to the Central Council which will serve as a coördinating agency. People will be much more likely to join their own state organization than the Central Council. So we want to make a central organization, composed of state units, each state to be divided into congressional districts; in each congressional district an active group of hospital board members, and nurses and others ready to recruit. We send into those congressional districts lecturers and all the assistance that we can give them. Public health nurses, hospitals and private duty nurses prepare lectures that they give in their hospitals, or just suggestions for lectures. Then when we in our central office receive a letter sent from a little place out in Wisconsin or Iowa, we will refer that young woman to her local committee, and they will get in touch with her and we will get in touch with her, and in that way we hope to really get them into the hospital training schools.

The expense of this movement is borne by the hospitals which have joined the Council, and they of course, receive the greatest benefits from it. But we believe that it will also help in raising the whole standard of Nursing Education by informing the public so that it will be better able to discriminate between good and poor schools for nurses.

(Olmstead, 1920, pp. 289–294)

The Selection of Students for Schools of Nursing and Problems of Adjustment

By Claribel Wheeler, R.N.

*Director, School of Nursing, Washington University,
St. Louis, Missouri*

The question of admission of students to our schools of nursing presents a problem which commands the attention of every thinking person responsible for the selection of such candidates. Secondary to this, and of almost equal importance, is the problem of assisting these students after entrance to adapt themselves to the unusual environment into which they have come.

The applicants must have had sufficient educational background and native intelligence to enable them to pursue the course to the greatest advantage; they must possess those innate personal qualities which shall render them adaptable and acceptable in their profession. In addition, they must be imbued with a steadfast purpose in entering the vocation of nursing.

I am convinced, from the statistics which have been made available to me from state boards of nurse examiners, and from some of our most representative schools, that the selection of candidates for the nursing course is not receiving the attention which it deserves. We are admitting to our schools hundreds of young women who are personally unqualified for nursing, many of whom never complete the course. The Grading Committee has pointed out to us the peril which now confronts us—that of over-supply. It has also given as the first answer to this question, more careful selection of applicants. Is it not more or less true, that hospitals have brought so much pressure upon schools to supply them with an adequate number of students to care for the patients, that the heads of such schools have been completed to take in nearly all those who have applied at their doors? The result of such a system is very wasteful and extravagant. Mr. E. Everett Cortright in his enlightening article in the May *Journal* recognized this when he said: "Nursing Education costs somebody something." He was also right when he concluded that this "somebody" is the patient in the hospital.

EDUCATIONAL BACKGROUND OF STUDENTS

The Grading Committee has made public the educational background of 63,000 students as found in our schools of nursing a year ago. This report is significant in several ways. It shows how many schools are just meeting the minimum legal requirement, and it demonstrates how short we have fallen from our ideal of a four-year high school entrance requirement. A surprising fact is revealed when it is found that some of the states with a four-year high school requirement do not rank at the head of the list which has been compiled by the Grading Committee. On the other hand, some of those with a low requirement stand at the top. It is encouraging, however, to see how far some of our states have progressed, and we may be justly proud of their record.

Although I sent questionnaires to all the states, only ten could furnish me with the statistics which I desired. The study which I have made of these ten states shows that there has been a steady increase in the number of high school graduates entering schools of nursing. Since 1925, over a period of five years, there has been an increase of 155 per cent in the number of high school graduates entered. This is, without doubt, encouraging; yet if schools of nursing are to attain the status of other educational institutions, obviously one of the first steps is to make the minimum entrance requirement at least a high school education in every registered school, and to live up to it once it is made.

In case we are able to effect a four-year entrance requirement in all states, in the near future, it will not solve the whole problem; there are high schools and high schools. There is considerable difference between a high school graduate who ranks in the upper third of her class in a city school and a graduate of the upper third of a second rate rural high school. A graduate of the latter may lack the power of concentration, and the ability to study intelligently. The student who has taken domestic science courses, or courses in commercial subjects, does not come with the same background as those who have had the regular academic course. Such students do not have an equal chance with their more fortunate sisters. The school is also confronted with the problem of teaching these students how to study, and they often require extra help in class work. It is difficult for them to keep up with daily assignments; the result is they are usually dropped in the middle, or at the end of the first term. Such students may rank normal in an intelligence test. The trouble lies in faulty teaching and lack of application on the part of the student.

WHAT IS THE CULTURAL BACKGROUND OF OUR STUDENTS

A factor which should be taken into consideration is the social class from which our students come. I have found no statistics in regard to such data concerning our schools of nursing. We often hear, however, that the strong wholesome country girl is the one who makes the best nurse. This is mere supposition. Here again, I do not believe we have sufficiently studied the matter. Intelligence tests given in the United States Army in 1917 showed that there was a definite relationship between types of occupation and intelligence. Men in occupations classed as unskilled manual work were found to rate decidedly lower than those in the learned professions. The relationship between parental occupations and intelligence of offspring has been demonstrated in such experiments as those made with school children in Madison, Wisconsin, and in the survey in Northumberland, England. It was found that the I. Q. of children of professional men was much higher than the I. Q. of unskilled laborers. There was, nevertheless, some overlapping in each group. This fact should be taken into consideration in the study of a problem such as ours.

INTELLIGENCE TESTS

Psychologists are coming to believe that one of the most valuable instruments of guidance, that has yet been devised, is the mental test. Since the French psychologist, Alfred Binet, was able, in 1904, to separate intelligently incompetent children from those who were normal or above, great progress has been made in mental testing. It has been definitely proven that many students who enter high school do not possess the intelligence to do work of high school rank.

Two years ago, Marian Faber and Louise Metcalf gave to the League the results of a study in mental testing in schools of nursing. Their conclusions showed that intelligence tests, properly administered, were invaluable in determining a student's native mental capacity, and were, therefore, useful in the selection of students and in determining whether poor scholarship is due to lack of intelligence, lack of application, or lack of interest. Not infrequently one discovers that students are doing work far below their mental capacity for such scope of effort. On the other hand, certain students by hard work and power of concentration do surprisingly well in relation to their capacity. Although the correlation between nursing practice and intelligence ratings is not satisfying, there seems to be a definite tendency to indicate that the better student in practice is the one who stands high in the scale of intelligence.

There seems to be an inclination among certain high school teachers and vocational guidance people to feel that the girls who are not particularly bright in high school, or the ones whom they would not recommend for college entrance, may do for the nursing course. This is an erroneous opinion, and most unfortunate. Without doubt, the fault is our own; we have not made the matter clear to high school officials. It would seem wise to establish a practice requiring students entering schools of nursing to possess the same degree of intelligence as those entering collegiate education.

There are other determinants of vocational choice besides intelligence tests which must be equally stressed, and which I shall mention later.

STUDENTS WHO RESIGN OR ARE DISMISSED

I have made an endeavor to study the admission of students to our schools in relation to the number graduated. In order to do this, I have taken the ten states which are fairly typical as they include all sections of the country, and represent states which have both large and small enrollments. In fact, some of the smaller states are keeping the best statistical records. In addition, I have studied sixteen representative schools. As the number of students admitted is not the same in each year, and I could secure only the number of those admitted and graduated, the figures give only a general picture; yet they seem sufficient to show what is happening.

The majority of students who drop out of the course do so in the first year, many of them during the preliminary term, although the process of elimination continues throughout the course. In the ten states studied, the number of students who had resigned or were dismissed varied from 21 percent to 69 percent with an average of 46 percent.

In the individual schools, there was a loss of from 12 percent to 60 percent with an average of 44 percent.

	States	Schools
Graduates	54 percent	56 percent
Resigned and dropped	46 percent	44 percent
Of those resigned and dropped:		
Resigned	64 percent	44 percent
Dropped	36 percent	56 percent

In the Washington University School of Nursing, where we could definitely trace through each class from the time of entrance until graduation, the figures are as follows:

WASHINGTON UNIVERSITY SCHOOL OF NURSING

Students admitted (1923–27)	293
Graduated	178—60 percent
Resigned	79—27 percent
Dropped	36—13 percent

The entrance requirement to this school is a four-year high school course acceptable for matriculation in the university. All individual schools studied had a high school entrance requirement, but this was not true of any of the states studied.

Reasons for resignation are varied. The most usual ones being: dislike of the work, unfitness for the work, inability to carry theory, illness, marriage, homesickness, unfavorable home conditions, infringement of rules, undesirability, transfer, and death.

New York State, which has a large number of schools, and consequently a large number of students, has kept such excellent statistical records that I am able to give you the following analysis for the period 1924–28 inclusive:

REASONS FOR STUDENTS LEAVING SCHOOLS IN NEW YORK STATE

Period five years

	No. students	Percentage
Went back to school	20	0.5
Went into other work	42	1
Death	47	1
Infringement of rules	93	2.5
Not desirable	149	3
Unable to carry theory	176	4
Personal reasons	231	5
Transferred	234	5
Misconduct	247	5
Not competent	374	7
Married	441	9
Dislike of work	482	9
Home conditions	485	10
Illness	867	17
Not fitted for work	1,040	21
Total	4,929	100

If we separate from this tabulation the number definitely not qualified, or those who possess undesirable qualities for the profession of nursing, we find that 38 percent come under this heading:

THOSE WITH UNDESIRABLE QUALITIES

Not fitted for the work	1,040
Not competent	374
Misconduct	247
Not desirable	149
Infringement of rules	93
	1,903 or 38%

In another state, covering a period of three years, the number of undesirables proved to be 27 percent. These figures lead to one definite conclusion; there is too great a waste in such a system. Ways and means should be found to insure a better selection of applicants.

It is difficult to make comparisons between a school of nursing and other schools as conditions are so different. I was interested, nevertheless, to compare our own school with other professional schools in the university. In the School of Business and Public Administration about 65 percent graduate, and in the School of Medicine about 67 percent graduate. In the former the students are all juniors and seniors, while in the latter they are graduate students. The schools therefore, which are most comparable to ours are the schools of Engineering and Architecture to which the students are admitted from high school. They graduate 87 percent of the students admitted, while the School of Nursing graduates 60 percent.

THE NEED FOR SOME MEANS OF TESTING CHARACTER TRAITS

If I were to pass around a questionnaire in this audience asking those present to give the causes of failure of graduate nurses whom they have known, I believe that the returns would show that the majority of such failures were not due to lack of theoretical or practical ability but to personality difficulties. It is, of course, a tragedy that anti-social or undesirable traits could not be discovered early in a student's course, and either corrected or continuance in the school discouraged. The need for some means of testing character traits of applicants is strongly felt by many.

A concrete illustration of the point that women may measure up in intelligence and still be unfitted for the profession of nursing comes to mind. Two young women with excellent educational preparation entered the school with which I am connected. One was a college graduate who had, for several years, been a teacher in a country school, the other was a young woman who lacked only a few units of credit for her A.B. degree. At the end of the first semester these students ranked at the head of their class in scholarship. Notwithstanding, they were both handicapped by personality difficulties. Much time was spent in conference with these women in trying to assist them to make the adjustment. However, greater contact with them in ward situations revealed that one was incapable of accepting suggestions from those in authority, that she was unkind, unsympathetic, and had an overbearing attitude toward her patients. The other student was utterly incapable of organizing her work; one patient would be well cared for while the others would suffer from neglect. It was necessary, after six months, to advise both students to seek other fields of work. Without question, we should have had either better knowledge of the character of these young women before they were admitted to the school, or we should have employed better means to help them make the adjustment after admission.

Edward K. Strong, Jr., Professor of Psychology at Stanford University, has done some work in this direction, in devising vocational tests which show a student's likes, dislikes, interest and lack of interest in certain things. These help to determine fitness for a certain kind of work. Theodore F. Lentz, Jr., Assistant Professor of Education at Washington University, in an article entitled "Character Research and Human Happiness" makes a plea for the financing of a scientific project in character research. May we not look forward to the time when the National League of Nursing Education may secure funds to undertake such a project? It is, perhaps, more needed in the vocation of nursing than in any other profession and offers a field of research presenting undreamed-of possibilities.

PERSONAL CONTACT WITH STUDENTS BEFORE ADMISSION

It would undoubtedly be a great advantage to establish some means of personal contact with students before admission to the school, either by an individual interview at the school or by a home visit. Some schools require the former, but there seems to be very little done in the way of visiting the prospective applicant in her home. This form of contact offers several advantages. Meeting a student in her home environment relieves her of any embarrassment or timidity, and it offers an opportunity to meet the parents and to discuss with them the question of the daughter's future. Many prejudices on the part of parents may be overcome in this way. This also affords an opportunity to look into the financial status of the family, and to discuss with them the cost of such a course. Students are very much handicapped when they enter the school with such limited resources that they are unable to dress in the same manner as their associates, or to take part in the social activities of the school.

The employment of a field representative who can make such personal contact with applicants, and who can (at the same time) visit the high school and have a conference with the vocational director or dean of girls in regard to them, would be a desirable addition to any school faculty. It would, undoubtedly, save the school from admitting many undesirable students.

PROBLEMS OF ADJUSTMENT

The more careful a selection of students, the less difficult will be the problem of adjustment after entrance. Schools of nursing do present problems in adjustment which are different from those found in boarding schools or colleges. Hospital life is rather unusual in character, and is entirely new to young women entering our schools. A student must adapt herself to strange routines, to a system of hospital etiquette which often seems meaningless, to working with all kinds of people whether pleasant or disagreeable. Here many a girl, who has always been the object of affection and attention at home, finds herself a member of a large group where no one receives individual consideration. With the exception of a very short vacation period, the student must live the entire three years under the regulations of the school. This may prove extremely irksome to her, and she may chafe under the restrictions which it involves. Having had her own way in most things at home, it is difficult for a young woman with boundless initiative and enthusiasm to work under the direction of others, unless she receives very wise guidance and direction. To one who has never been away from home, the adjustment to dormitory life with its many distractions is difficult. If a girl is attractive and popular, her room may be always filled with visitors, who prevent her from studying. In her class work she is confronted with an amazing number of new subjects. She must keep up each day with her lessons or she soon finds herself behind. She has no sooner become accustomed to the routine of study than she is introduced to the hospital ward with its bewildering number of sick patients, doctors, nurses and medical students, and is expected to adjust herself to this environment in a very short time. Such an experience is a severe tax on the emotional equipment of any girl. Obviously, there has been nothing in her past experience to compare with it. It is imperative, therefore, that students have a guiding hand and an understanding heart during this period of their course. Undoubtedly, too much is expected of the young students who enter our schools. Many are too young to assume the responsibilities which are often thrust upon them. It would be an advantage both to the student and to the school if the age requirement for entrance could be placed at twenty years. Ordinarily, students come filled with zeal and enthusiasm for the work they are to undertake. We must see to it that this spirit is not dimmed or snuffed out entirely, as is sometimes the case. The answer to this problem is adequate, wise and painstaking supervision.

VOCATIONAL GUIDANCE IN HIGH SCHOOLS

This discussion seems to bring us to the conclusion that there is need for better vocational guidance in high schools. Mr. Harry Kitson, Professor of Education, Teachers College, Columbia University, stresses in the May number of the *Record*, the importance of special preparation for those who are engaged in vocational guidance in secondary schools and colleges. Some large city systems have well organized bureaus of vocational guidance with a director and a staff of experts. Certainly all high schools should have a qualified person to advise the students. It is to such a people as these that we must go, to make known our particular needs. Steps in this direction have been taken in several places, the most noteworthy being the work done recently in the State of Washington by the League of Nursing Education. In consultation with high school authorities they have worked out a suggested course which is to be used in high schools for pupils who wish to become nurses. The program includes four years of English, two years of Latin, two years of modern language, one year of medieval and modern history, one year of United States history and civics, one year of chemistry, one year of biology or physics, one year of algebra, one year of economics, and one year of geometry. This curriculum has been sent to every high school, and to every school of nursing in the state. When such a piece of work has been accomplished in all our states, we will have done much in the way of solving some of our admission problems.

COST OF NURSING EDUCATION

Students in other professional schools pay fees which at least partly meet the cost of their education. In some colleges, it is estimated that the students pay about one-half the cost of their education. It may be true that students in the school of nursing pay a higher tuition than many college students, but this is true of only those who complete the nursing course. They do pay their tuition in long hours of service to the hospital. Those students who are dropped at the end of the preliminary course or during the first year, do not in any way meet the cost of their education. They represent a great expense to the school, or to the hospital which supports it.

In the Washington University School of Nursing, the average daily cost per student for the year 1929 was $2.66, $915.04 per year and $2,745.12 for three years.

The cost of students in the preliminary course is much greater than that of the older students, owing to the fact that that part of the work is almost entirely theoretical, and includes all the courses in the basic sciences, which are costly because of the character of instruction given and the equipment used. Probably a conservative estimate would be $3.00 per day for such students. This would represent an expenditure of $360 for four months of the preliminary course. Where from 20 percent to 25 percent of a class is dropped at the end of this period, one finds that a surprisingly large sum of money has been expended.

The majority of our schools of nursing charge no fees for this period although a few have always done so. At the University of Wisconsin, students pay the same fees for the preliminary course as other students in the university, including room, board, and laundry. This would seem a wise solution to the problem in a university school and it would appear equally just to require a good stiff tuition fee in hospital schools.

CONCLUSIONS

If we are to secure fewer and better candidates for our schools of nursing, and wish to eliminate the waste in our present extravagant system of nursing education, we must begin to pay more attention to the social, economic and intellectual background of our students. Those unfitted for the profession will have to be rejected through the use of intelligence and character tests. States must establish laws with a minimum entrance requirement of four years high school, and stick to this requirement. High schools, through their vocational guidance departments, must be informed as to our needs, so that they can intelligently advise young women who are thinking of entering our profession. Courses must be made available in high schools which will insure a better background for the nursing course. Students must meet a part of the cost of their education, especially for the preliminary course, by the payment of tuition fees, the same as other college students. Then, and only then, will some of the problems of admission and adjustment be solved in our schools of nursing.

(Wheeler, 1930, pp. 120–129)

Section IV
Ethics

Introduction to Ethics

*E*arly in the development of the Superintendents' Society, the leadership group recognized the need for a national association for the rank and file. Nursing leaders conceived such an organization, comprised of alumnae associations from different schools, as the appropriate body to initiate nursing's ethical principles. They saw a national code of ethics as the way to provide a foundation for professional conduct and rules of correct behavior in nursing. Alumnae associations fostered collegiality, dissemination of information, and unity among graduates. Prior to the establishment of those associations, graduate nurses remained isolated from one another and lacked the means for implementing ethical standards.

Ethical issues confronting the Superintendents' Society during its formative phase centered on applicants to training schools who had been dismissed for objectionable conduct from other schools, problems arising from the care of male patients, and the extent and nature of a disciplinary process for pupils. Later, the NLNE defined right and wrong with respect to interpersonal relationships, determined differences between ethics and etiquette, and described the characteristics of the desirable student. Although a national code of ethics was not adopted during the years 1894–1933, appropriate professional behavior remained an issue of concern among the superintendents over the entire period.

The papers in this section have been selected because they address ethical principles within the context of the goals of that time. Those goals included protecting patients from harm and promoting the moral integrity of the nursing profession.

How Far Are Training Schools Responsible for the Lack of Ethics Among Nurses

By Eva Allerton

Superintendent Homeopathic Hospital, Rochester

The subject assigned me by the Council does not admit of argument. It assumes that there exists a laxity of morals in some graduates from our training schools, and the question arises, to what extent are the training schools responsible for a state of affairs which we must admit exists to-day in the nursing profession.

We must take into consideration the fact that it is only within the last decade that women have come so prominently before the public as bread-winners. Not very many years ago the father, husband, or brother, dictated the mode of occupation for the female members of the household. If necessity demanded, a woman might teach school, music, clerk in a store, or sew; but she was daring, indeed, who ventured beyond these lines. In this age, without any special training to develop the stable side of character, a woman may support herself, or an entire family, by her professional work. Here she suffers from comparison with professional men, not only as regards the question of efficiency, but also in that of remuneration. This is largely the cause of so much adverse criticism of what is known as the "new woman."

While the public tolerates shortcomings in women who are engaged in other occupations, without any great amount of comment, it has fixed a higher standard of morality for the professional nurse. Why? Because her duties are of vital importance. She is brought face to face with the great problems of life, the mystery of death, and suffering in every form; she is taken into the home and confidence of the family where she is thrown into close relations with the inner life. Her duties are exacting, and if she fulfills her part and meets all the requirements she is often regarded as little less than an angel. If the reverse obtains, as is frequently the case, the faults and blemishes in her character appear more glaring than in any other class of professional women.

Fortunately or unfortunately, the criticisms we hear are those in regard to conduct rather than lack of skill or knowledge on the part of the nurse, except among one class of people known as the "newly rich," who apparently consider it a duty to find fault with any paid service rendered.

Now, to whom should the applicant for membership in our training schools be referred? Just here lies a great responsibility. I have made no attempt to learn in how many of the schools represented in this body the selection is made by the superintendent of the hospital, who may be a physician, a minister or a layman. In some institutions a committee, composed of physicians and lady managers, pass upon applicants; or a single individual, man or woman, as the case may be, is vested with power to act. This is all very well, provided the acceptance or dismissal of the applicant, at the end of the probationary term, is left with the training school superintendent, who is, of course, a trained nurse. Almost every superintendent here could tell of the great difficulties experienced in getting rid of pupils, who, from a moral point of view, are not desirable, though they may be adapted to the work by virtue of natural gifts and personal advantages. If at all pleasing in appearance and manner, and can cry becomingly, it is easy for her to obtain one or more advocates among those interested in the management, in which case it is made so difficult for the superintendent to act that she yields the point in despair; the pupil is allowed to remain in the ranks, and to graduate, only to bring disgrace and shame upon the profession.

We need a more uniform method of selection. Assuming trained nursing to be a profession is it not right and just that the question of fitness should be decided by members of the profession into which the applicant aspires to enter? Doctors, lawyers, ministers and dentists are passed upon by those who have been graduated in their own special line of work and who are, consequently best able to judge of fitness. Therefore it seems right and just that the matter should be left with the superintendent, who is, of course, a trained nurse.

The question of age is of prime importance. Every girl must have her silly age, and she should have passed this before she can be considered a desirable pupil in any training school. I think I may say that the majority of schools represented here, do not admit applicants under twenty-two years of age. I prefer to take them at twenty-five, when every girl may be judged as a woman, and it should not be found necessary to excuse misconduct on the plea of youth.

It is my judgment that the first steps to be taken toward elevating the standard of ethics in nursing, is to allow time for the development of the practical side of character. Have we, as women, the moral right to bring into this work girls of unformed character, thus to obtain, before they are able to resist its influence, a knowledge of the many phases of life so peculiar to our hospital work? It becomes the duty of the nurse to administer to saint and to sinner, the same kindly, courteous treatment. "Familiarity breeds contempt" and it is my experience that it also breeds toleration.

> Vice is a monster of so frightful mien,
> As to be hated needs but to be seen;
> Yet seen too oft, familiar with her face,
> We first endure, then pity, then embrace.

When we give to the nurse her diploma, we virtually say to the puplic: "Here is this young woman. We find her virtuous, truthful and faithful. Take her into your homes; trust your loved ones with her; place your confidence in her; she will not fail you or be found wanting." Do we always conscientiously say this? Do we not occasionally feel like saying: "We *hope* she will not fail you?"

We should instruct our pupils to consider character of first importance, then look to their profession. The school should retain only young women with vigor and loveliness of character. Selfishness, sensuality, greed and disloyalty are degrading, and to be deplored; gentleness and veracity, in word and act, must be absolutely demanded. The same ethical principles which govern the school should govern the individual.

It is the duty of the school to thoroughly instruct its pupils with regard to the use and abuse of certain drugs and stimulants with which, in daily life, they become so familiar. It should never be taken for granted that they realize their danger. Here again familiarity is a great source of evil. To the woman of weak character, the alleviation obtained by much means, when the mental and physical strain is great, makes the forming of unfortunate habits comparatively easy. Let us warn those under our supervision of the danger which is in store for them if they yield to this form of temptation.

She must also be prepared and fortified against the peculiar trials and temptations which will surely come to her after she leaves the hospital. Here our responsibility ends and hers begins: and though we are naturally solicitous as to her progress and success, and desirous that she perform her duties in a faithful and conscientious manner, we should not further be held responsible for the conduct of the nurse who goes astray from the principles inculcated during the years of preparation in the training school.

(Allerton, 1898, pp. 45–47)

How to Prepare Nurses for the Duties of the Alumnae

By Lucy Walker

Superintendent Pennsylvania Hospital Training School, Philadelphia

The first thoughts that arise in the mind when endeavoring to deal with this subject are: What are the objects of the Alumnae Associations? What are the duties of Alumnae? In order to answer these questions, a few of the many constitutions and by-laws were consulted, and there seemed to be but little variation in the articles dealing with "objects." They are all practically summed up in Article II of the Constitution of the Associated Alumnae, which reads: "The objects of this Association shall be: To establish and maintain a code of ethics; to elevate the standard of nursing education; to promote the usefulness and honor, the financial and other interests of the nursing profession." It would seem, therefore, that the principal duties of the Alumnae must be to aid in carrying out the various clauses of this article.

Only a few years ago, Nurses' Alumnae Associations were almost unknown. Each nurse, as she left her training school, found herself a struggling unit, with no professional code of ethics to guide her connection with other members of the profession. Naturally, her tendency under these conditions was to become a mere working woman, doing so much work for so much money, and thinking only of her own material welfare. As a result, the status of the profession was lowered, and many were thereby deterred from entering hospital training schools, who might have proven themselves most useful members. To-day almost every school has its Alumnae Association, and the majority of these have united to form The Associated Alumnae of the United States and Canada. Thus we have, in many parts of this great continent alumnae who have agreed to establish and maintain a code of ethics;

who have agreed to elevate the standard of nursing education; who have agreed to promote the usefulness and honor of the nursing profession, as well as its more material interests. In "union is strength" and it surely seems as though much must be accomplished in the near future, as it has been in the very near past. It is only requisite that the women who are daily entering our ranks shall be so prepared that they may have a true understanding of what their duties as alumnae are.

When a woman decides to study nursing she does so generally because she can secure for herself a profession in return for work done and without any first outlay of money. The number of those who enter training schools for other reasons is very small. They enter with but a vague idea of the duties they will be called upon to perform. Visions perhaps of smoothing pillows, administering medicines, reading to patients, etc., may have fired their enthusiasm, and they see themselves being and doing something noble. But, as we all know, while a hospital training school is admirably fitted for turning out well-trained and skillful nurses, it is not the best school for developing the special qualities essential to a woman who is to take her proper place in the world, or indeed in her own profession. The necessary routine of the work, the wholesale nursing, the strict obedience required, the technical skill gained long before the theoretical knowledge follows to render the work intelligent, all tend to make mechanical workers; the long, hard hours of enforced work tend to develop selfishness; the short time allowed for recreation, and the long time spent in absorbing ideas within restricted limits cause a narrowing of the mind. On entering a training school the first shock received by a would-be nurse, more especially if she has come direct from a home life, is the realization that she has lost her individuality. No one cares what she is or how she feels so long as her share of the work is accomplished. This, at first, seems cruel, but she often becomes hardened, and is herself as careless of the feelings of the next newcomer. Then, having a certain portion of the hard work allotted to her, to be finished within a given time, she is tempted to regard the calls of patients, or of other nurses, as so many unwelcome interruptions, and a disposition to be selfish and unfeeling comes to light. Again, she finds herself hedged in by rules of which she cannot see the use, and a rebellious feeling is apt to arise, followed by a certain changed attitude of mind towards the one in authority, whose duty it is to enforce such rules with the result that she who desires to be and should be the guide and friend, as well as teacher, is often regarded only as a hard task-master and an unmerciful judge.

The question as to how best to check these tendencies in the pupil nurse is a difficult one to answer. There is no present prospect for her of gaining the theoretical knowledge as the young doctor does, before entering the hospital wards. This in itself would be of infinite value as it would render the nurse's work both intelligent and interesting from the outset, and check the tendency to become mechanical. Neither is there any immediate prospect, in the majority of schools, of shortening the hours of work, or of giving more opportunity for recreation. It is, therefore, useless to discuss these points at this time. We can only acknowledge that the tendencies are there and that it is our duty to do what lies in our power to correct and check them.

And then the question arises, what does lie in our power? What can we do for these young women, who place themselves under our care in order to develop their best qualities? And how can we check the growth of other qualities which are not desirable? In a large hospital, the principal of the training school comes very little in personal contact with the pupils. It is difficult for her to learn their various characteristics, and to deal with them accordingly, because these are apt to be tucked away in some hidden corner, while in her presence. She is obliged to trust largely to the reports given her by the head nurses of the wards just as she is obliged to leave the practical training almost entirely in their hands. It is, therefore, necessary that the nurses selected for such responsible work, should be women above the average in every way; women, who realize the importance of their work and who are truly interested in doing their best for those under their charge. Their example and teaching mean much to the young probationer. By their watchfulness also and reports of the first appearance of faults, the principal is enabled to check the tendency at once, and perhaps to implant some good thought, or encourage some good resolution to take its place.

The rules, always so trying to the undisciplined mind, should be as few as possible, and only such as are absolutely necessary for the protection of the patient and the guidance of the pupil. If these rules were carefully gone over with the probationer and the reason for each explained it might possibly assist her to keep them cheerfully and willingly; and if each class could be induced to form their own class code of honor, it would be a good preliminary training for enabling them to assist in establishing and maintaining a code of ethics, when they become members of the Associated Alumnae.

Then, in order to prepare them for the duty of assisting "to elevate the standard of nursing education" must they not themselves receive the best education that we can procure for them? Not merely so many lectures and so many recitations, but a true education, "the discipline of the intellect, the establishment of the principles, the regulation of the heart."

During the pupil's first year it is necessary as a rule to teach her how to study and to supervise all her work most carefully, but when the year's work is satisfactorily completed, it is best to allow her to receive and digest for herself the knowledge placed before her; and although she may not appear to acquire knowledge so rapidly, she is acquiring with it self-reliance and a sense that she alone is responsible for what she gains or what she loses. The course of study should be systematic and progressive throughout the training and should embrace as wide a range of subjects as can be taken up with thoroughness and without over-taxing the mind; the chief aim being to cultivate a desire for knowledge and to train the mind, so that it may be able to assimilate and use with judgment, the knowledge when acquired.

To further prepare nurses for their duties as alumnae, it is well to instruct them in the history of nursing and in the efforts that are being made at the present time to further its interests. They should also be prepared to take their part in business and other meetings, and should be drilled in the usages of parliamentary law, and in the discussion of papers. During the third year of the nurses' training at the Pennsylvania Hospital a portion of their class-work consists in forming and managing an Association of their own. It is re-formed at the beginning of each class year, the members drawing up their own constitution and by-laws. The officers serve for one month only and the committees are appointed by each incoming President. There are two committees: the Committee on Nomination and the Committee on Arrangements. The Arrangement Committee selects subjects for papers and appoints members to write and discuss them. No restriction is placed on the choice of subjects. The Association is entirely self-governed, as the teacher never holds office nor does she know anything of the work done by the committees until they present their reports at the regular meetings. This form of class work has the following advantages: It gives the members ample opportunity to get over their "stage fright" before the time comes for them to speak in the presence of strangers. They learn to formulate their thoughts and opinions and to express them in a business-like manner. They also learn to express themselves correctly, which will be an advantage when teaching others. It teaches them to govern themselves and it certainly helps them to think of their work from the intelligent standpoint. They learn from their own mistakes, when the mistakes produce no serious consequences, and they gain some experience to guide them, when, their student days ended, they take their places as members of their own Alumnae Association and members of the Associated Alumnae. Most earnestly do we hope that the future members of our profession may be, above all women, high-minded, broad-minded, strong-hearted, striving not only to gain honor in their own individual work, but to heartily aid in "establishing and maintaining a code of honor; in elevating the standard of nursing education; and in promoting the usefulness and honor of the nursing profession."

(Walker, 1900, pp. 44–48)

Ethics to be Observed Between Training Schools

By Miss Laura A. Beecroft

Superintendent of Nurses, Minnequa Hospital, Pueblo, Colorado

"Ethics—the science of human duty; rules of practice in respect to a single class of human actions." This is Webster's definition of ethics. I think it is a good practice to go back to the root of things occasionally, and look at the foundation. We are all so apt to forget and when it comes to rules, we all add a little to fit our own case or strike out a little, until the original is entirely lost.

I remember when, as a child, I learned to sew, by making quilt patches. The cutting was the difficult part. It was too much trouble to hunt the pattern every time—as a result the patch soon was anything but a true copy of the original. Sometimes the pattern would get small pieces snipped off also, and it would not be exact. We do this same thing in our every day life—in our social and business intercourse— the little things that are so small and obscure at the time have the faculty of piling up, and as the old saying reminds us, "It's the last straw that breaks the camel's back."

I do not believe that any superintendent of nurses would deliberately neglect a human duty, or infringe on one of the rules practiced between hospitals. She simply has had so many other apparently more pressing needs on hand at the time, the true science of ethics has been obscured.

What are the rules that should be practiced between training schools? I must plead guilty to ignorance of those laid down by the founders of our training schools. If there are any written or printed, I have never seen them. The only knowledge I have is traditional.

Physicians begun long ago to follow the rules as laid down by Hippocrates, "Him who taught me this act, I will esteem even as I do my parents—he shall partake of my livelihood, and if in want, shall share my good. So far as power and discernment shall be mine, I will carry out regimen for the benefit of the sick, and I will keep them from harm and wrong," etc. The physicians of the present century have added many new ethical points of their standard. For instance, no physician must run down the character or work of a brother, if he does he injures himself. He must not neglect the patient for the sake of spite or hatred, but must bury these out of sight, giving all professional assistance needed. He must speak well of his Alma Mater or it in turn reflects back on him, and so on. Some one, writing in a medical journal last year, made the statement—"nurses are very narrow-minded, and since they had found out all sick patients insisted on having a nurse, they were also arrogant."

When nursing was first introduced into the hospitals, and such fearful conditions existed as history records, the necessity of having a certain class of women to help demonstrate the need of nurses was absolutely necessary. At that time, the human side of the people was aroused and many applications were received from good women—the best were selected and the others turned away as unsatisfactory. This was the origin of the first unwritten ethical rule between training schools, which was, as near as I can find out—any woman turned away from one school must not be admitted in another. It did not seem to make any difference what the cause of her leaving was. She could not reform, outlive, or outgrow the difficulty, she simply must not be reinstated or accepted in any other hospital if the head nurse of said hospital wished to be loyal to her profession. Some years later, some one seems to have had the strength of character to take another stand something like this, "We will admit nurses that have been in other schools, but she must come as a probationer and serve full time.

Since I have taken charge of a training school, I have found two other rules in existence that are just as objectionable as either of the above. 1st. Any pupil from any school, applying at our hospital, will be taken in. 2d. We will allow all time spent in any hospital, if two physicians recommend you to us.

There is a question that is coming before the Western State Examining Boards, Training Schools and Nurses' Associations,—these partly trained women—What are we going to do with them? This subject of uncompleted courses should be of interest to all of us. We tell the nurse she cannot nurse as a trained nurse unless she is registered. She applies to a training school to finish her work, and is told she must do three years' time, if she is given any consideration at all; and nine times out of ten, she does nothing but continue nursing, telling the physician and patient she has had training.

In Colorado, there are hundreds of these partially trained women. It is impossible for the Registration Board to get hold of them; they say, when brought to bay, we have had training and have said so, but do not claim to be trained, registered or graduate nurses. When taking the case, they may not make this distinction—what are we going to do? Take them into our hospitals and give them a diploma, thus having a lot of mediocre graduate nurses? In the name of Florence Nightingale—no. We have enough of that kind—graduated from mediocre schools now.

On the other hand, there are many emergencies which may arise for the nurse or woman who has started training in a certain school, which may make it impossible for her to complete her course in that institution. She may become bankrupt; break down in health; an unexpected illness in her family which may mean a change of climate, and again for personal reasons, it may not be best for her to stay in that school. Now, one of three things happens—she either gives up the idea of being a nurse altogether, or she goes out and enters the nursing field in competition with the graduate; or she makes an effort to enter a school that will allow her the time she has spent.

Second class registration and a local registry where such nurses could be registered, and the doctor and public both know just what kind of a nurse they are employing, is one remedy that is suggested.

I have adopted a plan of my own in regard to this class of women. When they apply to me, I send them a regular application blank with the regulations of the training school and a letter, requesting a letter from their former superintendent, also one from a reliable person who has known them during the previous six months. If the superintendent makes no formal charge, I then instruct them to come for two months' trial; at the end of this period, they must take the intermediate examination, if they want two years' time, or Junior examination if it is only one year. If their practical work is satisfactory, they are allowed the time accordingly. I feel if there is good material there, it is better to make good nurses of them, if possible, than allow them to go to the mediocre school or practice as non-graduates.

I would recommend a standard set of rules for training schools—these might be gotten up by the State Board of Examiners and the superintendents in each state. Every state should have its own standard, for different conditions make it impossible for the United States to make rigid nursing laws. For instance, there are in Colorado about one-tenth per cent of the institutions for learning that are found in New York State, hence the educational standard may be higher in New York than in Colorado; but per capita, we have as many people needing nurses. For we all know Colorado is the tuberculosis dumping ground for the union.

There are several other ethical points that might be discussed—the one of recommending mediocre graduate nurses to schools in distant states is sometimes met with. They say by their actions, Oh, well, they will have to keep her a year if they pay her transportation out there. Don't do it! You only injure your reputation and that of your school. The western doctors appreciate a good nurse and *know when* they get one. We might speak of the pernicious habit of running down other schools. Every school has its good and bad points, because you have an up-to-date operating room or a first class surgeon does not prove to me, your nurses will receive superior training. The training of the good nurse is done by the nurse in the ward and the teacher in the class room. No amount of lectures and fine stage play will make good nurses—they must get down to rock bottom and do the things for themselves. You must teach them ethics if you wish them to respond in like manner. You must teach your pupils surgical cleanliness if you wish them to be surgically clean; you must teach them to be thorough if you wish them to do first-class work, and it is the superintendent of nurses who does these things, that has the best school, and it will not be necessary for her to run down any other school to obtain pupils. What are the ethics or rules I would recommend to be observed between schools? Both the biblical rendering of the golden rule, also that taught by Confucius, "Do unto others as you would have others do to you," the latter "Do not do unto others what you would not have others do to you." If a pupil is leaving your hospital for good lawful reasons, let her understand you will recommend her to any school she may wish to enter, if she is being dismissed for cause, then make her to understand you will not recommend her. Do not take in any pupils that have been in other training schools without a recommendation from their former superintendent. Do not encourage migration between local schools, and lastly, let every superintendent teach ethics in her school and at the same time practice ethics herself.

(Beecroft, 1910, pp. 53–57)

Nursing Ethics and Discipline

By Charlotte M. Perry

The system of ethics which has obtained to a greater or less degree in the profession of nursing has come to us through a long heritage. By ethics we mean those rules which govern action relating to the whole field of professional duty, including discipline. The type is set in the Hippocratic oath, of which there are many variations. But even those who are most awake to the need of these modifications to meet the constant flux of social life know that for the nursing body the principle has always existed. There are those who inveigh against a too restrictive idea of the subject; who believe that when we begin to codify ethics we impede the way to a high and noble interpretation of professional law. When we come to teach professional ethics, one of the greatest difficulties lies in the confusion of mind which exists on the part of those who train the young in social ethics. Manifestly we must have some clear conception of the scope of professional ethics as it has been taught in the past, and of its present application, if we are to direct the vast army of nurses and institutions for the care of patients. If we confine ethics to social or professional customs which have become established by law or by the concensus of opinion; of, if we look at it from the moral standpoint, i.e., from human standards of right and wrong, we narrow its significance, though many will be content to stop here. But it can be shown how large an influence was exerted by religious bodies, especially in Germany and England upon our professional standards. It was from religious orders that the strictest system of ethics and discipline emanated. It is in religious belief and experience that we find the true exposition of morals as received from the Divine Lawgiver. In the evolution hospitals, history records the recognition of the ethical principle and of authority with its response in obedience (often self-imposed) from those taking upon themselves the care of the sick. There was the conventual system, when religious communities turned their houses into asylums or hospitals, or sent their religious out to care for sick and wounded. Religion formed the background. If one could not be cured, he could be enabled to die well. The obligation common to all with respect to the sick in these days is expressed in the Church's *oremus pro afflictis.* Her prayers for her afflicted ones reveal the neighborly and truly social desire to help those in trouble. And there is no real conflict between the strict discipline which has been a marked feature in the profession of nursing and the motive which every individual should entertain to spend and be spent for others. Our sense of duty is bound up with respect for authority.

In the changed social conditions of the present day, what is noticeable is the defective teaching in the homes of young women, many of whom, after arriving at the suitable age, feel drawn to the calling of a nurse, but who come to us unprepared and without those essential qualifications which might have been nurtured in the home. The benefit of early home training can hardly be overestimated. The laying of foundations is always important. The best preparation for the vocation of nursing is found in a wholesome development and right education of young life. So that although precedent has much to do with the formation of standards, the corollary of this is just as true, that times change, bringing new conditions which require alterations or fresh adaptations of rules. Superintendents of training schools are keenly alive to these changes, if not always mindful of the force of precedent. There has been wrought into our experience the sense that discipline is necessary for frail humanity—discipline in the early years, implying respect for parents and teachers; discipline in the formation of character, in the development of mind, and in the struggle to become masters of any line of work which we wish to make our own. The country at large is awaking to the serious bearing of the neglect of child-nurture, as is evidenced by the springing up of social organizations designed to secure more effective coöperation between the home, educators, boards of health and legislators, with the hope that their efforts may result in better citizenship, happier homes, in the health and efficiency of the individual. It has been plainly seen that the up-bringing is different from some years back, in a harmful sense. Parents have not exercised the authority it is their duty to exert. Young women are not only encouraged to choose their own course of study long before a right judgment is formed, but are allowed a large margin of

freedom in their manner of life and dress. Pleasure and indolence often
now rule the day where instruction and practical knowledge in the
home management were given and acquired. Habits of neatness and
economy were exacted from the child—and who will not see in this
the better way?

As a consequence of this failure in child-training, certain difficulties
confront our administration. There is not the hardihood, endurance,
nor perseverence to work upon. In the absence of this framework
of character, the ethical points which need insistence are too slowly
absorbed into the personality of the nurse. This re-acts alike on teacher,
pupil and patient, but most of all upon the latter, who, as Mrs. Robb
so forcibly put it, is susceptible more than we appreciate to impressions
often unconsciously made by the nurse, and who feels the lack of that
"spiritual and mental development or change taking place within us"
as a result of our training. There must be certain attributes on the part
of the person taking up the vocation of nursing—qualities of heart and
mind; and this in addition to the practical preparation she receives in
the home and through education. Unless the candidate has cultivated,
or is capable of being taught some of these distinctive traits, it is but
lost labor to persevere in the training. There are some forms of service
involving great responsibility, recognized by Church and State, in
which failure or laxity entail heavy loss, or bear weighty consequences.
Persons filling such positions must be reliable; must have proved their
metal. It must be conceded that accountability is attached to some
vocations above others. And we are assured that the observance of the
ethical principle is necessary to our professional organization; in fact,
a basic principle of the human race.

It may be well for us that we do not comprehend all that is required
of us when we appear at the bar of acceptance as a candidate for the
Training School. The ethical field is wide, the subject matter large, and
relations to others complicated. The category of desired characteristics
forms a long list—truthfulness, obedience, neatness, punctuality,
respect for superiors, thoughtful manner, control of the tongue, gentleness, dignity, self-respect, business capacity, good judgment, tact, quiet
observation, and the like. The selection of candidates has much to do
with successfully instilling ethical ideals. If the education could but
begin early in life, such preparation combined with what the boards of
education are doing for us in some states, anticipating subsequent
vocational training, would provide a larger number of suitable candidates. There are in thirty-six states Parent-Teacher Associations which

are doing a good work in this direction. Such subjects as "The Vital Relations between the Home and the School;" "The Education of Girls;" "Character-building by Parents," and others are discussed with far-reaching results. These organizations unite with the schools in giving preparatory education, and would doubtless join us in the endeavor to impress on those who look forward to nursing the noble side of the work—the opportunity for self-sacrifice—the fostering of a true sympathy for the sick.

There has been a great diversity of interpretation as to the application of ethical laws educationally as well as professionally. Educational systems have changed so frequently as barely to outlive the education of one pupil. A generation ago, high schools were dominated by colleges, and the course greatly restricted, with little or no reference to the work which was to follow. But the excellent advance made during the last decade has secured for us legislation, whereby our training schools have been taken into account, their interests studied, requirements more clearly outlined, and some undesirable elements of the past thrown out. Not only has education been planned in regard to general foundation, but has been arranged with special life-work in view, whether that be vocational or commercial. This has had a great deal to do with defining our professional regulations. Educational legislation has taught us our duty towards the pupil-nurse, as well as her duty towards hospital authorities, the medical profession, and the community. We give more because more is required of the pupil and of the graduate nurse after she leaves the hospital. Thus, education has stood for the good of the people. Such an educator as Dr. Eliot of Harvard sees in the existence of colleges and schools a higher purpose than that of mere culture. The college life must stand for moral leadership.

This superior aspect of ethics leads to the question of the application of discipline. A too repressive discipline is incompatible with that spirit of consecrated service and willing endurance which it is desirable to encourage in the nurse. It is also opposed to the idea of self-government which some schools practice, as may be the case where the nursing staff is composed of mature and cultivated women; although there are some who are of the opinion either that we are not ready for self-government, or that it is impracticable. The older interpretation of ethics and discipline have been compared with the present day attitude for the purpose of enlightenment. Changed social conditions and the educational systems of the day necessitate a study of the subject. It is a vast one. The educators of the country are engaged in a thoughtful investigation of general principles involved. In our professional dealings a few of these principles might be accentuated. The exercise of discipline should not be too autocratic. The personal element should be dropped out of sight. And though we exact an unquestioning obedience, and expect all discipline to be accepted in a military silence, there should be a court of appeal through which the offender may ultimately secure justice. This court of appeal may be composed of a training school committee which shall be representative, including trustees, doctors on the staff, and the superintendent of hospital and training school.

Before, however, we can have a universal standard of ethics, there must be a return to first principles, each educational unit represented by the classified schools must follow certain well defined laws of organization. In other words, each military campus must preserve its original system of rank, of authority vested in recognized heads. Florence Nightingale, in a letter written to Dr. W. G. Wylie, one of the founders of the Bellevue Hospital, enunciated the true principle that in the nursing and for nurses full control should rest with the superintendent of nurses. She speaks of the contrary custom in Germany as giving rise to a deplorable condition. She says that the kind of internal management which she recommends could not possibly result in any trespassing on the doctors' sphere, because superintendents of training schools are most careful to teach the right relation of the nurses to medical men, and to avoid confusing the two duties, medical and nursing. That nurses are taught that they are there solely to carry out the orders of the medical and surgical staff. That nurses are in no way under the medical staff as to discipline, but under their superintendent, who should be thoroughly trained. What she calls the hierarchy of the higher grade should know the duties of the lower grade better than the lower grade does itself; otherwise they will be unable to train. And every department of hospital corp, whether assistants, head nurses, night nurses, and the help, should be under her direction. Otherwise, discipline becomes impossible.

If the words of our illustrious pioneer are true, surely any undermining of authority works disastrously. Each grade should exercise only to a proper degree the delegated authority entrusted to it. In preparing women for the management of institutions, the error of overstepping rank should be emphasized more than it has been in the past. It is instruction which should be included in the course of training. Taking as an instance the first mentioned rank below the superintendent, the position of assistant is helpful in furnishing the actual experience in the duties which pertain to the office above it. If the relation of assistant to superintendent is clearly apprehended, there will be no tendency to teach independently, to weaken the superintendent's authority, to harbor wrong ambitions of preferment; and the military principle of observance of rank will result in harmonious working of the whole staff.

Again, there should be perfect comradery and good faith between the executives of the hospital. Otherwise pupils cannot be taught to render respect to whom respect is due. The medical and hospital staffs alike should be loyal to the superintendent of the institution or training school of which she has been placed in charge. Her credentials have been accepted, and idle rumors and criticisms should not be too quickly picked up and believed. There is an honorable and direct way of dealing with the difficulty of change of position. Evidence of unfitness for office ought never to be sought nor received from the pupil nurses, nor from ranks below the superintendent. This is a rule which will be readily acknowledged by those who have followed the same in ordinary social life. In the case of complaints coming from the offending party of too severe discipline, great care should be taken to submit the same to a properly constituted committee. The action of the superintendent should not be discussed in the presence of the governed. No chief executive of good standing would object to having her work scrutinized by those to whom she is responsible; even as a good bookkeeper desires at all times to have books open to investigation.

Thus in analyzing our difficulties we become conscious of certain defects in our social and educational systems, and in our internal management which affect our standard of ethics and discipline. There has been a lack of moral tone which we do well to rectify as far as in our power. We may ask, are we progressing toward a more perfect system, and are the imperfections noted due to the absence of clear teaching? The importance of the early years has been dwelt upon as affording opportunity for better preparation for the work of life, especially when that of nursing is in view. The inculcation of right principles it is hoped will awaken that quality so essential to the maintenance of ethical standards, viz., that reverence of which it has been said "it is deeply rooted in the heart of humanity: you cannot root it out. Civilization, science, progress only change its direction, they do not weaken its force."

(Perry, 1913, pp. 87–93)

The Purpose and Place of Ethics in the Curriculum

By S. Lillian Clayton

During the past few years many requests have been made that a book be written on "Ethics," to be used in our schools for nurses.

Hearing this request so often, one is led to inquire as to the reason *why* there should be such a demand. When a profession demands a book written upon any special subject, it is usually because there has been a great change of methods, or more scientific knowledge has been acquired, thus necessitating revision of the old matter, or entirely new material has been written.

Having this in mind, we ask, "Why is there a need for such a book?" There is no fundamental change today in our ideas of right and wrong conduct so far as that conduct is directed toward the individual, but with our complexity of social ideas has come a need—not for new books, but a reaching out for some standard of determining what *is* right and wrong. Such standards are not by any means fixed. We cannot hope to set forth standards which we shall be willing to accept twenty years hence, but what we wish is to determine where in our ethical ideas of twenty years ago there is need of revision, and the *purpose* and *place* of such revision in our profession today.

We are all familiar with the well-known fact, referred to so constantly, that as a profession, we are narrow in our ideals of relationships of one school to another, of the profession in one state to that of another, and of the profession as a whole to society. This has been a source of sorrow to those who have felt that they *have* met this obligation to their school, and to the immediate community, because of common traditions, and who have learned that the truest conception of right and wrong is gained by mixing with those traveling on one common road. Recently a prominent member of our profession, returning from administrative service in Europe, where she had been directing 80 American nurses, from different training schools throughout the United States, made a statement, setting forth the idea that the technic and skill of our American nurses was recognized by her, and by the Europeans as being above criticism, and yet, when placed before the world's gaze these same nurses were seriously criticized. Why? Because of their lack of ethics.

They would doubtless have been satisfactory when dealing with the members of their own school in their own community, but they had not learned the broader or social ethical relationships.

We see something similar in the family that has been trained to love and loyalty in all domestic relationships, whose conduct is above criticism when judged by abstract right and wrong, but who fail when the demand made upon them is, that they understand and appreciate the needs of the community. They have been so absorbed in self-development, that they have not recognized the claim of social obligations.

We know that no application of professional Ethics can, in any manner, take the place of those fundamental principles of right and wrong which have existed from the beginning of time, but as members of a common profession we can, with profit, apply some of these moral principles, not alone to the individual nurse, but to the community of nurses.

The *purpose* of ethics would be, first of all, to teach our students the application of ethical principles to their relationship with their patients. The *place* for this instruction would be in the beginning of their professional education, and as their conception of their own powers and responsibilities develops, such instruction would extend throughout the entire course of an ever broadening gauge. The subject matter of such instruction is already familiar to all.

We believe that the proper methods to pursue in moral education are essentially the same as those laid down for intellectual development in the schools. These should be closely related to the sciences. The broader we can make the student's knowledge of psychology, the more sure we shall be of her appreciation of certain facts of human nature and the laws governing them.

For instance, she will soon understand that ethics is the science of human conduct in personal relations, that we live in society, that unless this social law is obeyed, the family would not endure—then extending the thought further, she soon realizes that, just as she must obey the law of the family, so she must obey the law of society.

We must dwell upon the conceptions of modern thought, the universe governed by one law, the uniformity of nature, and the including of all human life under this law.

We have not, as a profession, sufficiently impressed upon our students the ethical responsibility existing toward society and toward the profession as a whole.

The older professions of law and medicine have made considerable progress in the development of their systems of ethics.

Nursing is a young profession, and can learn much from its elders. On the other hand, it is not hampered by tradition, which, while it lends dignity, frequently impedes progress. We have, therefore, opportunity to set up our own standards, thus showing the older professions that we have profited by the excellences they may have, but that we have added the results of our own experience and observation, and that we, in turn, will hand down to succeeding generations the aggregate of theirs and ours.

The thought of a profession carries with it the idea of personal service; a relationship different from that offered in commercial life, and, when considered from the nursing point of view, shows a personal relationship that is three-fold.

The purpose of the study of ethics to our profession should be to place before the student the underlying theory, upon which these laws of conduct toward the community, as well as the individual are based.

We can only discover truth by a rational and democratic interest in life. Our interest must extend outward to the community, to other schools, to the nursing profession at large. I would urge that the ethics taught in our schools include these broader relationships, as well as the personal, basing such instruction upon the truths proved by science, that the great forces governing human conduct are the same as they always have been. Is it not true that out of the desire for the welfare of those we know, develops the broader desire for the welfare of our community.

We do not desire to teach *new* motives, but how to maintain and develop advantages already acquired.

A sound system of ethics is desirable in order to give greater definiteness to our aims and methods. Happily we do not have to wait for a perfect system to be placed before us, until we begin.

What place in the curriculum shall this instruction occupy? The teaching of ethics should be based upon psychology, sociology and history, beginning in the preliminary course, and occupying a definite place throughout the three years. There should be no separating line between the training in technical subjects and those dealing with the moral or ethical.

The true code of ethics is based upon a knowledge of the working of one's own mind, the development of society, the events of the past as found in history.

Students as well as children can be led to make their own decisions as to conduct through their knowledge of these fundamental laws.

The purpose of ethics in our schools is to give depth and breadth to our relationship to the individual, the public, and the profession, and we see that the place it occupies is a large one—beginning and ending with the pupil's stay in the school, and that it permeates all phases of the school life.

May we not hope that the result in the lives of our graduates will be that described by Prof. J. R. Seely as the highest type of desire to work for others, known as "the enthusiasm of humanity," and a full realization that civilization grows largely in proportion to the willingness and ability of men to coöperate; and, as coöperation demands great moral qualities, shall we, as a profession, not be definitely aiding the cultivation of these qualities?

(Clayton, 1916, pp. 252–256)

Report of the Committee on Ethical Standards

By Louise M. Powell,
S. Lillian Clayton, Chairman

At the annual convention of the National League of Nursing Education held in Kansas City, 1921, a Committee was appointed as an advisory committee on Ethical Standards. The idea of the Board of Directors being that there should be a group to whom State Officers or others could go for consultation if necessary.

The Chairman was appointed to select her own Committee. Miss Louise M. Powell consented to serve on this Committee. It was very difficult to secure other members. Consequently it was decided to call upon others if the occasion arose.

During the year, a number of requests have come for information as to whether the National Organization had a code of ethics and if so, could it be sent to that particular state, in order that the State code could correspond to the National. A number of Alumnae Associations have written, saying that they were forming a code of ethics for their own Associations. The principal conclusion the Committee formed, after receiving these communications, was that the nurses throughout the country are desiring something concrete which they may accept as a basis for professional conduct.

The Committee, upon further study of the subject, finds that most professional groups, also most business and industrial groups, have such standards of conduct in written form, setting forth the principals of ethics underlying their own particular profession or business. In many cases this printed form is presented to individual members at the time they join the Association, which represents their particular profession. The principles of ethics thus presented, are, of course, but a written statement of all ethical instructions received by that individual during her years of preparation, or in the case of business and social groups, the principles are founded upon trustworthiness, efficiency, etc.

In any case, the membership in the groups is secured because of the individuals ethical standards as well as his or her professional or business standards. The American Academy of Political and Social Science presents the following list of organizations having ethical codes; Ethical Code of Lawyers, the Medical Profession, including Physicians, Dentists, Nurses and Pharmacists (I do not know from whom they secured the nursing ethics), Engineers, Architects, Teachers, Librarians, Ministers, Social Workers, Journalists, Editors and Accountants, also various kinds of business organizations.

The ethics of nursing are taught in all our training schools, but although so much has been presented concerning the subject, never have these subjects been put into such form as to make one feel sure that all nurses had the same ideals for their professional conduct.

This Committee, therefore, recommends:

That a Committee be appointed to prepare a statement of the Principles of Nursing Ethics.

That the personnel of this Committee consist of representatives from the American Nurses' Association, the National League of Nursing Education and the National Organization for Public Health Nursing.

That the recommendations of this Committee be presented to the Joint Board of Directors at its annual meeting, January, 1923.

That the recommendations when accepted be presented to every member of the organizations and to every person who in the future shall join any one of the National Nursing Organizations.

Furthermore, that every Superintendent of Nurses be asked to make her students familiar with these principles during the time they are in the schools of nursing, as a part of the regular instruction in Nursing Ethics.

These recommendations are based primarily upon the fact that nurses throughout the country are devoting themselves to this problem thus indicating a definitely felt need.

Second, the National Bodies are the logical sources of standardization.

Third, the Committee has made somewhat of a study as to the value of such codes of ethics to the members of other professions, and we believe that if they are appreciated by such organizations as have been mentioned previously in this report, they would also be welcomed by the nurses of the country. We are living in the midst of social customs that are elastic and in times when standards are varied. Therefore, anything that can be done in the way of standardization will, we believe, do much toward maintaining our ideals of the past and adding to them much that is good of the present.

(Powell & Clayton, 1923, pp. 27–29)

Teaching of Ethics and Ethical Problems

Reported by Laura M. Grant, R. N.

Director of Nursing Service, Lakewood Hospital, Cleveland, Ohio

Judging by the stimulating reports given and suggestions made at this conference, ethics continues to receive much serious thought from those responsible for the ethical guidance of the students in our nursing schools, and still occupies an important place in the curricula. There seems an alertness to the importance of this subject in every quarter and this was particularly evidenced in our own group by the number attending and participating in the discussion.

The courses vary in name, length, and content. "Ethics" or "Professional Problems" seems to be the usual title given to any course in practical idealism, the latter apparently having the preference.

Only one outstanding school reports no course at all, namely, the Yale School of Nursing, but it seems fair to assume that its students with their greater maturity, their probable background of courses in sociology, psychology, and possibly of philosophy, their "hand picked" faculty, do not stand in the same need of such a course as the younger students of other schools who have not had the same basic preparation.

The courses outlined seemed designed to stimulate the growth of personality in order to enable the young woman to function effectively in the practice of her profession, to think independently and constructively, to accept responsibility for her own conduct, and to fit her to meet the problems arising in the hospital, home, or her own life.

The subject matter covers a wide range. The difference between ethics and etiquette and between general and professional ethics seems to be stressed quite generally. Emphasis most often seems to be placed on the historical background and traditions of nursing; the changing emphasis in nursing education, and on the future trends in nursing.

Special topics for discussion cover such points as: 1. the broad underlying principles of her profession governing her relations to the patient, the doctor, and other professional workers, etc.; 2. her ideals on entering the school and the necessity of keeping them alive; 3. her professional, social and civic responsibilities; 4. nursing organizations; 5. nursing legislation; 6. nursing literature; 7. business methods; 8. problems of supply and demand; 9. development of new standards; and 10. vocational guidance.

The case study, individual conference, and informal class discussion seem to be the favored methods of teaching.

The student must be encouraged to express her own opinions, to bring questions for discussion, to seek information for herself by visiting persons and organizations, to consider definite problems, to make her own judgments, and to formulate her own code of ethics.

Other factors noted as influencing the ethical development of the student might be summarized as follows: 1. selection of the faculty; 2. early elimination of the undesirable student; 3. extra-curricular activities.

(Grant, 1927, pp. 229–230)

Interprofessional Relationships from the Viewpoint of the Superintendent of Nurses

By Effie J. Taylor, R. N.

Professor of Nursing and Superintendent of Nurses, Yale University School of Nursing, New Haven, Connecticut

The subject which is announced in the program for this morning's discussion is an exceedingly broad one and may lead through its ramifications into deep and abstract philosophies. We may, however, think to dispose of it by a series of practical opinions such as the various subtopics on the program would indicate.

You will note I have said "think to dispose of it," and I have suggested an element of doubt after a good deal of thought and after having experienced for almost a quarter of a century the ups and downs, the joys and sorrows which follow as a result of satisfactory and unsatisfactory interprofessional relationships in large and to possibly a lesser degree in small institutions for the care of the sick.

We are hearing a great deal today about this term "relationship"; family and domestic; parent and child; student and teacher; parent and teacher; capital and labor; civic, state and federal relationships; and the subject which is occupying so large a space in our newspapers throughout the world and occupying the time and thought of our statesmen is our international relationships. What does it mean and what can we do about it?

The first part of the question depends for its answer on various philosophies and the second part relates to our personal obligations in interpreting those philosophies and in creating new standards of conduct to meet our more progressive steps in life. Mrs. Woodhouse has presented some of the general principles of interprofessional relationships which I believe do not vary in substance wherever human beings are living together.

I believe the application of the basic principles are as essential in the home and in the school as they are in the shop, in the institution, or in the government of our country, and stated in their simplest terms they are concerned with making provision for each human being to attain his highest and best self and giving him the opportunity to contribute his creative thought, whether much or little, to the experience and for the good of mankind.

This relationship which gives the human being his natural right to develop to his highest capacity is the fundamental principle in democratic thought and rightly and wisely applied should tend to the highest degree of group order and control. In the individual it should lead to self-discipline and moderation rather than to license and excesses.

The application of such principles in the home in the early life of the child does not presuppose a relaxing of supervision, but rather a speeding up of an understanding supervision and a withdrawing of authority and dominant control. Supervising and directing the development of an activity is something quite different from inhibiting or forbidding the development of the activity. With the prevailing new thought towards education and discipline it is probable that oft times the pendulum has swung to its extreme angle, and instead of replacing the former idea of autocratic rule and authority by intelligent direction and supervision, children have been permitted to drift fitfully along, unguided and undirected.

The nursery and elementary schools in some measure are making up for the failure in the home to bridge the change in thought, but they cannot do so entirely, and as a result serious problems of adjustment are being presented continuously to our higher educational institutions. As hospitals have a place in the system of professional education, these basic things are of as great importance to them as to other professional schools and colleges, and therefore they are vitally concerned with what happens in the early life of the child.

In schools of nursing we are compensating for our urge to change by making the error of fathers and mothers. We know that the old-time military discipline will not [sic] longer be accepted. Young people are absolutely against it. It does not fit in with their ideas of progress. Their background has not prepared them for that which we accepted without a challenge. In its old form it does not coincide with their experience. They have always exercised the right to question. They are living in an age when rights and privileges are dominent topics for consideration. They see no reason why they should follow an order or rule because it is an order or rule. In consequence we find ourselves facing innumerable new and teasing problems to study (I had almost said settle), and I believe we must admit that much of the fault is ours. In our anxiety to seem progressive, to show our interest in modern ideas of freedom and liberty, we have retrenched in our authority at this point and that, and have also gone to the opposite extreme, with the result that many of the objectives we formerly sought to gain through military discipline we have lost sight of entirely. Thus the achievement in the care of the patients is often less good than should be reasonably expected from thoughtful students. Neither the time at my disposal nor the topic to be discussed permit me to follow this discussion to a conclusion other than to say, we have suppressed our ideas of military discipline, but have not made adequate substitution for that discipline through a better understanding and a closer personal supervision of our students while they are giving bedside care to the patients in the hospital wards. Most of their inefficiencies, I am convinced, are due to our inadequacies in presenting to them their obligations in so high a vocation as nursing rather than to their unwillingness to accept responsibility of a nature they are competent to assume.

Only a short time ago in discussing the subject of "personal and professional relationships" with a class of students, the question of what the student owed to the patient, the institution and to the community versus what the institution owed to her, gave me much food for thought. In a later conference with an individual student she said: "I believe it would have been better had we known those things earlier. I think we would often have reacted differently." Now it is quite interesting to note that many of the points in question were not new. They had been discussed in some very early classes, but the experience of the students was probably too limited for them to make the necessary application. At that time the students were presented with the facts, at the later date these facts were worked out through their experience with the aforesaid result.

It is evident that our present personal relationship to our students is less restrained and therefore more wholesome and natural than formerly, but it is still less perfect than it should be and apparently less valuable to the students. A careful study in detail of student, school and hospital relationships would seem to be essential before we can presume to form with precision satisfactory policies for the conduct of the school within the hospital.

Desirable interprofessional relationships are determined by an understanding of "obligations and claims" or "responsibilities and rights," through adjustments and cooperation. The students in the school of nursing and in the school of medicine have certain obligations to the institution as factors in fulfilling its function and certain claims on the institution for the part it contributes to their education. They have on the one hand obligations and responsibilities, but on the other hand they have claims and rights. These obligations and claims are inherent in any organization and in any community. Perhaps because our hospitals were organized on a military basis to meet essential needs and service was the dominant note, the relationships have always been more or less determined on the basis of "obligations and responsibilities" rather than on individual "rights and claims" or, better still, on an accepted consideration of each in fulfilling its specific aim.

The central figure in the administration of a hospital is the hospital superintendent, sometimes a doctor, sometimes a business man and often a nurse. In the administration of the majority of institutions that officer represents every other department to the board of trustees. In about two thousand hospitals in this country there are schools of nursing established each with a principal or superintendent of nurses (though sometimes the superintendent of the hospital occupies both positions). I have not the figures from which to quote but I am confident that only a small proportion of these schools have direct representation from the school on the governing board. It is therefore assumed that the superintendent of the hospital is the official administrative head of the school of nursing, and the superintendent of nurses must depend upon him for her opportunities to develop the school. As most schools are organized as a department of the hospital and make up the nursing service, practically speaking this organization is correct. But obviously it is not quite just and the education of the student is a secondary consideration. The school under these conditions is represented by someone who knows technically little about it except that it adequately or inadequately meets a need in the institution. I am of the opinion that this condition would soon be changed if the superintendents of hospitals were women and the heads of the nursing schools were men.

A few days ago I had the privilege of attending a dinner where equal rights, including equal pay for men and women, were discussed and I was more deeply than ever convinced that a major problem in considering interprofessional relations between men and women in hospitals is "responsibility without representation" and equal work with unequal pay. There is no doubt that in many institutions a serious handicap to establishing happy and satisfactory interprofessional relationships is found in an inequality in the salary scale. The recognized heads of the professional departments are paid both out of proportion to each other and to the various other members of the related staffs associated with them. This accounts, in some measure at least, for the tremendous turn-over which is seen in hospital personnel. No business concern or industry could exist under such conditions. Well-prepared and efficient people cannot long be persuaded to remain in institutional positions. I firmly believe that good relationships will never be established till more intelligent consideration is given to the appropriation of salaries and till individuals, whether men or women, are adequately paid for service rendered in proportion to their responsibilities and their ability to meet them, and till a more businesslike attitude is assumed towards the economics of living.

The medical department in a hospital has always claimed and assumed a priority over nursing, and tradition has accepted the claim. There is a sense in which this claim is just, for nurses are dependent on physicians for direction as to what therapeutic measures they will administer to patients and must needs follow with accuracy whatever is prescribed as treatment. Nurses are also dependent on physicians for diagnoses. This priority, however, is carried to the extreme when it enters into personal relationships and when what is traditionally called "hospital etiquette" provides for a subservient attitude on the part of the nurse to the physician, whether chief or interne, whenever they are associated in the hospital wards. My personal feeling about this traditional form of "hospital etiquette" is that it belongs to the past. Thinking men and women are emancipated from such ritual, and only those who are handicapped by an inferiority complex will allow such formalities to be reflected in their personalities. True politeness, however, and consideration for others is as much as obligation and a mark of culture today as in years gone by. In our emancipation from form and ceremony and our growing interest in real, practical and perhaps more material things, we have sometimes forgotten that courtesy and kindliness always go with good breeding and culture, and that "hospital etiquette" and common ordinary politeness and consideration for others are one and the same thing. The old form which required a nurse to pop up from her chair whenever a doctor entered the ward and stand with her work in her hand, or remain idle and speechless, is a relic of militarism and autocracy and has no place in a well-ordered and democratic institution. At the time I believe it is equally out of place for any individual, whether man or women, to remain in his or her chair when the occasion calls for another type of response. This one need not emphasize for a cultured person always senses the fitness of things. I have in mind, at the present moment, a woman who never fails to rise and find a seat for one of her colleagues or for anyone, man or woman, who enters her office. She is as deliberately unconscious of what she is doing as she is deliberately unconscious of taking up her pen to write. This is the kind of courtesy and politeness which should prevail between individuals wherever they meet. Further gestures and exaggerations of priority and personal right to ceremony are entirely irrelevant. These ceremonials are equally inappropriate between nurses in the nursing school and have no permanent value. Emphasis placed upon kindliness, courtesy, consideration for others and respect for knowledge and experience will prevent and safeguard any tendency to discourteous and undignified behavior. Instead of aiming to develop an attitude of fear and formality in students and staff through these artificial responses an attitude of frank spontaneous behavior should rather be encouraged by persons who hold important official positions.

The nursing staff too often has been accused of assuming an attitude of control and superiority over other professional workers in the hospital wards. This attitude no doubt was developed when the medical and nursing departments held the prominent places of responsibility; but now, dietitians, nutrition and social workers have also found their places and are filling many pressing needs. Patients are treated by diet more often than by drugs, and dietitians are as essential as nurses in helping to carry out these therapeutic measures. A close relation should exist between these different workers and they should all feel equally at home in the hospital wards. The dietitian was introduced to the hospital as an instructor in the school of nursing but I believe the best relationship exists where the dietary department is centered in the general administration and is not a department appended to the nursing service. At the same time, because the wards under our present organization are administered by a head nurse who is also responsible for the care of the patients, every worker coming into the ward should seek to function in cooperation with her, as good fellowship will exist only where teamwork is the first objective.

No individual in any department has the right to use the prestige of his office for personal power over others. Similarly no individual has the right to rise on the shoulders of his associates. This is not infrequently done in institutional work. Credit for a piece of work should be given to the person who creates or initiates it. This attitude of mind is really a test of a big man or woman as it is a temptation in group life to adapt for one's own use the ideas of others particularly if the other individual has not the opportunity to carry them through to completion.

To present the foregoing thoughts in summary, as seen from the point of view of a superintendent of nurses, the most satisfactory interprofessional relationships will prevail: when the school of nursing has the opportunity to develop its educational policies unhampered by the immediate economic needs of the hospital; when there is developed a closer and better understanding of the obligation of the student to the institution, the institution to the student, and each to the cause for which they both exist; when representation always accompanies responsibility; when adequate and equal pay for equal work is given consideration in every department of the institution; when better teamwork for the care of the patients exists between the various associated departments in the hospital without undue emphasis placed on the priority or prestige of any group; when common sense, politeness and courtesy replace the traditional formality of ceremonial "hospital etiquette;" and when policies are discussed and established for the general welfare of the institution in departmental group conferences.

(Taylor, 1929, pp. 208–213)

Through Better Selection of Students

By D. Dean Urch, R. N.

Director, Highland Hospital School of Nursing, Oakland, California

This is not a report of what we are doing to improve practice in nursing through better selection of students, rather is it a discussion of certain trends and possibilities along this line, as well as suggestions regarding some of our obligations and responsibilities to our profession, to the public and to the young women seeking admission to our nursing ranks.

That the selection of better students and better methods for the selection of students will improve the practice of nursing goes without saying. You cannot make a "silk purse from a sow's ear," nor "bricks without straw." You cannot make a professional woman from one who has the mentality and emotionality of a child.

We cannot build up a strong, professional group by filling our ranks with the failures from high school and college. If you ask what I mean by better students, my answer is, women who meet the commonly accepted requirements of professional practitioners, viz., cultural background for nursing with the innate capacity to learn how to solve problems, make judgments, and assume the responsibilities and risks of acting on their own judgments. Certainly they should be above average in native intelligence.

Women who come to the nursing school should have had a good, broad, general education—at least full high school and preferably one or more years in college—they should be physically and emotionally equal to the stress and strain of nursing, and should have the social background which gives poise, graciousness, refinement, courtesy, tact, and acceptability to patients, they should be women who have certain personal qualities which make it possible for them to become increasingly altruistic in motivation, viz., restraint, self-discipline, urbanity, dependability, and devotion to a cause. We now have many such women but all who enter our ranks should measure high on such a scale.

We need, also, to take into account the various types of nursing which students will do after graduation, i.e., public health, teaching, head nursing, bedside nursing, and so on. Criteria set up by which to measure efficiency in teaching do not always measure efficiency in giving bedside care to mental patients and vice versa.

I do not need to remind this audience of our well-known tendency to select and keep in our schools the students who submit to drastic discipline, who satisfy doctors, patients, head nurses, and the immediate needs of the hospitals rather than those who exhibit the qualities of leadership, who disturb the even tenor of the hospital by having ideas and opinions of their own, and whose trend is toward expressing them. The seemingly desirable submissiveness which adds to the smoothness of the hospital routine is almost sure to be a handicap in the later professional career outside or even inside the best hospital.

The two most outstanding points to consider in the selection of students are (1) that we select those who have the innate aptitude to do the nursing work that the community needs and wants, and are capable of finding happiness and satisfaction in doing it; and (2) that we develop more scientific methods of selection for prospective students, using available criteria and tests and working out such new ones as we need. We are fortunate in having experts in various fields of education who know pretty definitely whereof they speak in matters of intelligence testing, health testing, even in measuring emotional and social qualities.

I am sure that every member of this audience is familiar with the work of our Grading Committee, with the various types of testing done in colleges and other schools, and with such studies as the one made by R. Louise Metcalfe of the "Achievement of Nurses in Relation to Intelligence List Ratings," given before this group four years ago. Some splendid work has also been reported in *Born That Way* by Joseph O'Connor, and the March, 1932, *Trained Nurse and Hospital Review* gave "Some Technics for the Selection of Students" by Dr. Rohiback, quite worthy of your consideration.

We are not alone in our attempts to find better methods of selection of students. Teachers' colleges and medical schools are experimenting in better selection of members of their profession. The University of California is trying out aptitude tests for admission to its medical school. Teachers College, Columbia University, announces a new college for 1932 which will constitute a new type of teacher-training institution. One of the outstanding characteristics of this school will be its rigid selection of students. I quote from the announcement:

> Fine courses and excellent faculty avail little without the proper type of student body. It is impossible to hope for fine, inspiring young teachers if the personnel of the student body is selected from those who are mediocre in talent and personality. The best training in the world will not make a fine teacher out of inferior human material. Mediocrity is today the curse of our teaching profession. It is also important for the students in the new college, that the student body itself be of highly selected character. A student learns more from his fellows than from his teacher. The reactions of one student upon another in a very real sense is an important part of the curriculum. We might term this contact of student with student as educational living.
>
> Rigid but sensible methods of elimination will be pursued in the selection of individuals who give promise of developing desirable leadership in the field of education. In order to secure young persons of proper qualifications, the coöperation of teachers and executives working with high school and young college students will be sought. The chief bases of selection will be sound scholarship, promise of growth in the field of education, and desirable personal qualities. These will be determined by selective entrance examinations, personal interviews, and statements from former instructors and others well acquainted with the prospective student. The student body will be chosen from a wide geographical area rather than restricted to a local area or section of the country.

Some such clearly defined plan as this could well be set up, by those controlling our nursing schools, for the selection of only those students who possess the qualities which are thought to be indicative of the successful nurse. The qualities this teacher group emphasize are "high mental ability, worth-while achievement, good character, abundant physical and mental health, sufficient energy, a pleasing personality, wide cultural interests, good habits, high ideals and sincerity of purpose."

It is evident that no one trait is sufficient to consider. It is equally evident that we need to use all the resources available in studies already done, in school records, and in gathering opinions of people who know the candidate and who also know the traits essential to good nursing. How many teachers in the United States are cognizant of the traits we deem essential in the individual who is capable of making a good nurse? Are we frankly facing the fact that the public teachers direct into nursing the girls who are failures? And are we doing anything about that? Local Leagues could well have conferences with public and private school teachers and get this information over to them. We could also circularize the teachers with material along this line. And furthermore we could decline to accept these lower levels in our school.

I should like to emphasize some of the available material regarding candidates we can and should secure from the school files. Most of the schools of the country have assembled for their students the I. Q.s, results of arithmetic ability tests, reading ability, number sense, extracurricular activities, health record throughout life, muscular coördination, bodily repose, posture, endurance, responses toward novel situations, response to other problem solving ability, achievement, home influence, occupation of parents, and so on. Time spent in going over such data would undoubtedly result in the refusal of many of the misfits and would be very well spent.

My second emphasis is our obligation to supplement these investigations by tests such as health and other aptitude tests and make them before the student goes to the expense of entering the school. The I. Q. is relatively easy to get. Health examination should include an x-ray of chest, Wassermann tests, examination of the feet, throat, heart, lungs, urine, eyes, and metabolism if indicated, and an examination by a good psychologist. Aptitude tests, such as described in O'Connor's *Born That Way,* and others already worked out to test nursing traits, can be used. Research might well be done to develop more such tests.

Every principal of every school of nursing in the United States could, if she would, when selecting each prospective student, put to herself these questions:

Is she the type of young woman I would like to take care of me if I were ill?

Would I choose her to teach health to my daughter?

Would I be proud to have her be a member of my profession?

Would I invite her to be a guest in my home?

Has she the mental capacity necessary to learn the sciences necessary to intelligent understanding and practice of nursing?

Is she physically and emotionally equal to the stress and strain of dealing with human beings when they are at their worst?

Is she adaptable enough to adjust herself to the fifty-seven varieties of duties a nurse must perform?

Then if our principals would use all the materials available, viz., school records, health examinations, tests for intelligence, social background, emotional reactions, adaptability, and the like, to make the selection as scientific and impersonal as possible, much could be done to eliminate the waste in time, energy, and money which is spent on misfits. Approximately fifty percent of the students who enter the nursing schools of the country do not graduate. No one knows just what percentage of those who do graduate are failures. By a failure, I mean one who is unable to earn her living doing a needed type of nursing work in a manner that is acceptable to the ones she serves, and at the same time find personal satisfaction herself in doing that work.

These misfits are not only very expensive (in time, energy, and money) to the nursing school faculty and the hospital, but to the students themselves. I am fortunate in having a member of our Committee on Admissions who repeatedly remarks (when discussing a questionable applicant), "I think we would be doing this young woman a grave injustice if we allowed her to attempt nursing. It isn't fair to her to lead her to believe she can succeed at nursing." This doctor expresses a point of view too frequently overlooked. I wonder how many of the unemployed nurses in this country could have been saved from nursing if they had been more carefully selected.

I quote from O'Connor's *Born That Way*:

> Not only does the inapt girl lose the position which depends upon her acquiring dexterity or succumb to jaded discouragement, or continue as a slow, mediocre plodder, but she may even approach a nervous breakdown because of the too great dependence of her welfare upon achieving an intangible aptness. She sees life's conflicts approaching and overwhelming her feeble efforts more rapidly than she can pick up characteristics which others unconsciously possess . . . . Such a worker, ill adapted to her task, but driven to it, daily, develops not only physical signs of overfatigue, but symptoms associated with mental disorders. The misapprehensions of such a girl often differ little from those of some mentally diseased hospital inmates, who display as one of the first auguries of the impending breakdown, a suspicion that unknown persons have selected them as their particular victims. Delusions of persecution!

I said, a moment ago, that no one trait should be the determining factor. Some years ago any earnest, respectable young woman, who was willing to give good hard service seemed most acceptable. Then we began to stress intelligence. Now, if we are going to produce nurses to meet all the nursing needs of the community, will we not find it desirable to give considerable thought to the ranges of intelligence, to emotional stability, to social background, to pleasing personality, and to worthwhile interests. For many types of nursing work we unquestionably need intelligence of college level, but shall we then decline the otherwise desirable young woman whose I. Q. is 104? Certainly she must reach 100 or over. Students of psychology tell us that many of our splendid public school teachers come from the just-above average of intelligence. What they lack in native smartness they make up in industry, application, earnestness of purpose, character, and the like.

O'Connor found that some college graduates with splendid records made dismal failures when they attempted to do office work. Would it not be better for our profession to have certain schools in which to prepare the teaching-executive groups, and others for the bedside workers? And then select, evaluate, and direct applicants into the appropriate school? We shall need for our future nurses a goodly share of the 1,500,000 especially gifted children found by the White House Conference, and many of the 38,000,000 average, but unless we look to our laurels, we will find some of the 5,630,000 handicapped on our hands—and whose fault will it be?

Professor Allen Nevins, writing of Mr. Harding in the *Dictionary of American Biography*, joins President Hoover in regarding that unfortunate individual as more sinned against than sinning. Sinned against by the American people. "A heavy responsibility, for his record," he declares, "falls upon the party and nation which elected a man of moderate abilities, weak judgment of character, excessive amiability, and total lack of vigilance to so exacting an office." In like manner the "unemployable and misfits" in our profession lie heavy on our consciences. Now would seem a propitious time to do something. To make hay before the sun of "economic prosperity" begins to shine. Much is being done by some schools, but as long as every misfit who is turned from or out of one school can find another school which will confer its diploma on her, we are not getting very far. We need a nation-wide drive and the understanding support of all the people— physicians, teachers, parents, and others. And particularly nurses! And still more particularly, principals of nursing schools.

All the other things discussed here today, improvement of nursing methods, more adequately prepared faculties, improvement in the educational process, improvement of educational facilities for workers in service—are of little use if we admit the "leftovers" in high school classes, those who have failed at teaching and in other fields, the people who cannot afford a college education, and those who seek a living with a small honorarium, instead of a school.

I should like to summarize my remarks as follows:

1. We should select fewer students, therefore we can select more carefully.

2. We should select our students objectively, impersonally, scientifically, without regard to getting the hospital work done.

3. We should set up appropriate, unambiguous, clean-cut criteria, by which to judge nursing traits.

4. We should select only those students who are adapted to nursing.

5. We should work out new tests with which to measure nursing traits.

6. We should use all available materials in the files of schools from which students come, and secure opinions of teachers who are informed regarding nursing traits.

7. We should consider no one point, such as intelligence. Health, wholesome personality, good disposition, earnestness of purpose, social background, and other qualities are quite as essential.

8. We should spend more time on the selection of students and thus save on trying to make nurses of the misfits.

9. We should inform the public, especially teachers and parents, the necessity of high, or above average, intelligence and other qualities essential to nursing.

10. We should secure the coöperation of physicians, hospital executives, women's organizations, teachers, parents, boards, and the general public.

(Urch, 1932, pp. 185–191)

Section V
Image

Introduction to Image

Florence Nightingale's work in the Crimea and later her influence during the American Civil War established nursing as essential to saving lives and preventing disease. Her educational reforms for nursing education brought the modern nursing movement to America in the late 19th century. As the Nightingale-influenced schools opened, women, for the first time, learned how to nurse. They combined the importance of sanitary reforms calling for pure air, food, and ventilation with knowledge of the human body and disease. Late 19th-century hospital reforms, often attributed to new discoveries in science, also owed a tremendous debt to the work of trained nurses and the new schools. As nursing care in hospitals and in private homes steadily improved, trained nurses became increasingly popular. Hospital boards discerned that training schools would be a benefit to the institutions because of the economical and improved services performed by pupil nurses. Over time, the trained nurse replaced the untrained nurse of the past.

However, for years to come the memory of the untrained nurse lingered in the public mind. Visions of the slovenly, unsavory character of the nurse, frequently referred to as Charles Dickens' character, Sairy Gamp, remained. They had earned this distinction when untrained nurses, often themselves patients, vagrants, or prisoners, cared for the sick in hospitals. Popular images of women with questionable ethics and morals plagued the training schools' drives for new recruits. Despite this negative characterization, women influenced by the late 19th-century woman's movement and women from the rising middle class who needed work accepted the new image of the trained nurse. As a result, more and more women with family and cultural backgrounds that promoted higher education filled the new training schools for nurses.

Women of high moral character and ideals who displayed intelligent, strong, and efficient attributes enhanced the image of the "modern nurse." This more positive characterization combined the ideal woman with professional knowledge to reveal a picture of the "ideal nurse" (Davis, 1907). Yet the positive image of the trained nurse did not alter the opposition and prejudice experienced by superintendents in the 20 years following the opening of America's training schools. It became apparent to those leaders that a unified organization was needed to confront the battles they faced. For the next 40 years, the Superintendents' Society and the NLNE continually addressed and sought to understand the different images of the nurse.

Images of nurses and nursing affected generations of men and women in their selection of careers and support of the profession. The image of nursing has been inseparable from the image of women. Even though men trained as nurses in the few schools that opened for them during the late 19th and early 20th centuries, their legacy remained hidden in this predominantly women's profession. The very role of the nurse, considered for so long a natural role for women, remained a constant remainder that nursing was women's work. Few people challenged society's role expectations for men or for women.

The belief that some women were born nurses inhibited the idea that nurses needed a formal education. Nurses struggled against society's dual role expectation of an ideal woman who stayed home and raised a family, and the "new woman" who worked outside the home and supported herself financially. During this period, higher education for women became a feminist struggle of great significance. Nursing educators, whether associated with the woman's movement or not, struggled with the same issue of higher education. Colleges and universities helped superintendents meet educational goals. They offered faculty greater control of curricula and demanded more academically qualified teachers. An atmosphere that combined liberal arts, humanities, and science courses found lacking in hospital-based schools, attracted students. Nursing schools that affiliated with universities and colleges challenged the traditional apprenticeship models found in hospital schools and promoted nursing's *professional* image.

Long hours of clinical service coupled with unsupervised night duty, too few hours for recreation, inadequate housing of pupil nurses, and too few jobs after graduation led to some of the derogatory images the organization had to overcome. Strengthening nursing as a profession rather than a vocation meant moving education out of the hospital and into the university. College students did not experience interrupted classes, for example, as did their counterparts in hospital schools.

World War I accentuated the romantic ideals of women healers associated with the heroic deeds of Florence Nightingale and other battlefield nurses. During this period, women clamored to enroll in new schools created to meet the increased demands for nurses. As shorter training periods became solutions for increasing the supply of nurses, the need for educated nurses once again provoked challenges for the profession. The NLNE mounted recruitment campaigns projecting a positive, intelligent image of the nurse.

Throughout its 40 years, the Superintendents' Society and the NLNE gained many friends outside of nursing who fully supported their efforts. Since this section looks at image, it is appropriate to include a speech by the non-nurse, Frances Payne Bolton, who was one of nursing's most important supporters. Her philanthropic work supplied the profession with money, political support, and a valued image.

As society's need for nurses changed, the image of nursing continued to change. The development of technological advances, complex cures and treatments, and new roles for nurses created opportunities for the emergence of a new, enhanced, professional image. The following papers depict the response of the Superintendents' Society and the NLNE to the evolution of this image.

What We are Overlooking of Fundamental Importance in the Training of the Modern Nurse

By M. E. P. Davis

Whenever it is suggested that I attempt to formulate ideas and put them on paper, I am at once reminded of the remark of a noted actor who said: "It is so *easy not* to write a drama that I wonder so many persist in doing it. My present attitude may look like that same foolish persistence in deliberately making effort in the least easy direction. A little explanation will perhaps disabuse your minds of the fear that you are to be "victimized" listening to a tiresome paper setting forth arbitrary views. When I, with the other members, was asked to suggest a topic for discussion at this meeting, I took it literally and at once jumped to a conclusion, and made a snap diagnosis.

I had a little conversation with myself, and I said, "This is a delightful innovation. The Council means to select the most interesting subjects, send a list to each member, or better, publish the list in the *Journal,* so that each may come prepared with her pros and cons gathered from her experience, more or less convincingly expressed, according to the degree of her positive belief in, or her disapproval of, the points under discussion, stimulating others by her personality to a fuller expression of their opinions, so that new ideas, bare facts or actual experiment may become common property."

Now here was an opportunity to get views on what has long appeared to me an all-important point, the systematic development and coordination of the trinity of the pupil, which we are careful to speak of, as the cooperation of head, hands and heart (the intellect, the physical and the humanities). I forthwith grasped the opportunity, posted my topic to the Secretary and thought little more about it, till I was notified that the Council thought the subject interesting (or mystifying) enough to select it as a subject for discussion, and agreed that I would be the proper person to put the matter before you, the natural inference being that I knew what I was talking about. I *do* know some of the things, and wishing to know more, consented—not to write a paper but to introduce the subject, "What We Are Overlooking of Fundamental Importance in the Training of the Modern Nurse."

Our dear friendly critics tell us that we are giving the head undue attention and are overlooking the humanities, and, in suggesting improvements in the education of the nurse, make capital out of the perpetual iteration that the nurse is selfish, mercenary, unsympathetic or wants time to eat and sleep while the world is suffering and do not hesitate to say that in the *tout ensemble* of the finished product the humanities count for more, judged by lay standards than technical knowledge or manual skill. Dr. Richard C. Cabot in an address before the New England Society, "For the Education of the Nurse," voiced this universal criticism when he made a plea for what he called "Comfort Nurses, Those Who Fit In," thereby emphasizing and endorsing that criticism. Not that Dr. Cabot is altogether one of the cult who is clamoring for less technical or practical training, but for *more* coordinate development of the head, hands and heart, with emphasis perhaps on the heart qualities.

He enumerated among other desirable teachings loving service, sympathy, unselfishness, tact; and singled out tact as the virtue *par excellence* in the nurse's equipment, which he stated *should be* because it *could be* taught. Perhaps it can, but not separated from the whole mental development, which requires a much more strenuous educing and a firmer grasp on the underlying principle which governs motive than we have hitherto been able to secure. But at no stage of the development would I select tact—desirable as it is—as the pivotal virtue in a nurse's manifestation of her mental attitude, because it is a product or exponent of a happy mixture of head and heart qualities graciously expressed through the physical. The regrettable thing is that Dr. Cabot forgot to tell us *how* tact could be taught; of course all the critics *know how,* but they leave it in that delightfully tantalizing state of uncertainty that makes one so indignant when criticized, for the superintendents, or some other body of teachers, of training schools to tackle and evolve on a practical basis.

In view of the prevalent attitude and our own recognition of the need, is it wise to longer ignore the demand and cling to the old idea that routine, discipline, environment, contact, precept, example, or even high intellectual attainment, is the only ground on which the mental attitude can be approached or the only way through which a change or development of the personality can be effected? It is about as wise, I should say, as for the schools to adhere to the manner of teaching which obtained twenty years ago. Granted that the ideal woman is she who takes the correct attitude toward the issues of life, and regulates her conduct by her standard of character, and that the ideal nurse is but the ideal woman *plus* her professional knowledge, how is the ordinary probationer or pupil to be brought to recognize this underlying principle from which to work toward ideals, and develop character that will regulate conduct at all times, even when the safeguards of discipline and supervision are no longer operative? How are we to get at this? We reach the mental only through the physical; *i.e.,* we judge the mental attitude by the physical act. For example, if one takes the physical attitude of courage and maintains that attitude, the physical expresses "a bold front," as we say.

We are overlooking then the culture of this physical expression. We are overlooking the important part the instrument plays in this coordination and cooperation of the trinity. We must teach the pupil the right use and the possibilities for greater usefulness of the instrument with which the work is to be performed. We might at least teach her to adjust the instrument at the angle of most correct expression, which will be the angle of easiest performance of the physical act. Whether she stands, walks, sits or bends, let the body be so adjusted, the position so normal, that the least exhaustive demand be made on strength, power of endurance or the proper functioning of the body. This will produce a correspondingly easy mental attitude, less friction, less fault-finding, fewer lions in the way. Teach her how to concentrate her whole attention to the thing in hand. "This one thing I do," and it is done well. One thing at a time. Don't let the mind get separated from the body, nor from bodily work, when the work is being performed.

Teach her how to relax. We all know the recuperative power of a few minutes' sleep. A few minutes' relaxation is the best substitute when sleep is not possible. Drop everything, every tension, every care, and come as near the unconsciousness of sleep as possible. Let us hear the conclusion of the whole matter, with all our teaching let us endeavor to teach the pupil to get wisdom, which is to "know herself."

(Davis, 1907, pp. 104–107)

Factors of Elimination in Schools for Nurses

A. REASONS FOR PUPILS LEAVING SCHOOLS FOR NURSES BEFORE
   FINISHING THEIR COURSE OF INSTRUCTION.
B. REASONS WHY ELIGIBLE PUPILS DO NOT ENTER SCHOOLS FOR
   NURSES.

By Mrs. E. F. S. Smith

To so small an extent is this paper original with me that I may, with perfect propriety, I believe, present it to you as a valuable compilation, containing as it does the opinions of many representative women in the nursing world.

Upon receiving from Miss Wheeler an invitation to prepare a paper on the above-named subject for this occasion (a highly appreciated honor, I assure you) I at once addressed letters to superintendents of nurses in various states, asking for contributions, and it is with great pleasure and also with a feeling of security from personal criticism, I now present them to you.

Illinois sends this:

> One of the reasons for women not entering Schools for Nurses is, that due to the great and rapid increase in the number of Schools for Nurses, *efficient teachers have not been procurable.*

The data in Illinois stands like this: Between 1880 and 1890 there were eight schools for nurses established; between 1880 and 1900 there were thirty-two more schools established; between 1900 and 1910 there were something like fifty-three more schools established. Data from Missouri and other states might show this rapid increase, and also that the actual count of pupil nurses in the smaller schools is larger than the number in the larger schools. We might compare this with a part of the arterial system, namely; there is more blood in the capillaries than there is in the larger vessels near the heart. With less efficient teaching in the large number of small schools, we have lost out in having a great number of the best young women apply.

Another reason is that there are so many more openings for women, with better financial returns in a shorter length of preparatory time, with shorter hours on duty and much less responsibility.

The tendency of the day seems to take the easiest way; not necessarily the most complete and finished work as a result.

Still another reason is that the discipline in a majority of homes is very lax, and transferring the young woman from the home to the hospital where there must necessarily be some degree of discipline, means that it is distasteful, and they will not stand for it.

Due to the great number of schools, it has been necessary to take in a great number of young women regardless of education, age, and general fitness, in order simply to get the work done.

The result has been of course that the hospital has gained by a smaller pay-roll but that the nursing profession has been engorged with women who should never have been placed in the position to be made responsible for duties which they could not in any way measure up to.

AND HERE IS A VOICE FROM COLORADO

(*a*) During four years as superintendent of nurses, and four years as teacher in training school, I have observed that where probationers have been carefully selected, about 10 per cent drop out during the three years, because of ill health, insubordination, and inability. The number leaving training school because they do not like the work, is surprisingly small; I should think about one-half per cent. During the first year the percentage of elimination is higher; during third year very low, so that I think 10 percent for an average is a fair estimate.

(*b*) Reasons why eligible pupils do not enter schools:
1. Because of long duty hours, and physical strain of nursing for three years.

2. Prejudice against nurses as a class.

3. Notion that nursing is a menial occupation. The latter objections are dying out, and will eventually regulate themselves, but the first needs strenuous effort and agitation from the nursing profession. It is a crime to exploit our young women's physical strength by the long hours on duty that our hospitals demand.

INDIANA HAS THIS TO SAY

I believe the greatest reason for the better educated girls not entering the schools is on account of our low standards of education for admission. Many parents object to their daughters entering the profession because they look upon nursing as belonging to the ordinary class of working girls.

State registration is slowly correcting this impression, but we have not outlived the Sairy Gamp age.

I have lately been very much impressed with this phase of the question by some young high school graduates coming to me for advice. They wanted to enter training schools but were opposed by their families, and urged to be stenographers, or domestic science teachers, as work in these lines was of a higher quality, and much more respectable than nursing.

Many girls take to these lines of work of their own will, because they can get through in a much shorter time, and get to making money; with many this is a necessity and not a choice.

The great prosperity of our country for the past few years has made it unnecessary for many girls in the families of our great middle class to become self-supporting.

The chief reason for pupils leaving the schools is perhaps the failure on the part of so many schools to give what they promise. Many enter too young, 17 to 18 years of age; others enter with a sentimental idea of nursing; the long hours and hard work soon dispel that idea, and they leave,—cured.

I will add another reason for pupils not remaining in schools, which is the lack of properly qualified women at the head of many of our schools; I know this is the case in our state.

OF COURSE MISSOURI HAS SOMETHING TO SAY

One contributor says: I have thought that our surroundings have had a great deal to do with our shortage of probationers. High school and university graduates have been accepted as probationers here, but have stayed only long enough for their trunks to arrive so they could send them back.

These did not like the surroundings. We hope to have large classes when we move to the new hospital. In a good many hospitals poor food, lack of training and long hours will cause the pupils to leave when they realize they are not getting what should be given them.

A great many eligible young women do not know anything about training schools.

From another contributor:

Two reasons for pupils leaving schools:

1. Improper housing conditions in many schools. In boarding schools and colleges, the dormitories are given special attention as to cleanliness and the comfort of occupants. Why should Training Schools for Nurses be any less particular, and even more so, because it is the only home the pupil nurse has for three years of her life.

2. Because so little attention is paid to the social welfare of the pupil nurse. As a general thing she must seek her own means of entertainment. The lack of direct personal and sympathetic association and especially the lack of at least some small social relaxation such as is needed by any normally constituted young person.

Reasons why eligible pupils do not enter schools.

1. Because nursing is pictured to the laity as a drudgery; the high school and the college graduate think only of the practical work, not of the possibility in it for teaching, and work in the many different lines now opening up to the profession.

2. Because as a rule eligible pupils are discouraged by friends who picture the life as one of confinement, with few social pleasures.

Another contributor writes thus:

I have had no experience in pupils leaving here for other schools, but have had many applications from pupils seeking to enter here, after spending some time in other training schools, and since we have had our laws regarding registration this number has increased.

The reason they give me when I question them is, "We are not getting what we expected nor what was promised us."

"Why did you enter that school?" "It was recommended to us by our pastor or our physician, and we thought it was all right, but we have since learned that it does not come up to other schools."

Reasons why eligible pupils do not enter training Schools: I believe that young women generally know very little about the work, its advantages, its usefulness, and where the education may be obtained. If we could have all applicants educated in the requirements of state laws, and a knowledge of the reputable schools, before they enter, and not leave it for them to find out in some round-about-way after they have been in school for from six to eighteen months, we might be able to keep out of our profession those who are now finishing in poor schools because they do not come up to the requirements of the better schools.

And here is another opinion:

I think the greatest reason why pupils leave training schools is principally due to poor selection on the part of the training school superintendent. I have found the number of dismissals, also resignations, much less since raising our standards.

As to the second question, I would say this applies to the raising of the standard of the training school.

Briefly speaking then, the first question could be answered by requiring a higher standard for pupils, and the second by demanding a better standard for training schools.

I quote from another Missouri Superintendent:

I must confess that the reason most frequently advanced for lack of pupils does not appeal to me, that is, the hard work and long hours. The work seems to me so much less hard and of a much more interesting nature, because of the more thorough theoretical training, and certainly the hours are not what you and I had.

I truly sometimes wonder if they are not given too much time for other things and thus fail to become absorbed in their work. I grant you it is a hard life and one becomes very narrow who has no outside interests, but has it not been your experience, that the nurse who goes out least and has fewest friends close at hand, is the one who is most satisfied in her work, as well as the one who is most satisfactory.

It seems to me that I have never found such difficulty in putting the nursing spirit into any group of girls as I have met with here, and taken as a whole I have never worked with a more intelligent group, but very few of them put much enthusiasm into their work. My explanation for this is that they have had too much time for outside things.

ANOTHER VIEW

1. Lack of ability to keep up with the work. Lack of desire to submit to discipline. Failure after the first year of training to develop in

correspondence to their unceasing responsibility together with an inability to see the necessity of so doing. During the first year they retain their enthusiasm, submit to the necessary discipline, but after that time there seems to be an inclination to "rest on their oars" with the air of having accomplished their object, instead of realizing it has scarcely begun. Overwork, with too little regard for a nurses' health; undesirable quarters; insufficient, nourishing food; insufficient diversion during her "off duty," too much menial work; too long hours; lack of proper instruction.

The last contributor to this paper has this to say:

1. The probationary period. Too little attention is paid to the probationary period. A great many probationers who would have made excellent nurses, have been lost to the profession because of lack of encouragement and attention during this period. A probationer should be made to see the better side as well as the more unpleasant.

2. Pupil nurse's service; In the course of the service of pupil nurses many things arise which discourge them, some for which they are at fault and some for which they are not responsible. Discipline should be administered with great intelligence and care. Expulsion from school should be reserved for extreme cases.

3. Age of admission: It has been the practice of training schools not to admit pupils until they are 21 years of age. This leaves a number of years between the high school and the training school periods during which habits of study may be changed. If the student could pass from the high school into the training school, this of itself would increase the effectiveness of the work, and would establish the importance of the service in the eyes of the public and of prospective pupils. Furthermore, under the present arrangement the way is open for the admission of pupils who have been failures in other walks of life or who enter the work in default of something to do.

4. Instruction. The approximation of the high schools and training school courses would make it possible to develop the modern tendency of more definite pedagogic instruction. The course could easily be lengthened, the didactic and laboratory instruction made more comprehensive and the time of the students' service be far better utilized in the direction of providing ample time for study.

(Smith, 1913, pp. 54–59)

The Responsibility of the University School of Nursing to the Individual Student, the Hospital, and the Community

By Mrs. Frances P. Bolton

Two university schools of nursing have sprung into being since the last national nursing convention. Very quietly, two great universities have welcomed the profession of nursing and have taken the small-seeming yet infinite step that separates the departments of nursing within medical schools, women's colleges, etc., from the free, independent, self-determining school, a step which marks the beginning of a new era and consummates the dreams of half a century.

There is no need to trace for you the evolution of nursing through these fifty years, no need to point out the glaring faults of apprentice training which has been made so clear by the Rockefeller Report, as they do the desperate need of hands, as well as the economic necessities of hospitals which have themselves evolved from being places to care for the sick poor into institutions to meet the needs of all classes, including the clinical requirements of medical schools—all this is too vividly a part of your lives to need any portrayal. Indeed it is still all too widespread an actual fact But regardless of the time that must elapse before all hospitals adopt adequate training-school standards the fact shines out clearly that nursing training has come into its own and has taken its place in the field of education.

To insure ourselves against possible misapprehension let us take a moment to clarify our minds as to our conception of education. Modern education in the United States has tended to become merely the means of making the individual economically productive. Little emphasis, if any, is placed upon the development of the individual as a human being, as an all round, balanced citizen. Facts are crammed into the head at high pressure, and the mind that can evidence its ability to contain these facts is retained within school and college regardless of the character and heart and capacity for future growth of the individual along the lines of human development. This is not the interpretation that we can tolerate when we say with deep joy that university schools of nursing have placed this specialized training in the educational field. *Education* as we understand the word is *preparation for life*, and in a full, rounded, contributive life, the economic factor—though necessary—is but a fractional part. Therefore, we mean by education, the process of developing all the faculties of the body, mind and spirit and of preparing each individual for that special place in the kaleidoscope of life for which he is best qualified.

Nor is there any desire upon the part of any one connected with the establishment of these two university schools to confine the training of nurses, even in the distant future, within university walls. The mere physical limitations preclude such a possibility. Yet it is readily seen that nursing training has been definitely recognized as of educational value and in consequence even the smallest training school acquires a new dignity and assumes a correspondingly greater responsibility.

As we step over this threshold of opportunity it behooves us to take an accounting, to analyze our hopes, to face our responsibilities, not because these have changed, but because they have been deepened and broadened and heightened. Every hope and every dream for the development of nursing through a more satisfactory method of training is based upon the cry of suffering humanity, upon the need of adequate care of the sick. The increasingly heavy demands of institutions and communities for nurses and for good nurses have made a situation that unfortunately has not simplified the problem. In order to secure numbers, compromises have been made on every hand, and these compromises have, in a measure, defeated their own ends.

The Vassar camp that the war gave us brought into the profession a large group of intelligent, purposeful young women, and the two years of their experience in the various hospitals of the country showed them and us how much we need women of their stamp, and how little we are really meeting standards of balanced training even in our best schools. It showed us also that nursing has a direct appeal to the very finest women of the country, not just to such occasional individuals but to large groups. The problem is—how to secure their interest.

The university training school is the direct and definite answer. By placing nursing training in the educational field it immediately becomes of new interest to the young woman seeking to prepare herself for a broad life of self-dependence and service whether she choose a university school of nursing or a regular hospital training school. If she chooses the regular hospital school she will seek out the one whose standards approximate most closely to university standards. Further than this training school committees and hospital trustees will realize that only a well balanced basic training will bring them the greatly needed students and the community will see that such standards of training alone will protect it from inadequately prepared nurses.

Because of the ramifications of the influence of these schools of nursing it is my desire to try to interpret something of the sense of responsibility to the students, to the hospital, to the community, resting upon those intimately connected with their establishment.

What is the human material coming to the modern training schools? Half a century ago the women who went into nursing were of mature years, with an understanding of life, its complications, its possibilities. Their bodies had already been through tests of strain, their minds had met disillusion, their hearts had experienced both sorrow and joy. They took up nursing because they had learned to value human life. Today the student nurse is still in her teens, her body is in the process of maturing, her mind is but beginning to find itself, her heart is still in a state of emotion. She is wholly inexperienced, life looks very wonderful, rosy, filled with every brilliant prospect. She dreams of the joys of an ideal service to humanity, she sees herself as a ministering angel. Of course she has no sense of the value of human life—how could she? She is too recently awakened for that, too throbbing with her newly discovered and still intangible sense of womanhood. Coming as so many do from communities where social life is tied up with the church, the breaking off of that association, combined with the fact that hours are of necessity such that new church affiliations are difficult to make, the student feels deprived of a normal outlet and divorced from accustomed counsel. She has become one of a group and for a time she loses herself, sensing little but her aching body, her dazed mind, her curiously cold heart. Perhaps home-sickness has seized her in its clutch and utter darkness surrounds her; but that must not be allowed to keep her from her work. Who cares whether she is lonely or not? Who knows that every breath she draws hurts because it is not home air? To whom does it matter whether every experience brings with it a shock that life and death are so different from what she had imagined them?

Months pass, she becomes more accustomed. She has learned something of nursing procedures, her duties have taken on definite responsibility, too great, perhaps, for the time of preparation, considering her youth. Night duty! The terrible stillness with the strange, weird sounds that the sick make during sleep or in the long hard hours of wakefulness. The creeping cold, the insidious temptation to allow her normal desire for sleep to slacken her attention, conquered by an extra tour of the beds with a whispered word of reassurance to the patients whose dread of the long dark, increases rather than dispels her own. The lowering of her threshold to all the weaknesses of her nature, and oh! so little understanding of that nature or life to help her. Only those in whose lives is the memory of such experience can fully appreciate how it shakes the very foundations of being.

She goes from one service to another, finding some intensely interesting, others indescribably horrible. These follow so quickly one after the other that she has no time to digest them, to assimilate them. Always the pressure of work, mental as well as physical, for she must stand well in the classroom if she is to complete her course.

Fun there is, too, the happy intercourse of a sort of boarding school life with new friends and an enlarged horizon, though here, too, are shocks and re-adjustments—always with the background of sickness. So she comes to the end of her three years when she goes out into the world to serve humanity.

We all agree that the university school of nursing has a very great responsibility to these young things, all of them, everywhere, for whatever is set up within university walls will be followed in varying degree by all training schools. Youth is a fervent, vital, thrilling time, but it cannot evaluate life and service. Its ideals are in the clouds, its feet have not yet reached good mother earth. What must be a part of these years of training to protect the girl and to return her enthusiasm and her desire into the right way?

First—She must be given certain ideals for the understanding of positive health of body, mind and souls, and those ideals must be made so practical that they become a modus vivendi as well as a norm by which to judge deviations. Second—She must learn to value human life and to appreciate the privilege of service.

To make these things possible, her education must be based upon what the community expects her to know rather than on what any particular hospital can give her, which involves living and working conditions that will enable her to build up proper habits of study, work and play, with protection against too heavy responsibilities before she is prepared for them. And further than that she should be taught to appreciate that all this is justified only on the assumption that it will enable her to render more worth while service.

Medicine and surgery have been occupied with the study of disease in order that society might be protected against the scourges civilization brings with it; all the energies of the profession have had to be expended in the effort to find the causes, supply antidotes and remedies, and to effect cures. So great has this task been that there has been no time left in which to study health. Only very recently has there been intruded into the minds of certain medical groups the idea that the future medical school must offer its students the opportunity to study and practice health principles and function. The public wants health, and its demands are growing more and more insistent. Especially is this true of women, for their function is to bear children, and they want healthy children. The external appearance of physical strength which is apt to be man's definition of health, has no attraction for woman. She wants that which will give her the endurance she needs to bear and rear children, and to take her place in the larger world that modern life has opened to her. She wants knowledge not of the abnormal, the diseased, the evil, but of the laws that govern health and happiness. Man by his nature is a fighter and the crisis toward which he moves is death, either for himself, or the other fellow. Woman in her nature is the creator and the supreme experience of her life is birth—so her demand for a better understanding of life is one that cannot be stilled— nor can it be satisfied with panaceas. Necessary as it is that medicine should study disease, germs, serums, etc., is it not time that health be made a subject of intensive study and that a definite application of its principles be made possible to all men and women?

If there is any one group of people more than another that should radiate health it is nurses. If you have had experience of illness you may have been cared for by a nurse who was always tired, worn, depressed, or you may have found the radiating smile, the bright eye, the clear skin, the steady strength of buoyant health. If you have experienced both, you know how great a factor this health quality is in determining the atmosphere of the sickroom, and you may also be able to weigh its direct contribution to the reestablishment of health.

To my mind one of the first responsibilities of university schools as standard making bodies is to change the attitude of all concerned toward this matter of health. The first step in this as in all things is to do away with ignorance and in its place to put, not only knowledge of health principles and law, but the demonstration of these by every student and every nurse, twenty-four hours a day. This is not an easy matter, for its requires teaching for which few are prepared. It would appear that the medical profession has little to offer us in this emergency for, as we have seen, its emphasis is placed upon disease, its nature and its cure, and for all the theoretical knowledge a doctor may possess of the functioning of a normal body, he has little understanding of how to have health and how to keep it, as it is outside his sphere, and he seldom applies the principles he may have known to his own body. Teachers of health for our young students should have thorough scientific knowledge of structure and function, but more important still they should know how to apply this knowledge, how to make it practical, how to teach it, *how to live it.*

Shall we find what we seek among the so-called physical culture teachers? Have they a sufficient background of anatomy, physiology, biology, chemistry, psychology and function to answer our needs? Just a course in gymnastic exercise will not be enough for our purpose, though even this is better than no emphasis at all on the student's own well-being. But perfunctory gymnastics do not insure health. And there is a definite feeling among gynecologists and obstetricians that there is every possibility of injury from the athletic form of exercise now in general use in girls' gymnasiums. A practical working knowledge of the natural laws of internal cleanliness, circulation, respiration and their daily use, combined with an understanding of and obedience to the laws of the inter-relation of mental and bodily function, and a realization of the limitless possibilities for self-control, self-development, self-mastery, that is the background necessary for health, that is what we want for the student. If she can be given a comprehension of the marvelous mechanism that is the "house we live in," and appreciate through actual experience to the wonderful kindness of nature, she will have a reverence for her own body that she can acquire in no other way, and through that, a reverence for the bodies of others, and a sense of the sacredness and value of human life.

In order to accomplish all that we want through this education for health it must include the *practice* of the principles involved: bodily function, mental development and character building. "Character," says Stanley Hall, "can be defined as muscle habits." So by beginning our teaching with the body structure and function, applying those same great principles to the mind and through both to building character, by giving them such knowledge we shall be protecting them from themselves and from the temptations that freedom from the usual restraints has involved them in—and we shall be giving them a vision of the sacredness of that which we call life.

Again I feel impelled to insure ourselves against possible misunderstanding, through differing definitions. I do not use the word "knowledge" in the sense too often used in health matters by those who decry the "knowledge of life" that the young people have indiscriminately gleaned from heaven alone knows what sources, for this is not knowledge, it is information without wisdom. Knowledge is two sided—it gives understanding because it gives both good and evil. It is based upon a true picture upon science, upon reason.

Because our students today are so young it is clearly our duty to counteract the effects of their contacts with the results of the misuse of function by giving them a vivid picture of the results of right living, right function and a real capacity for happiness—that they may find knowledge.

Hospital atmosphere is another great factor in the life of a student, and it involves all the individuals who play a part in the network of its machinery from the trustee to the garbage man. If the members of the board of trustees are too concerned with other affairs to study hospital problems, if they place an over emphasis on financial returns, they quite definitely contribute an attitude that, as it goes down the line, grows into a curious disregard of the real center of activity, the patient, and he becomes a victim rather than the hub of the wheel. The medical staff plays a very important part in this intangible but powerful factor in determining the type of student that is developed. Men who have not certain fineness of feeling, who lack the humanities, exude a certain hardness and cruelty that leave a trail of acute mental suffering among the patients, and indirectly teach those qualities to the students. No amount of lecturing on hospital psychology, nursing ethics and the like, be that lecture ever so marvelous, will efface the effect of making rounds with a man who discusses the problem at the bedside, who intrudes the personal element, or who stoops to suggestive inuendoes. Men of this caliber are unfit to teach. We hope they are very much in the minority, and we trust that the medical profession of the future will be able entirely to exclude them from its ranks. The influence of men who, as the writer of The Corner of Harley Street says: "Take off their hats" to the marvels of the human body and the laws that govern it, who have found a reverence for nature in all her manifestations and who value human life because of that reverence, have an immeasurable influence over the student, as well as radiating it into every corner of the hospital.

Surely our university schools of nursing should face frankly this responsibility in the matter of teachers and insure their students against the unconscious influence of a bad atmosphere, securing for them the benefits of the good.

Girls who choose nursing as their career, though they may have but a vague idea of what they are involving themselves in, very definitely know that they must do without certain light hearted fun that their friends are experiencing. They give it up very cheerfully, feeling that they will find compensation in the sacrific. But we who have the planning of those years of training must keep ever before us their need of normal, healthy, happy playtime to balance the exactions of their discipline. This regulation of the free hours is as important in its way as is the proper arrangement of theory and practice, and hand in hand with it comes the necessity for pleasant, wholesome living conditions. This does not mean luxury, but it does mean that the residence facilities shall be such that each student's rest time shall be protected from interruption and that she has an environment that spells health and happiness. The idea of self-sacrifice for a principle is a most estimable one, and, as I have said, there is quite rightly an element of it in every student's heart, but if she has to stay herself upon it in order to keep up her courage, in order to bear the pressure of overwork, or inadequate playtime, improper housing conditions, etc., she is in danger of being possessed by the idea that she is a martyr, that her life is nothing but sacrifice. Surely this is far from the actual fact. I feel certain that not one of you but knows that there is nothing so overwhelmingly soul-satisfying as the experience of saving life and leading a human being back to health! So let us not run the danger of the student starting her nursing life with the wrong conception. Let us so adjust her work, her rest, her play, that she will recognize the privilege that is hers in being able to train herself to serve humanity, and through that service to find an abiding happiness.

The actual educational responsibility of the university schools of nursing can scarcely be over-estimated, nor the extent of their influence upon other nursing schools. Curriculums will be based more nearly upon what a nurse sould have as equipment rather than upon what any one hospital is able to give her. The Boards of the hospitals giving the practical training will make superhuman effort to secure the funds necessary to the proper balance of the student's work, once they see the need.

It would be unfair to the student not to give her a realizing sense of the opportunity that is hers—not to have her appreciate that the only possible justification of this additional expenditure in all its ramifications is the assumption that she will be able to render better service not only during her student years, but in all the years of her active nursing life.

The primary cause behind all medical and nursing schools, the *raison d'etre* for all hospitals, is the poignant need of suffering humanity. The patient is the center and from him radiate all the spokes of medical education, diagnosis, treatment, care, etc., that reach out to reconstruct this Wheel of Life. All hospitals, large and small, exist primarily for the care of the sick, and each makes its particular contribution, but those that are definitely teaching institutions assume an added responsibility for they must set standards, they must be the living example of all that is best in medicine, surgery and nursing.

This constitutes a dual problem: Adequate care of patients and balanced training for the student, and if either has to be temporarily held in abeyance it *must* be the student's training.

It is in the nursing department that the dual problem is most acute. To give adequate care to the patients and at the same time have the student body free for the theory and practice of nursing procedure is not an easy task. Unless there is a force of graduate nurses to supplement the student service one of two things must happen: either the patient will not receive proper care, or the student will be on the wards over the time required for her education, and will have an unbalance of services. Naturally it is the student not the patient who suffers, this must be so, and should be so, no one could possibly wish it otherwise. But with the assertion that a university school of nursing makes nursing training an *educational* matter comes the necessity for enough supplementary nursing service in the hospitals involved to do away with the over use of the student.

The economic factor is, unfortunately, all too often the deciding one, and it is well that, as one of the results of the Rockefeller Committee report on training schools, we of the laity have been made to realize that three years in a hospital has not necessarily meant a well-organized, well-balanced training. We found to our horror, those of us who did not already know it, that R.N. after a name does not necessarily guarantee us against the perfectly honest but inadequate nurse whom we have called in, in our need, to care for our children, who has had but a week's pediatrics while in training, and no contagious work at all! We have been rudely awakened and made to see that it has been somewhat our own fault, we have been blind to the fact that as trustees, we were misusing some of those precious hospital years from sheer ignorance of the problem. It is very human to search about for an alibi. And I think we often hide from ourselves behind the feeling that somehow we should have been informed, that you of the League[1] should have taken us more into your confidence, that we might have helped you bear the burden, and so hastened the day that has begun to dawn.

As I study the history *you* have made I am thrilled beyond measure at your endurance, your patience, your steady determination to establish adequate nursing standards. I doubt if there has ever been a more consecrated body of women anywhere and your achievements make me proud to share your womanhood. I have the joy of possessing an N. O. P. H. N. pin, and you of the League have given me the privilege of an equally intimate comradeship. I am happier than I can tell you to have this opportunity of expressing in person my deep and lasting appreciation of your graciousness. The fight for recognition that you have had to make has developed among you a wonderful *esprit de corps*, something that women need. To my mind you have in conséquence two clear responsibilities, one to the rest of us, one to yourselves.

Your fifty years of studentship in the art of working together for an ideal have given you an experience that all women need. Can you not pass on to us some of the fruits?

The other responsibility consequent upon your long struggle, is one of self analysis in an attitude of the utmost selfishness. Is there not always danger that too concentrated an *esprit de corps* confines growth and so starts involution? Is this not the moment for you to catechise yourselves both as individuals and as a group as to whether you have not come to the end of the old revelation where your God was, and had to be, the God of battles, whether you do not stand upon the threshold of the new world where God is not only a judge but a father, a mother and a son? In this world it is no longer brother against brother, sister against sister. Will you not consider, among other matters requiring your deliberations, whether you cannot find a larger development for the future of your profession through a greater intimacy and an actual working hand in hand with the steadily increasing numbers of sympathetic and educated laity?

The problem of securing a well-balanced basic training for the student nurse is so involved with that of securing sufficient financial

---

[1]National League of Nursing Education.

support for hospitals that I see no better way to attain it than to share the burden with the financially responsible. It is a matter of educating enough people to see it your way, and it is infinitely better psychology *to work with* people than to insist upon their doing something *your* way. Once men (or women) realize that they run the risk of having a nurse in a time of stress who is inadequately prepared simply because of the hospital she trained in hadn't funds enough to relieve her of enough ward work to permit her to get the training she went for, they are going to put their right hands into their pockets. But so long as they have a feeling of suspicion about it all, so long as they imagine that "what the nurses want" is an "easy road," or something equally ridiculous as it is false, just so long will they refuse to make it possible.

The only way I can see to dispel these illusions is for you to open your hearts to them. You have only to do this to reap the fruits of your long years of labor and of ceaseless struggle for the ideal that is a light in the darkness of suffering. Not one of you but shares in the responsibilities now resting upon these new branches of education. You have cherished the hope, you have laid the foundation stones and put up the framework and you must help to build the walls. Each one of you has the power to influence many separate individuals, each case you have, each day you spend at your work will be a definite help or hindrance to the development of these and other schools. You are just as definitely a part of this visible evidence of a new era in nursing as any member of the faculties, and you share with the trustees the responsibilities they have assumed of interesting the young women in nursing as a career, of safeguarding them during training, and of interpreting nursing in all its practical value and its beauty to the community.

This matter of securing students is one that is of greatest moment, for without students there can be no university school of nursing or any other. And they must be of good quality, capable of appreciating the opportunities of such a standard-making school.

The hospitals in which university students will receive their practical work have a right to expect them to have an appreciation of this high quality of service, of the privilege they enjoy in participating in the work of the hospital, being co-workers with trustees, doctors, etc., in the wheel of relief of pain and the study of disease and cure. We must never lose sight of the fact that we share the hospital's responsibilities for the care of the patient, and our students should feel the challenge and the opportunity.

Further than this it would seem that the time has come when the actual economic value of the instruction, the teaching equipment, the living conditions provided by the hospital and the university should be more definitely realized by the student. She should see that if she wants the dignity of her profession recognized educationally she must begin to pay for what she receives in something other than service. If her time is so arranged that her service to the hospital is in very truth guarded for her training, she in turn should recognize its value and joyfully pay as students in all colleges do.

This is one of the matters requiring much thoughtful consideration on the part of the hospitals and the schools of nursing and other hospital training schools. It involves the coordination of the groups other than undergraduate students, those of affiliates, of special post-graduates and of regular graduate service. It is not possible to discuss it at this time, but it would seem pertinent to emphasize the sense of responsibility carried by the university schools in this phase of the problem.

In closing I have only a word to say in the matter of responsibility that these new schools recognize to the community at large. As I see it, it is twofold. The first consists largely in those matters we have already discussed: the selection of the best human material, safeguarding them, developing them as human beings and assuring them a truly sound fundamental training in those essentials of nursing that are generally termed basic, that they may be truly fit to go out into the community as women trained in the care of the sick.

Just at this point I want to say a word about the university student not as yet touched upon—the postgraduates. There is a great need of supplementary and additional education for graduate nurses who have suffered from the failure of the apprentice type of training, and it is the university school of nursing that should recognize a definite responsibility to the community to insure these women the chance to secure instruction in those branches they have missed, as well as to provide the training required in so many of the special fields now open to the nurse. These special fields are numerous and a nurse must have, besides a sound basic knowledge, an additional technical training in public health, industrial nursing, tuberculosis, etc.

Finally, it would seem that university schools of nursing have a definite responsibility and a somewhat unique privilege in the matter of interpreting nursing, not only to the student and to the active nurse, but also to the community, that there may be brought about a more general understanding of what nursing is, its ideals, its aims, its principles, its opportunities.

The community should be given the chance to see its own responsibility in the solution of the problem of securing adequate care for the sick and the further education of the individual for health. This can be best interpreted by the schools of nursing within universities as their very position within the seats of education gives them a certain impersonalness that is essential, and this gives them a further duty: to secure a more general recognition of the many fields now open for the nurse, dissimilar in external form, called by various names, but all based upon the need of the suffering and the clamorous demands of all humanity for health.

(Bolton, 1925, pp. 131–142)

Address

By Mary E. Gladwin, R. N.

President, Minnesota League of Nursing Education

There seems to be a well-founded belief that we are nearing the end of the preliminary period of modern nursing education. The grading project is the ceremony which marks that end. Certainly, no preliminary students could display more anxiety or dread at the inevitable conference with the principal of the school, than do the schools at the outcome of the first grading. They fear, and with reason, that their whole future is at stake. Indeed, certain small schools have gone out of existence rather than face the ordeal.

The dread is easily understood. No matter how confidential the result, low rank means fewer applicants or applicants of inferior quality. Intelligent mothers who have read an account of the grading activities are beginning to ask, "Are there too many nurses? Is there a future of well-paid work for my daughter, if she follows her desire to study nursing?"

The grading of schools is a grave enough issue in itself, but in addition, it is closely related to other questions of equal importance. Hospital authorities are uneasy because of a possible increase in the running expenses of their hospitals. With the increase in competition and specialization, with the insistent demands for more complex and costly equipment, the financial burden is already a very heavy one. No hospital superintendent can face addition to the load without concern.

With the increase in the number of specialties and specialists, the demand for more costly equipment, and the magnificence of today's building plans, has come to the patient and his family a tremendous and crushing increase in the cost of illness. There is nothing harder, in all the world, than to face unrelieved suffering and possible death for one we love because of inability to pay for the best service. We are rather callous about this omnipresent condition. We talk of "the ward purse and the private room aspirations" as though there were no tragedy behind the curtain. We see desperately anxious people, vainly spending every cent they have in the world. Even though life itself is spared, they go back home to what? Weakened health, no nest-egg for the future, no possibility of keeping up life insurance, the provision for another illness or old age swept away, the education of the children restricted, the comfortable future of their anticipation changed to one of dread and anxiety.

In the readjustment, the revolution, which must come in nursing affairs, we can not afford to lose sight of the hospital and the patient or of the truth that what we are doing affects thousands of young women who fear that their livelihood is threatened or at least involved.

Thus we come by slow steps to what is for the League of Nursing Education the crux of the whole matter, the education of the pupil nurse. The words, "The Education of the Nurse" have long been a battle-cry, a signal to gird on one's armor and to sharpen one's weapons. It would be a pity, if after these many years of struggle, we were no longer willing to fight for the faith that is in us, but a still greater pity if we had not learned to fight with broader understanding and greater charity. Our struggle is not against people but against wrong ideals, outworn traditions, misinformation.

The Sunday edition of the Chicago Tribune devoted several columns to Glen Frank and his work as President of the University of Wisconsin; it quoted him as saying "Human history presents unanswerable proof that only through the open and unhampered clash of contrary opinions can truth be found." So one may take comfort in remembering that if our struggles were over, if we could expect no more opposition or conflict, if there were to be no further "unhampered clash of contrary opinions," our work would be finished and we would be on the downward grade that sometimes comes to all human effort.

The logical place to begin preparation for what is before us is an intensive study of the history of modern nursing; not the sort of thing which led an irreverent young thing, at a recent commencement, to whisper to her neighbor just as the orator of the occasion got under full sail, "Good Lord, Florence Nightingale again!", but an analysis of the various steps in our progress, the position we now occupy, and our future possibilities in the light of what has gone before. Before coming to any decision about our future plans, we should know about the origin of the nursing movement, its successive steps, and the reasons underlying its successes and failures. The physical disabilities which the years often bring are not isolated phenomena, having no relation to earlier years and neither are the problems of the nursing world isolated having no connection with the past. They have the most intimate possible relationship with all that makes nursing history.

As our President said a few minutes ago, we are still thinking of nursing education in terms of long ago, at least, many honest people who are discussing nursing education are doing it in that fashion. They are unaware of the great changes that have taken place in even the last five years. We need to show them a comparison of hospital equipment and nursing procedures of the period, let us say, just after the Spanish American War and then those of today.

The method of the amateur detective in the "crime-a-month" books is admirable for our purpose. The treatments and procedures of ten, twenty, and thirty years ago in one column and those of today in the adjoining one; the diets of that day against those of today; the serums, vaccines, solutions given intravenously against those once given. Any typical chart reveals the enormous progress made in medicine and surgery, and the corresponding changes in the work of the nurse. The change in the treatment of medical patients, in even two years, is rather astounding and yet it is hard to convince some of our friends of the necessity for better educated young women whose intellectual and mental faculties have already been fairly well trained.

The distinction between medical and surgical patients seems to be rapidly disappearing or at least these are becoming purely arbitrary terms. The surgical patient is given so many medical tests and so much medical treatment before and after operation that it looks as though the services would soon become interchangeable. These are very significant features of the hospital life of today and prophetic of the conditions of the future. It would be folly not to look forward and make ready for the changes almost upon us.

One of our important tasks is that of making our connection with general education a little clearer. It is instructive to take a casual glance backward. The Great War is by no means responsible for all the things that have happened but it is a convenient milestone. Since it ended, certain marked stages have been apparent in educational thought and pronouncement. First, educational experts warned us that we were in danger of becoming an eighth-grade nation. As if in answer to these warnings, we were almost immediately treated to the spectacle of youth clamoring by the thousand at the doors of our colleges and universities, until, strange talk for a democracy and savoring of privileged classes, suggestions were made that higher education be restricted.

Now, it appears, it is the content of the curriculum, the methods of instruction, and the preparation and education of the teachers which are the subject of controversy among educators generally. All of this is of importance to us. It means that the concept of education is changing—*has changed*. Education is that process which enables a man to adapt himself to his environment in such a way as to make the most of his abilities or to make his environment fit his own development.

There is a curious truth about nursing education which should not be allowed to drop out of sight. Nursing schools were not organized, are not now organized, with possibly one or two exceptions, in order to provide fitting, well-paid work for young women. Even though the gracious and kindly women who were instrumental in founding the Bellevue School talked and wrote of their hope of founding a real college of nursing, that was the contributing cause not the primary reason for the organization. The school was founded for the purpose of rescuing the sick poor from the abhorrent and intolerable conditions in which they were found.

Schools were founded and are organized and increased in size today for the same reason, for the purpose of filling the need of the hospital so that its work should be done. No one would venture to assert that with this there has not gone a great deal of kindness and helpful unselfish interest, but the fundamental fact remains. Many of us are in charge of schools. We are enrolling a September class. Do we ask ourselves "Should we admit all those applicants when we are told that there is an oversupply of graduate nurses?" No. The members of the faculty ask each other, "How many pupils do we need?" Somebody calls attention to the fact that a goodly number dropped out of the last preliminary class and "we must be sure to have enough students to see us through next summer's vacations."

Of course, the oversupply of nurses is an economic problem which will right itself in time as all questions of supply and demand do but the way in which this may be brought about gives us food for thought. It may mean a serious decrease in the number of applicants or a deterioration in their quality. In some of our ways, we resemble the proverbial ostrich who buries his head in the sand under the delusion that he is successfully hidden. Our greatest problem isn't the oversupply of nurses but that so many inferior nurses have already been graduated from our schools. There isn't a school in this country which has been in existence ten years which has not given diplomas to students who should never have received them. These students were kept in the school by the stress of circumstances, because the principal did not know how to get her work done without such help as they could give her.

We have arrived at that period when it is essential to our future stability that we exercise much more care in the choice of applicants. During the preliminary period, we should painstakingly weed out the undesirables. The decision should not rest upon the judgment of the principal of the school. It should be the concerted action of the faculty as a whole. After the decision has once been made that the student has no aptitude for nursing or has not the moral qualities to make her desirable, then no pleading on the part of relatives or friends, no begging for another chance, should influence us. It is a waste of time and effort to keep her. In the end she has to go and the school is censured for having retained her so long.

If the League could work out the terms of an agreement whereby superintendents would pledge themselves not to admit a pupil who had been dismissed from another school for good and sufficient reason, it would be of the greatest assistance. Recently a pupil was dismissed because her practical work was poor, her theory worse, patients complained that she neglected them and was unkind in manner and words, and she was caught and confessed to stealing; and yet within two months she was admitted to another school and is now working toward her diploma and ultimate registration. A few nurses of that type in any community do us incalculable harm and lower the moral tone of the whole profession.

It seems to be the fashion to deny that there ever was a shortage of nurses; but I remember that in the years just after the Great War I worked in four or five states and that as I went from hospital to hospital, superintendents complained that they needed more pupils, had no waiting list, and were often obliged to keep poor pupils because they had no applicants to fill their places. We are now reaping the result of those years when we were driven by circumstance to retain and then to graduate poor nurses.

I remember that Miss Anna C. Maxwell, whose loss we mourn because she was such a friend and exemplar for all who longed to do good work, told me in 1921 or 1922 that she had always had enough applicants so that she could always supply two or three small schools with those she did not need but that then she had barely enough for her own school. These are some of the conditions with their results that we should study carefully in making plans for the future. It isn't any marvel that the quality of our nursing sometimes deteriorated. The evil did not disappear when applicants became more plentiful. We have only to remember how often we hear superintendents say that they would not have certain of their own graduates as special nurses.

At present the grading of schools of nursing is our most absorbing topic. We are conscious that it isn't just placing the schools in classes or groups that is of importance; it is *the grading in the individual school* that must follow the work now being done. The value of the various services and their relation one to another needs to be estimated, so that when a senior nurse goes to a floor she does not find herself doing just the same sort of work that she did in that place in the early part of her first year. Our present method is for the most part as absurd as it would be for a college student to plan to take classes anywhere in the four years' course, so that he would go to a Freshman class, then to one in the Senior year, and follow that by something he liked in the Sophomore course.

We have made many steps forward. First came the demand that heads of schools have better general education and definite preparation for the work they have chosen. Then came adequate laboratories and recitation rooms with qualified instructors. Now we are putting emphasis on better teaching on the floors, more and more bedside demonstration and instruction. In the work of the future, all supervisors must be teachers and as a consequence must be better educated and better prepared.

I was much impressed by what the President said of the little hospital of fifteen beds and the things which happen within its walls, but let us make no mistake, the things which happen in the little place are more easily perceived because of its size. Similar things often go on in the larger hospital. The pupils are moved from pillar to post not to round out their services or to give them the right sequence in their work but to answer the need of the various departments of the hospital. The entire system of practical work should be revolutionized and put on the educational basis which for the most part it now lacks.

In the years to come, there will probably be more than one type of school. It is quite evident that the school should be more independent and in many instances an entirely separate organization. In that same article in the Chicago Tribune about Glenn Frank, to which I alluded a few minutes ago, the statement was made that the President of the

Wisconsin University was asking the voters for millions of dollars with which to carry out his plans. The inference was that the millions would be forthcoming not because the voters understand just what it is all about but because they have confidence in the sincerity and integrity of purpose of the man who has the courage of his convictions. When after careful thought and study, with no ulterior purpose, the necessity of endowing schools of nursing in order to safeguard the welfare of the patient of the future is established, the money will be found.

Upon reaching Chicago Sunday morning, I found myself increasingly nervous at the prospect of addressing you with so little preparation, so to turn the current of my thoughts for a little while, I bought in the station Hackett's *Life of Henry the Eighth*. It is a gorgeous book, an enthralling picture of Tudor days. I couldn't read fast enough but there was one place that brought me to a full stop. When Henry the Seventh died, he left an endowment so that masses should be said for his soul as long as the world lasted and Christopher Columbus had calculated that the end would become in one hundred and fifty-five years—*as long as the world lasted!*

Many of us have labored hard in this field of nursing education. We have spent years in the work which our hands found to do. We have fought many battles. Sometimes we have lost and again we have been victorious. Now we see that much we thought permanent must be torn away, very soon it will go into the discard. But after all, isn't that what good and honest work is for, to make better and finer work possible? It is not meant to stand as long as the world lasts. If all our effort means simply that another generation can profit by our mistakes and labor, and go on to the victory which has been denied to us, then it is all worth while and we should rest content. Changes come and go; it is only the spirit that lives.

In that book of Mr. Hackett's, he describes the deathbed of Henry the Eighth and talks of the succession of the boy king Edward. He ends with, "And the trumpets sound with melody and courage." Today at the beginning of this new epoch in nursing education marked by the grading of the schools, we hear the silver trumpets of the past, the melody growing fainter but the courage transmitted to those younger people who are to follow us with a new melody as with hope and purpose they move forward. "And the trumpets sound with melody and courage."

(*Gladwin, 1929, pp. 28–34*)

Professional School or Trade School?

By Isabel M. Stewart, R. N.

*Professor of Nursing Education, Teachers College,
New York, New York*

However conscious we may be of the deficiencies of some nurses and nursing schools, most of us are on the defensive at once when nursing is referred to as "a woman's trade," or when nursing schools are found in some of our State Departments of Vocational Education listed with industrial schools. This is no fault of the Statement Departments or of the Federal Board of Vocational Education, which administers the Smith-Hughes funds. These organizations naturally assume that institutions asking for financial assistance from funds specifically assigned to vocational secondary schools for training in industrial, agricultural, and other occupations are willing to accept this classification and all the implications which go with it.

The question which we have to answer is whether the rank and file of nursing schools really are on a professional basis, or whether any considerable proportion of them are of the general order of trade or technical schools. It is quite evident that there is a good deal of confusion in our thinking on this subject, and that we do not all understand clearly what is implied in the use of terms "profession" and "professional school." Indeed some schools calling themselves not only professional schools but university schools of nursing, state frankly that a substantial part of their work is secured from secondary schools and is paid for from Smith-Hughes funds. Such schools would undoubtedly feel deeply injured if they were told that they are operating under false pretenses. They are quite convinced that they have a right to the title of "professional school" no matter what their actual educational standards may be, and it would be difficult to persuade them that a good honest trade school which makes no such pretenses might be infinitely superior to them in its educational work.

For the sake of our own integrity and also to aid in the clarification of our educational objectives, would it not be well to face this matter without emotion or prejudice, first trying to determine what the outstanding characteristics of a professional school are and then making an effort to measure ourselves by these standards?

While no hard and fast line can be drawn between schools of the trade school or sub-professional type and those of professional type, there are certain differences which are generally recognized just as there are certain fairly well marked differences between the occupations usually classed as professions and those which are classed as industrial, commercial, mechanical or domestic occupations. Some of these differences are inherent in the nature of the occupations themselves, and the demands which they make on the individual practitioner. Some of them are largely traditional, and are a matter of degree rather than kind. It may be helpful to begin by summarizing some of the points which are usually made in defining the duties and obligations of professional practice.

The laws of the United States define a profession as "a vocation in which a professed knowledge of some department of science or learning is used by its practical application to the affairs of others, either in advising, guiding or teaching them or serving their interests or welfare in the practice of the art founded on it." Many other definitions might be quoted. Analysis of those definitions will usually point to certain general demands and qualifications, some of which are listed below:

1. Professional occupations are primarily concerned with human beings, their behavior and relationships.

2. The situations they deal with are usually rather complex and the activities highly variable in character. It is not possible to predict the demands which will be made on the worker, to anything like the same extent that they can be predicted in a trade.

3. Professional procedures cannot usually be mechanized or routinized. They often have to be improvised to meet the situation. There is a constant demand for individual judgment, and adaptability on the part of the worker, especially in crises or emergencies which are likely to be frequent in professional practice and which often demand decisions involving vital human issues.

4. Professional workers usually work individually with little direct supervision. They must therefore possess a fair amount of initiative and must be able to assume individual responsibility when necessary.

5. Professional practice is constantly changing and therefore requires constant study to keep abreast with the new knowledge that is being discovered and with new methods of practice.

6. Professional practice requires a fair degree of maturity and a high degree of personal integrity and social responsibility. The service given is always expected to be the best of which one is capable, regardless of the remuneration received. It is assumed that business or personal considerations will be subordinated to the interests of the client or patient, and that public good will come before private gain.

Is nursing, then, a profession? Few of us would dare to claim that all graduate nurses meet these standards but we should have little difficulty in picking out a good number of representative nurses who are practicing nursing on this general level. As a matter of fact all members of even the old and established professions do not measure up to all these standards but the obligations are recognized even though they are not always honored.

How do these standards affect the standards of professional education? First it is obvious that any professional school which aims to produce workers to meet such demands, must secure candidates of potential professional calibre. No matter how excellent the educational process planned or how rich the educational resources available, it is quite impossible to produce a genuine professional product out of coarse grained or warped, shoddy or cheap human materials. Professional schools usually try to secure candidates who bring a fairly high standard of preliminary education and who also give evidence of having a good cultural background, sound character and a personality which makes for good human relationships. No schools of recognized professional standing now accept students who have not graduated with a satisfactory record from high school and most of them require from two to four years of college work for admission. It is usually stipulated that this preliminary education shall be of a liberal rather than a vocational character. This means that commercial subjects, for example, would not be accepted as a substitute for "the humanities" in the high school or college course. To secure applicants of good intellectual capacity, many professional schools now admit only those who are drawn from the upper quarter or third of the high school or college class. Other schools apply special intelligence tests on admission to exclude students who are mediocre or who seem to be poorly adapted to the demands of the profession they desire to enter.

Having considered the human material to be prepared for professional practice, the next thing is to consider the educational process itself. Here again the standards tend to be more exacting in the professional school than in the school of the sub-professional type. This does not mean that the methods of teaching are necessarily superior in the professional school. Excellent teaching may be found in many trade or technical schools and poor teaching may be found in many professional schools. However, the general level of intellectual work is expected to be higher and students are expected to get farther below the surface of things in a professional school. The following assumptions are commonly made in regard to schools of this type:

1. A longer period of definite, organized pre-service preparation is required, practically never below two years and often from four to six years.

2. The general content of the professional curriculum is expected to be more substantial and the subject matter more difficult and also more concentrated than that required of trade school or secondary students. It is also expected that it will contain more of the so-called "liberal" or "cultural" elements.

3. A larger proportion of time is usually spent on the underlying sciences or principles than on technical skills, and there is likely to be less repetitive training to secure a high degree of skill. Future growth and competence are not so likely to be sacrificed to immediate wage-earning ability.

4. Students are expected to be able to make their own application of principles, and not simply to follow rule-of-thumb directions or specifications. They are supposed to work with greater independence than students in secondary or trade schools.

5. Students are expected to get a broad enough foundation to build on in the future, and to acquire the habits of study and research which will enable them to add to this foundation.

6. Their programs of study are heavier as a rule and it is assumed that they have passed the stage where they need much supervision or assistance in their studies.

7. Methods of discipline are suited to adult professional students who are expected to assume a large measure of responsibility for their own conduct.

8. In the requirements for graduation the test tends to focus more on fundamental knowledge and reasoning ability than on a high degree of technical skill or on the completion of a specified period of attendance.

9. The members of the professional faculty are expected to be highly qualified from the standpoint of general and professional education, and to have ample time not only for preparation and study, but also for some creative work in the form of writing, experimentation, etc.

Judged by these standards it is doubtful whether more than a very small proportion of nursing schools in the United States could be classed as full professional schools. A good many would be semi-professional rather than professional in type and probably over half would be definitely sub-professional. On the lower levels there is no clear difference in standards between schools which are supposedly training professional nurses and those which are training attendants and child nurses. The educational requirements, grade of instruction, etc., are practically the same though the period of training is longer as a rule for the trained nurse.

While most of us will agree that this is a very unsatisfactory situation, there is no reason why we should be unduly discouraged about it. Admitting that nursing is "an emerging profession" and that very few nursing schools have yet achieved full professional status, it is encouraging to realize that a fair number are in the process of becoming professional schools in reality as well as in name. It must be remembered also that other vocations such as teaching, are going through the same process but most of them are a little farther ahead than nursing schools in getting their educational standards established and recognized. However, there are still some states where courses for teachers are provided in connection with secondary school programs, where the training is exceedingly superficial and where full high school preparation is not yet required for those entering teacher training institutions.

It seems probable that in nursing as in engineering, agriculture, business, home economics and several other vocational fields, certain schools of a sub-professional type will be needed for the preparation of those workers who do not assume full professional responsibilities and whose nursing duties are of a more elementary and limited character. It would be reasonable to expect that the trained attendant and the child nurse might continue to receive instruction on the secondary school level and that public systems of vocational education might provide some of the facilities for such instruction. It will be generally agreed, however, that the preparation of professional workers should be definitely placed above the secondary school level and that every effort should be made to clear up the present confusion between these two groups and their preparation.

Knowing that professional preparation presupposes full secondary education, it would seem to be very unwise for any school to establish a combined high school and nursing course, if it really wants to be considered as a professional school and nursing course, if it really wants to be considered as a professional school and if it wants to attract applicants who are high school graduates. It would also be unwise to require such students to return to a high school for any part of their professional preparation. Most students feel that they want to go forward rather than backward when they reach this stage in their education and they quite justly expect that a school which offers professional training will be able to supply the necessary facilities for such training.

While it would be ungrateful not to recognize the assistance which has been given in a few places by high school, the progress which has been made during the past few years to improve standards in nursing schools, should surely lead us to assume that all but a very few are now past the stage when they need to call on high schools to help them out. It is possible that in some of the states where educational standards are a little more backward and educational facilities less accessible, instruction in the elementary sciences and dietetics, may still be very difficult to secure. In such cases special arrangements might be made to use the equipment and the teaching staff of a good technical or general high school for a limited period of time until the nursing school can strengthen its own educational facilities.

It would be very unfortunate, however, if such temporary arrangements should lead to the impression on the part of secondary school teachers and others, that the work of nursing schools belongs on the secondary level. This is likely to happen especially when the teaching extends beyond the subjects of the preliminary course and includes clinical and other definite professional subjects. Most of the preparatory subjects might be considered as belonging either to general or to professional education. While it would be necessary for full professional standing to have them taught on a junior college rather than a secondary school level, and highly desirable to have them taught in direct connection with the student's practical experience, there may be exceptional situations in which it is preferable to get this teaching from a high school or a secondary vocational school rather than from an unprepared or over worked nursing staff.

The essential thing is that no agreements should be entered into which would tend to fix such connections in a permanent way or to establish them on a state-wide or a nation-wide basis. The whole movement toward the professionalizing of nursing schools might be seriously retarded and affiliations with higher institutions made much more difficult than they now are, if state or local departments of education, which are concerned particularly with secondary vocational education, should advertize widely or actively encourage combination high school and professional (?) courses for nurses, subsidized from Smith-Hughes funds. If individual nursing schools accept such aid for the teaching of the basic sciences or dietetics, the subjects should be definitely stated, so that there should be no misunderstanding about the extent or the nature of the teaching contributed by the secondary school.

It may be well also to remind those nursing schools which are anxious to establish connections with universities or to secure definite recognition as university schools of nursing, that subjects which have been taught by secondary schools and on the general level of secondary school work, are not usually credited by universities and that connections between secondary schools and nursing schools would raise very definite questions about the professional standing of the nursing school and its right to be considered as a university school of nursing.

In conclusion, may we say that without in any way disparaging the ideals and standards of industrial and commercial vocations and others of a non-professional character, we believe that nursing by its nature and traditions, belongs with the group of professions, rather than with the group of trades, mechanical arts, domestic, clerical, or business vocations. If this is true, then it is reasonable to assume that the preparation of the nurse should take on more and more of a professional character and that the manual, mechanical or technical elements in the training should not be allowed to submerge the intellectual, social and human elements. If the nurse is considered primarily as a technician or hand worker, dealing with inert materials or with automatic machines it might be quite proper to give her much of the same kind of preparation which is given in a trade school to a skilled artizan; but if her work is mainly with human beings and with social situations, if it involves decisions requiring a fairly wide range of knowledge, then she needs a very different kind of preparation, more like that of the teacher and social worker.

The trouble is that so many people are willing to pay "lip service" to nursing as "a noble profession" and at the same time use all their influence to secure the elimination of practically all the intellectual, scientific and humanistic elements in the nursing curriculum, leaving in the main only routine rule-of-thumb practice. Any good trade school makes a definite effort to include some liberal or cultural subjects in its program, for the benefit of the individual student if not for definite vocational use. Even this concession to the broader educational aims would not be considered necessary or "practical" in many nursing schools. Our philosophy is plainly in need of some reconstruction as well as our educational programs. Those who are responsible for nursing schools surely owe it to themselves and their students, to state their aims and purposes more clearly, to define their terms and titles honestly and to make their training consistent with their professions and convictions whatever these may be.

(Stewart, 1929, pp. 131–137)

The New Epoch in Nursing

By Annie W. Goodrich, R. N.

Dean, School of Nursing, Yale University,
New Haven, Connecticut

I should presume that there was only one answer to these matters which Mrs. Burgess has so ably presented. Dr. Davis has already given that answer, education and a committee.

I speak in all seriousness. I did not suppose I should ever live to see the day when it could be said with any possible degree of accuracy that nearly enough nurses had been produced to meet the community's need. There is, it is true, a gloomy side to this picture, but there is also a happy one. At least it assures us that the nursing needs of a community may eventually be met by trained women. And if we have many problems yet to work out, I am sure you will agree with me that all of these problems have been faced and in some instances the means for dealing with them have already been instituted.

It is, I believe, true that we have reached a new epoch in nursing, and that is in itself an inspiring fact. We have passed the day when our objective is limited to the acquiring of the technical nursing procedures demanded by curative medicine, and we are now concerned to evolve the content of nursing education demanded by the field of preventive medicine.

At this late hour I cannot attempt to discuss the great problems that the facts presented by Mrs. Burgess reveal. I can only briefly and sketchily touch upon certain points which I think important for your consideration. I said we needed education and a committee, and I said it advisedly. I believe that what has been developed in a number of localities should be universally and rapidly produced, namely a committee or council of persons to consider the health and sickness needs of the community, and the means by which these needs can be completely met. Such a council should be as representative as is the council appointed, shall we say, for the development and execution of a community chest. I am of the opinion that women should predominate in the membership. The council would function through committees, outstanding amongst which would be a committee to determine upon the machinery and the personnel required to meet the needs as presented through a study of the community, and a committee to study the professional preparation of the required personnel with due consideration of the educational resources not only of any given locality but of the state and the educational system at large.

Let me digress for a moment to consider this question of education. We often hear discussed, sometimes acrimoniously, sometimes encouragingly, the question of college education. What do we mean by "college education"? What do we imply when we say "degree"? We are simply summarizing the fact that to-day there is a body of knowledge that bears distinctly upon human life, that any such body of knowledge has a direct relationship to the profession with which we are concerned, that every day, even every hour, in the great laboratories of science that knowledge is changing. What created thing could be of greater importance than human life, and who is more concerned with the development of that creation than the nurse, except the parents, and even they can't escape the nurse; they may occasionally escape the physician, but to-day they rarely escape the nurse.

We must require of our women in the future two languages, the language of the people and the language of science. That nurses have learned the language of the people is evidenced by the group meeting here to-day. This great body of nurses could not have come into existence in these few years had they not ministered in some way to the people, and what is true of this continent is true of every other continent. But if we are truly concerned with our field of work we must speak also the language of science.

I agree with Mrs. Burgess that if we face the facts, our problems will not be difficult of solution, for the problems of nursing and nursing education do not differ from those of almost every branch of life activity. Business has found it necessary to relate itself to education, to wit, the Harvard, Columbia and other university schools of business, and has rapidly amassed a body of knowledge that relates to the conduct of business and through which it is hoped to make business methods economically sound. Many other branches might be cited, all of which I contend are secondary in importance to our field of work, because we are assisting in the creation of future citizens.

Another committee I wish to mention is that of publicity. For a number of years we have been striving to bring before the young women of the community the importance of nursing, and this we must never cease to do, but a change of emphasis is called for. If nursing does not commend itself to parents as a desirable field for their daughters, and it does not, we must seek the reason. What is it that makes parents averse to letting their children enter nursing? Is it that the field itself is of such little importance, this bringing to light the ills of human beings and striving to avert or heal them,—is that an insignificant social contribution? I contend it is not. I contend it is one of the most important contributions.

We must make the community see that if the conditions are such in nursing and nursing education that the profession is not attracting our best educated women, then conditions must be changed. This means a study of the hospitals in relation to nursing education. Are the hours what they should be? Is the educational content what it should be? Can the parents be assured of conditions which will give their daughters that kind of joyous service Dr. Frank discussed last night? If not, why not?

There is another matter of importance for the council. What are we doing for the sickness and health needs of the small communities. We are informed that there is an over-supply of nurses for the cities, but that the small community and the rural areas have not an adequate supply. In this case should the local hospitals maintain schools of nursing and if so under what conditions? The small hospital offers certain advantages sometimes lost in the larger institution. Preëminently it demands an approach to and consideration of patients which is highly desirable in a program of nursing education; it provides for more personal understanding and direction of the student; it permits of more extended and thorough knowledge of the case; the atmosphere more nearly approximates the home environment of both patient and staff; it is believed that the students, limited in number, are a desirable factor in these small institutions; upon graduation, if their professional preparation is sound, they can serve equally well their own or the surrounding rural areas, or in the larger city with which they will be familiar through their preliminary and later affiliated courses.

It is important therefore to establish a program of centralized instruction particularly in the sciences, through which a recognized hospital in a given community may be assisted to maintain a school with justice to the student of nursing and the public that she is later to serve.

I have inspected hundreds of these small hospitals and know that many of them are beautifully equipped; that the clinical material offers under the right auspices excellent experience. It is perfectly possible through the ever increasing number of universities and colleges, many of which are already offering courses in nursing, to provide through extension courses a pre-nursing science course. So I hold a brief for the small hospital school if the education in these institutions is based on a sound foundation, which is a scientific foundation.

This is a brief consideration of some of the problems and the ways in which they may be solved. We need the right kind of publicity; we want to awaken in college girls an interest in nursing; we want the women of the community to appreciate its importance; we want the hospitals to shape or reshape the conditions in nursing so they will appeal to the type of student that we need. I believe there is no question that these changes can be brought about.

No one can attend these meetings without being impressed with the extraordinary growth of the nursing field. I refer not to its numerical growth but to the broadening view and the tremendous enrichment of the field evidenced by the papers presented and the subjects discussed.

We have no reason whatever to be discouraged. We are, I believe, at the turn of a road, but we have come to this with a far wider vision than has before been possible.

Let me briefly review our professional history. Guided by laywomen, nurses went into the hospitals something over fifty years ago and cleaned up those institutions. You have only to read the history of Bellevue and Blockley to appreciate the great change in the methods of caring for patients. In those days the hospitals were for the pauper class alone. They were called asylums,—idiot, lunatic and pauper asylums,—terms no longer in use, an indication in itself of social evolution. Hospitals to-day take care of all classes of people. It is no longer a disgrace to go into the hospital for medical and nursing care, quite the contrary, although I must admit I recently heard of the case of a young husband who suffered a serious mental reaction which was finally traced to his distress that should his boy be born in a hospital he could not in after years point to the home in which he was born. This well illustrates the change that has come about.

Women have had much to do with these changes, and I see as the next step, as I hope you do, women going out into the streets, into the factories, into the tenements, into the prisons, and making those same changes in the community that have now been achieved in the hospitals.

If I have brought back but one impression from my journey to the Orient the inspiration which I received from it would have compensated for every day of absence. Let me preface my explanation by the following: Last year on their way home from the International Congress of Nurses held in Montreal, some of our foreign friends visited the United States. One of the things which impressed them was the absence of fences or high walls between the beautiful places in many of our smaller towns. They said, "These beautiful places unprotected and not overrun by the public! I should think you would like more privacy." It recalled a journey through southern England where we chose the old-time coach rather than the automobile in order that we might look over the walls surrounding the beautiful estates. The social significance of this change did not at first enter my mind. Light began to break when I reached China but it took the hours of meditation of the homeward voyage for the inspiring implication of this social evolution to dawn upon me.

Of the Great Wall of China we had for many years heard. In Peking we found the wall of the Tartar city, and the wall of the Chinese city, and as an outstanding building our attention was called to the Forbidden City. Wherever you go in Peking you will see the walls, the towers, the golden roof of the Forbidden City, a magnificent series of buildings for the use of the imperial group and their entourage, protected from all intruders by two walls and a moat. The Forbidden City is to-day a dead city, a city of the past with grass growing between the pavements, its buildings open now for a few coppers to any who choose to go through them. But there is another series of buildings which you will also see, the beautiful green enamel roofs of the Peking Union Medical College and Hospital,—buildings reproducing the best of Chinese architecture. Around these buildings there are no walls, and under these roofs may be found both the wealthiest citizen and the poorest outcast in Peking. Never have I seen better equipment, better medical care nor nursing care than I saw in the Peking Medical School Hospital. In no other hospital have I been where there was a periodic health examination of every single individual in the institution. I presume we could never grasp at what cost medical men and nurses have helped China produce this, but this is not the point altogether. The point is that here you have a picture of something that is happening in this world of vital importance; here you have convincing evidence of social evolution.

We may have a long road over which to travel. We must make communities see that they must support the hospitals and not lean on student labor. We must so adjust our program of nursing service that the unneeded contribution of the private duty nurse can be applied to the greatly needed bedside nursing of the sick in the hospitals. The best bedside nurse instructors will be the successful private duty nurses, but in order to obtain their services in the hospital their hours of duty must be such as will enable them to enjoy their work. We must see to it that the advancement in their salaries will relieve the economic pressure. All this is perfectly possible for such a wealthy nation, and only through such adjustments shall we create a democracy in which we can believe.

Heartened by that wonderful picture of progress in far off China, let us press forward, and obtaining the aid and assistance of the women of the community let us seek to achieve this program of social betterment.

(Goodrich, 1930, pp. 84–89)

Section VI
Power

Introduction to Power

*F*rom its inception, the Superintendents' Society pointed to the establishment of a national organization for nurses as a priority. The disregard for standards and unrestrained growth of unsound training schools fueled the chaotic state of nursing education and gave the matter of national unity increasing urgency. Responsible nurse leaders recognized the dangers inherent in permitting the erratic situation to continue and consequently exercised their power to institute change.

Alumnae societies established in the various training schools increased nursing's influence and served as a basis for implementing a national organization. Alumnae associations provided the means for reaching nursing groups and eliciting their support in moving the profession forward. Networks among those associations became a powerful force in shaping nursing's image and promoting nursing as a suitable career for women.

Nursing organized to gain empowerment and control its own education and practice. Similar to the work of other late 19th- and early 20th-century reform groups, organized nursing promoted the health and welfare of the public. At this time, several municipal women's groups, such as the Chicago Women's Club, Health Protective Association, and State Charities Aid Association, advocated reforms that improved sanitation, work environments, and living conditions. Similarly, the muckrakers' activities exposed corruption in various industries and in the political arena which further generated public support. Thus, in keeping with the day, nurses seized the opportunity to move ahead with their reform agenda. Nursing organized to gain control of the profession knowing that nursing reform meant health care reform.

By the time the Superintendents' Society organized in 1893, autonomy in planning nursing's future had been effectively recognized and advanced by the early nurse leaders. Visionary in its need to set standards for nursing education and practice, the Superintendents' Society and later the NLNE became powerful champions of society's right to qualified nursing care.

Nursing realistically prepared to defend its position in the face of anticipated negative reactions. Opposition originated with those who were most threatened by the prospect of high standards—the proprietors of disreputable training schools and correspondence courses. Responding to this challenge, organized nursing initiated power strategies such as circulating publicity to gain support of the public, apprising the general nursing community of the need for a unified commitment to proposed initiatives, and establishing committees to carry out designated goals.

The papers that follow illustrate nursing's understanding and effective use of power in managing the profession's growth and development over the period 1894–1933.

Training School Alumnae Associations

By Miss Palmer

*Late Superintendent of the Garfield Memorial Hospital,
Washington, D.C.*

In gathering up material for this report on alumnae associations that I have the pleasure of presenting for your consideration this morning, I have succeeded in obtaining from various sources a list of one hundred and sixty-four training schools; twenty in Canada[1] and one hundred and forty-four in the United States.

To the superintendent of these schools I addressed a circular card of inquiry and received personal answers from one hundred and nine. The remaining fifty-five did not respond.

In a number of instances I had sent communications to hospitals having no training schools, and the superintendents or matrons of these hospitals wrote me very courteous letters, informing me of my mistake. I think I am justified in concluding that those superintendents who did not respond have no alumnae to report, and are not interested in the subject, for in almost every instance of superintendents reporting no organization, some explanation is offered or regret expressed. A number of schools in this list have not yet graduated a class; in others the number of graduates is small and very much scattered, and in several cases superintendents were waiting to obtain information on the subject at this meeting before taking active measures for organization.

I have made no attempt to classify these schools with reference to their eligibility for membership in the Superintendent's Association, excluding, however, the schools connected with asylums for the insane, private hospitals, and the theoretical schools.

---

[1]The laws of Canada require a special permit from the government for the organization of beneficial societies of any kind, with a fee of one hundred dollars.

I wish to say further, in explanation, that the list of schools prepared by Dr. Billings for Burdett's Hospital Manual numbers only forty-nine in the United States, so that I feel quite sure my list includes all the larger or more important schools, and a fair proportion of the small ones.

Taking, then, one hundred and sixty-four as the number upon which this report is based, I have twenty-one training schools with alumnae associations or clubs organized and in active operation, with constitution printed.

Ten training schools, with alumnae associations in process of organization, constitution *not* printed, making a total of thirty-one. Seventy-eight training schools reporting no organization (but showing interest); fifty-five not heard from, making a total of one hundred and thirty-three.

I have received copies of constitutions of twenty-one societies, and these I have divided into three classes:

First—Those organized and managed entirely by graduates, which are alumnae associations proper.

Second—Nurses' clubs, admitting to membership pupils of the school of graduates of other schools.

Third—Religious societies, with a number of the officers, clergymen or members of the training school board.

Those included in the first class have practically a common object and the same form of government; differing, of course, in detail to meet the peculiar requirements of each society.

The object of these associations is for the union of the graduates of the respective schools, for mutual help and protection; to promote social intercourse and good fellowship; to provide friendly and pecuniary assistance in times of illness or death among members, and to advance the interest of the nursing profession.

Several societies pledge themselves to support the directory and school.

Only those graduates in good standing in the profession are eligible for membership.

Fees vary from five dollars to fifty cents a year.

The officers are a president, a vice-president, secretary and treasurer, who are elected by ballot, at the annual meeting, to serve for one year, or until other successors are chosen.

Several of the societies have two vice-presidents, two secretaries—recording and corresponding—and two treasurers, the treasurer proper, not a member of the society, and a sub-treasurer, who is a member, and who performs the duties usually belonging to the treasurer.

The duties of the treasurer proper are to have charge of the permanent or invested funds.

The president presides at all meetings, and in her absence the duties of her office are performed by the vice-president.

The duties of the secretaries I need hardly explain. In the majority of cases the officers form the executive committee, and transact all the business of the association. They investigate all charges against any member, and she is given opportunity for defense before being expelled from the society.

Several of the societies have a board of trustees composed of gentlemen, whose election is permanent: one member acting as treasurer, already mentioned. This board invests the money of the association, and advises the officers of the society, when necessary.

Where a society has received legacies, or owns real estate, I should suppose a board of this kind would be necessary; but in small associations, having only a contingent fund, it would seem to me better for the governing body to be composed entirely of members of the association, and the form of government to be as simple as possible.

The executive committee, composed of the officers, would certainly be an easy and comprehensive plan to adopt, when a society is forming. Meetings are held monthly or quarterly, usually in the training school parlors. Notice of meetings and special business is sent by mail at least five days in advance, by the secretary. Papers, discussions, lectures and social intercourse are the usual features of the meetings.

In a number of societies the election of officers is by ballot, sent by mail; in others, voting is by members present, and the number necessary for a quorum differs.

The benefit fund is composed of all moneys not appropriated for the necessary expenses of the society obtained from initiation fees, yearly dues, donations and bequests. One has both a sick fund and an annuity fund, the latter being made up of all that is left after expenses and benefits have been paid.

One has a beneficial society that is a separate organization, with an additional fee of six dollars, although all of the alumnae are eligible for membership.

The amount allowed a sick member from the benefit fund also varies; in some cases the amount is limited to ten dollars a week; in another, it is left to the discretion of the executive committee, and when feasible the nurse to be cared for at the hospital, the society bearing the expense.

Married members, supported by their husbands, are not entitled to benefits.

Nearly all have honorary members, who pay no dues, and have no vote, but are allowed to speak in meeting.

One has honorary members who pay an annual fee of ten dollars, ($10.00) and life members who pay fifty dollars ($50.00).

There are minor points of interest in all the constitutions, but they are too many to enumerate at this time.

Of the clubs, there are only four, and they differ from the alumnae associations, principally in their rules for membership. Pupils, as well as graduate nurses, are eligible for membership, and can hold office, and the superintendent of the school is the president.

Two of these clubs require no regular membership fee, but the expenses are met by voluntary contributions. These clubs have no benefit fund.

One requires an annual fee of six dollars for graduates, and three dollars for pupils, but this club has a benefit fund; its primary object being the care of sick members.

There is one Directory Club, open to all graduates of regular schools, but with a membership of eighty-nine names only three are from outside schools. This, I will mention, is in connection with the Rochester City Hospital.

All of these clubs are well organized, but would, I think, be required to make some changes in their constitution in order to be eligible for membership in a national alumnae association.

Of the religious societies there are two, and like the clubs, changes in the constitution would be necessary before membership in a national alumnae could be considered. These societies are in connection with church hospitals, and should be classed properly with guilds. They unquestionably hold an important place in the schools with which they are connected.

There is a Graduate Nurses' Club in Boston admitting to membership graduates from all schools in good standing. Its object is largely instructive and social, and it is exceedingly popular, and to nurses in the city falls the need, in a measure, of an alumni association in connection with their own schools.

The organization of alumnae associations in connection with training schools is comparatively a new movement, and general interest has been stimulated by the agitation of the subject, both in Chicago and at a meeting of this Society a year ago.

I do not consider it necessary for me even to touch upon the advantages of such societies to nurses, the object of this paper being simply to show the material available for a national alumnae.

In conclusion I want to urge upon the superintendents of schools that have not yet taken steps for organization, the importance of immediate action in this matter.

Organization is the power of the age. Without it nothing great is accomplished.

All questions having ultimate advancement of the profession are dependent upon united action for success.

The Directory question, the Uniform Curriculum, the Rejected Probationer, every subject that concerns individual graduates, as well as schools, can only be reached through this channel.

The superintendent can do so easily, what is so very difficult for the graduates alone to accomplish; and she is the proper person to make the call for the first meeting. Even if she is not a graduate of the school, the hospital and the school are mutual points of interest to the older, as well as the younger graduates, and all would recognize her as the proper leader in the movement.

Do not wait for large numbers before taking action. A little society of ten members, let it be largely social, if you will, forms a nucleus, that time will develop. One superintendent, a New England girl, trained at the Massachusetts General, who went west some years ago, "to grow up with the country," reports a small school, with an alumnae of three members. That is the proper spirit.

If you have not a large school, make the most of your small one. Remember that it is only through organization that individual members can be reached, and their co-operation in progressive movements be obtained, and that without their support and their good influence with the public we lose an immense power.

I sincerely trust that when this association of superintendents holds its next annual meeting, schools reporting "no organization," may be very much in the minority.

(Palmer, 1897, pp. 52–56)

A National Association for Nurses and Its Legal Organization

By L. L. Dock

In the course of preparatory work needed to present the subject of a National Association of Trained Nurses, it will be found, I think, that attention must first be given to the general structure, laws and powers of the Government under which we live and hope to unite. Next, that the plans of organization of other national associations be considered and compared. It is necessary to know what legal supports may be obtained for an association such as we wish to form, and it is useful to know something of national associations already existing, what machinery they have, and how it works; how their purposes compare with ours, and what means they take for accomplishing them; how much power and influence they are able to exert, and how prestige and dignity are best obtained.

After this ground has been pretty well gone over, our knowledge of our own needs and present conditions will lead us naturally, and with little further trouble, to the lines upon which a national organization of nurses can best be founded, and will also indicate, with a good deal of certainty, the shape it will take and the functions that it may be expected to possess and acquire.

It is not necessary to describe to you the national organism, the union into one common country of States possessing many attributes of sovereignty, the subdivision of States into counties, and counties into townships; but it may be well to recall the main characteristics of the law-making power, the limitation of Federal and the scope of State law. You remember that the States are so many governments within a government; that, to quote Mr. Bryce, "the Nation is a State, which, while one, is nevertheless composed of other States even more essential to its existence than it is to theirs. The States have over their citizens an authority which is all their own, and not delegated by the central Government." By the Constitution, the law-making power of Congress is limited to certain subjects which are of common interest to the whole Nation, and which I need not here enumerate. By it, also, such independent powers are prohibited to the States as would bring them into conflict with the National law. "All other legislation and administration is left to the several states without power of interference by the Federal legislature or Federal executive." Or, in the words of the Constitution, "the powers not delegated to the United States by the Constitution, nor prohibited by it to the States, are reserved to the States respectively, or to the people."

Beyond these specified powers no legislation can be had from Congress except by amendment to the Constitution. It is of the greatest importance that this limitation of federal power be clearly kept in mind, for in it lies the key-note to the general scheme of national organizations of private individuals in the United States.

In the Dominion of Canada, to quote Mr. Bryce further, "the distribution of matters within the competence of the Dominion Parliament, and of the Provincial Legislature respectfully, bears a general resemblance to that existing in the United States. But there is this remarkable distinction, that whereas in the United States Congress has only the powers actually granted to it, the legislatures retaining all such powers as have not been taken from them, the Dominion Parliament has a general power of legislation restricted only by the grant of certain specific and exclusive powers to the Provincial Legislatures."

The British Parliament, again, "is, in the sphere of law, an omnipotent body." It has power to make and unmake any law upon any subject. "In point of legal theory, it is the nation," and therefore possesses that entire sovereignty which in this country is held by the people. It is, of course, not to our purpose or advantage now to discuss the relative merits of different forms of government, nor to argue as to which would be most convenient for the solution of our special problems. We simply care to consider the practical fact, that owing to these differences in the governments of countries, private or personal associations formed under them respectively will also differ in their plans of organizations. For instance, the Royal British Nurses' Association holds its royal charter under the Great Seal of the United Kingdom, and looks forward to act of Parliament to fix the status and protect the certificate of the graduate trained nurse, precisely as the medical acts establish a standard and furnish a protection for the medical profession of that country. But American nurses cannot expect the national government to do anything of this kind. Such legislation as is deemed wise or helpful, in aid of any of our higher standards can only be sought through state legislatures.

Now, if we take a general survey of national associations, be they philanthropic, professional, or labor unions, there is found a strong general likeness between them all as to form. All pattern more or less closely after national outlines, according to the country in which they flourish. With us, this general structure may be diagrammatically represented as a tree, of which the national or central body forms the trunk, the state associations the branches, and the city, town or county associations the twigs. The W. C. T. U., one of the most thoroughly organized bodies in the world, follows state lines in every country with minute exactness, while its International or World's Union is formed of the chief officers of each nation. Thus organized it is in the best position to exert influence and bring pressure to bear at any given point.

Of the labor unions may be taken the International Brotherhood of Locomotive Engineers as a good example of dignity and conservatism as well as of compact organization. This union covers Canada and the United States, with an exceedingly strong and close network, and has "a legislative board in every State, territory, and dominion, which shall have power to take charge of all matters coming before the Legislature wherein the interests of the Brotherhood of Locomotive Engineers are involved," and also its committees duly appointed to confer and arbitrate all questions arisng between the railroad officials and their employees.

The Association of Collegiate Alumnae has a director in each State. The American Medical Association is composed of National, State, county, town, and city societies, all bound together by the code of ethics. Here and there, especially in the older States, minor variations exist which do not materially alter the general scheme. Later on we shall need to consider more fully the organization of the American Medical Association.

In these different bodies the unit of representation varies somewhat. In the State it is the township. In the Women's Christian Temperance Union, the small local union—the nucleus of which will be a church congregation. With the Brotherhood of Locomotive Engineers, it is the railroad division. With the Association of Collegiate Alumnae it is the associated alumnae of certain specified colleges. In the conventions of the Church, the parish is the unit of representation, and with us it would be, indeed could only be, the incorporated alumnae associations of such training schools as were recognized for this purpose by the general association.

We now conclude our brief survey of surrounding bodies by observing how the machinery (which we have found to be so nearly alike in all cases) works. The most striking characteristic of all alike may be said to be, without doubt, a systematic division and sub-division of work and responsibility. The central bodies having limited legal or extrinsic powers, find their chief strength and security in moral force. They lay down principles; keep an outlook over the whole country; support ideal standards; deliver messages embodying the objects and purposes to be worked for and the reforms to be undertaken. The State organizations take up each one its share of the actual burden of the whole. They are working bodies. Each one conducts, according to its best ability, its separate part of the whole campaign. If a closer network of organization is to be built up in the State, if State laws are to be invoked, if State schools (of course I mean schools within the State) are to be brought into line, or standards worked up, it is the business of the State association. While in the small component parts, the twigs, be they railroad divisions, parishes, alumnae associations, county societies, or what not, all the close individual work is done, which is of all the most important. Here must be carried on the small, fine work, often trivial or petty, often wearisome and discouraging, always laborious and painstaking, seldom appreciated, never realized outside, the work of keeping high individual standards, of applying individual discipline, and of encouraging individual enthusiasm and strong purpose. Not long ago a well-known man said at a public dinner that the essence of sound government is held to be that "the Nation should devolve all that it can upon the State, the State all that it can upon the county, the county all that it can upon the township, and the township all that it can upon the individual." And in the articles of a labor organization, already referred to, we find these words: "It is to be hoped that every precaution will be taken to ascertain, beyond a doubt, the merits of each individual, as regards *ability* and *character,* remembering that upon these two rest the honor and universal acknowledgement of our organization." In these examples is laid down the principle which must be the motive power of every kind of co-operative work, if it is to be successful, namely: The supreme ultimate importance of the individual; and with us, if we become an organized body, the primary source of strength must lie in the associated alumnae of our schools. Their work will be to keep watch over the professional standing and general character of future candidates for membership in our organization.

Among their unpleasant, but necessary obligations will be these: "To exclude or expel unworthy individuals, to censure or warn backsliding members, to expose, so far as can be legally and honorably done, such wrongs and injuries done to our best standards as they may encounter, and to check harmful tendencies as they may meet them. Their responsibility will be tremendous, but they will be equal to it, if they will do their duty.

Let us now suppose for a moment that a national organization, following the lines here suggested, was on the point of completion, what might we reasonably expect from it? For a long time, without a doubt, little or nothing tangible. I know that in our profession there are many who imagine that some magic power lies behind the word "organization," and that the declaration of a pass-word or motto, and the adoption of a badge will settle at once all troublesome questions, and fix the status, privileges and responsibilities of the trained nurse. They believe that kaleidoscopic transformations in nursing work are possible when an association of superintendents meets to exchange views. They write anxiously to the magazines to inquire "why do not the superintendents fix a standard of work; establish a uniform curriculum; do this and that?" Or to say "the superintendents ought to abolish quack training schools; ought to do thus and so" as if they understood the superintendents to be absolute monarchs. These women will be disappointed and offended, when, the day or the year after joining an organization, they find themselves pretty much where they were before as regards grievances, imperfections and irregularities. They will then lose heart and blame the officers of the organization; they will fall away and advise others to do the same. But it is not likely that any of you entertain such delusions. You know that the growth of such a common feeling of loyalty to our work and responsibility toward one another as we need to cultivate is a slow one, not to be hastened, but to be fostered through years with painstaking care; that radical changes are not to be brought about in a day, and that reforms that are worth anything have to be worked for long and arduously.

You all realize that what we may hope to do now is, not to change at once all the conditions of our training and work with which we are dissatisfied; not to fix at once a final and satisfactory standard of excellence, not to establish immediately a complete and perfect curriculum of study, but so to unite and fraternize all the best of our profession that they will learn to stand together, move together, work together. Then in the future we may safety expect them to progress in the right direction, to acquire influence, moral dignity and force as a body, and to undertake successfully the solution of those varied complications which we can now see time and circumstances are fast bringing into nursing questions.

It does not seem as if there was any real ground for faintheartedness over our outlook. The record of what has actually been done by other bodies in other lines of work forbids it. I would suggest that those who are dubious or unbelieving study the history of, say, the better class of trades unions, the work of the Women's Christian Temperance Union, of the Federation of Women's Clubs, of the Association of College Alumnae, of those associations which unite the members of the different learned professions, and I believe their doubts will be dispelled.

Of all the organized bodies about us, the one to which we would naturally most closely conform in general outline is the American Medical Association. Founded in 1846, it was at the outset framed broadly, as was not only advisable, but necessary. A rigidly exclusive association could not then have represented the whole medical profession, but must have failed in its purpose, which was to furnish a leaven for the whole, not only to separate from the rest the small portion already leavened. With no such thing in existence as government control or guardianship in educational matters, and with the rush of settlement in a vast new country, a thousand pressing and instant necessities ran away with standards for the time being. A crop of medical schools sprang up like mushrooms, unfurnished and unendowed, but the best that could be had at the moment. The foundations of the American Medical Association were laid with stones that would be rejected to-day. The lines loosely drawn then are now being tightened year by year. Standards first fixed at what was possible are being brought up to what is desirable.

Year by year, now in one State, then in another, the influence of the Medical Association has been bent toward securing better conditions. It is a mistake to suppose that the medical schools as such have been the leaders and standard bearers of the medical profession. It is notable that reforms and advances in schools of medicine have come as results of unceasing pressure brought to bear by the profession through the Medical Association. They have not originated with the colleges and universities. The schools do not precede the profession in the march of progress. They are led and urged on by the concerted purpose of the organized profession.

The association worked steadily, first, for better preparatory requirements; then for a lengthened term; a lengthened course; a year added; then another; then better post-graduate work, and so on; also in the States it labored to secure the passage of beneficial laws. In looking over its ordinances, you will find resolutions on the order of this one which I quote at random: "Resolved, That the faculties of the several medical colleges of the United States be recommended to announce explicitly in their annual commencement circulars and advertisements that they will not receive certificates of time of study from irregular practitioners, and that they will not confer the degree upon anyone who may acknowledge his intention to practice in accordance with any exclusive system." And of this: "Resolved, that each year, until otherwise ordered, the president-elect and the permanent secretary shall be directed to appeal in the name of the association to the authorities of each State where no State Board of Health exists, urging them to establish such boards."

I have gone over this ground because I believe that in certain features there is similarity between the medical and the nursing worlds, and to illustrate the suggestion that a full study of the history and transactions of the American Medical Association would be most instructive and helpful to us in working out our own.

The plan of organization of the American Medical Association is roughly as follows: The National body is composed of delegates, invited members and permanent members. The delegates are sent from State societies and from local societies which are recognized by representation in the State society. Members by invitation are reputable men from districts having no representation, being vouched for by a certain number of members. They have no votes. The permanent members are all those who have at any time been sent as delegates. This provision for permanent members has manifest advantages, and would be a good point for a nurses' association to imitate. They remain members while in good standing with the local body which they first represented. They, also, have no votes. The National Association drew up the code of ethics, the "Ten Commandments" of the medical profession, the acceptance of which is obligatory upon all members.

The officers of the National Association are such as are usually found like bodies. A very important feature of the association is the judicial council, entrusted with the duty of deciding all questions of an ethical or judicial character coming before the association.

The State societies are made up of delegates from town and county societies. In minor details the State associations vary, while in essentials they are alike. They all subscribe to the code of ethics, and make it obligatory for the local societies to do the same. I have not be able to study the different State medical constitutions, nor do I suppose it necessary for our purpose to do so, though it would be interesting. If we organize in any like manner, instructive and pertinent points from them all can be looked up by nurses in the different States.

Pennsylvania, for instance, allows permanent members to vote, though they are not eligible to office. The State is divided into six censorial districts, and censors are appointed to examine the laws and regulations of the local societies, and to endorse them to the State society when approved. The censors also act in ethical questions similarly to the judicial council of the National Association. The State constitution fixes the conditions and qualifications under which the local society may organize, states the conditions which disqualify individuals for membership, and defines the functions and limitations of local societies so fully as to amount almost to making their constitutions. Upon the local society rests the obligation of censuring or expelling any member who is convicted of violating the code of ethics.

Now to come down to the practical consideration of an organization among nurses, the first question asked is, naturally, "Who shall be included and who excluded?" In a letter from one of the most prominent among you the following words, in effect, have been written to me: "I will be glad of anything that elevates nursing; but if your organization is only going to be a grand *leveling* process, I do not feel any sympathy with it." Nor would any of us, certainly, if we felt that the "leveling" was to be *downward*. My correspondent's dread of leveling shows that she fears the nurses who stand high must be degraded to the level of those who stand low, for I know she would feel only pleasure if she thought that those who stand low would be elevated. What needs to be answered, then, is not her indefinite thought that organization involves leveling, but her definite fear that leveling must be a downward rather than an upward tendency. Is this the case, and must a national organization among nurses result in general deterioration? I cannot think so, nor believe that you can. This idea of leveling is something of a bugaboo, at any rate. Before the law all nurses, wherever or however trained, are on a level now, and if we will ever look to the law to break that level we can invoke it much more successfully as an organized body than as an unorganized mass. Outside of the law, human nature forbids leveling. Could all nurses, or all schools, be leveled to-day, to-morrow some would be up and some down. This, of course, is by no means an original observation. There are no dead levels, but there are planes; and organized forces, the world over, stand on higher planes than the unorganized. Compare organized and unorganized labor, military systems, educatonal systems, and in our own small province compare the working efficiency and moral force of one of our training school alumnae societies with the chaotic and forceless condition of unassociated graduates of similar schools.

My correspondent will probably say, "Is it not organization I object to, but having that organization include anybody and everybody."

For many reasons it seems best to organize as broadly as possible. We need to avoid the appearances of being a clique. It will be easier in the future for us to draw the lines closer than it will be to regain the support of some whom we have alienated at the outset. As I reminded you before, the American Medical Association formed on very broad lines, and found it necessary, in the course of its history, to make many concessions. We labor under the very serious practical disadvantage of having no recognized standard of work or requirements. The Association of Collegiate Alumnae organized on the basis of certain degrees given by certain institutions. Everyone knew exactly what that meant, and the line was drawn at new institutions until they had come up to the mark. We cannot do that, and our only guide in selection can be that general personal knowledge of schools which we may all have.

Yet, while we wish to be guided by liberal ideas, our organization— if we form one—must stand for something definite—must express, at least, an approximate standard of attainment, or it will be chaotic and without influence. At the present time it will probably be best to include in a national organization the graduates of those schools whose superintendents are members of this society, provided they have already associated themselves into their alumnae societies. If they have not done this, the necessary unit of representation will be lacking, and however higher their schools may stand, it will be readily seen that until they form local bodies, no part can be taken by them in a national body.

Having started on this basis, which on the whole is tolerably comprehensive, other schools may be admitted by the rules of the association.

The admission of new schools will be an important and abiding question, and the committee charged with this duty should be a most carefully chosen one. The Association of Collegiate Alumnae had a good deal of trouble at first with irresponsible nominations for the admission of new schools. In 1892 the Committee on Colleges presented a report suggesting that in the future a method be adopted which would prevent application from without the association, and the following resolution was adopted: "New institutions shall be nominated for membership in the association by any five members of the Executive Committee, who shall represent five different institutions already enrolled as corporate members of the association." In proposing the above the report goes on to say: "The committee have had in mind two distinct ends, regarded by them as of equal importance. First, to provide for the Association a safeguard against irresponsible nominations which force the Executive Committee to an examination of the institutions in question, and to a definite decision concerning them; and second, to afford by this new method of nominations as full an opportunity as possible for a wise extension of the corporate membership of the Association." To adopt at the outset some such plan would probably save us trouble.

Having decided what schools as such may be eligible for membership, let us glance at the plan of organization, beginning at the small end. It will be seen to be quite necessary that the associated alumnae of such schools form comprehensive local societies similar to the county or city society of the Medical Association. Nurses scatter over the country and move away from the neighborhood of their own schools, and it should be made possible for all who are eligible to join a local society in whatever part of the country they are, just as church members take their letters about and connect themselves with churches wherever they go. Besides this, if a nurse is a thousand miles away from her alumnae society she is completely removed from its discipline and influence. If then she commits some breach of professional honor, who is there to check or censure her? Such a case could only be reached by a local society covering the whole ground within certain limits, to which all eligible nurses within those limits should connect themselves.

They must have their officers, laws and by-laws, business meetings and plans of interesting and holding their members, and for maintaining a standard. They should be incorporated. They will elect delegates to the State societies. The State societies will be incorporated under State laws, elect officers, hold stated meetings, and supervise the whole field of nursing in the State. They will elect delegates to the National Association.

Now to look over the general plan again with reference to the actual steps in organization, we begin with the central body and work outward.

The first thing to be done would be to call a convention for the purpose of preparing a constitution. Let us suppose that this society of superintendents, first, calls upon the alumnae societies of, let us say, the twelve oldest schools whose alumnae are organized, to send, each, one delegate from among private duty nurses; and, second, elects an equal number of its own members to meet with them as a convention charged with the duty of preparing a national constitution.

This constitution should indicate, among its other articles, the requirements for admission of new schools, the plan of representation by delegates from State societies, and, in a broad way, the essentials of the State constitutions. Preliminary articles drawn up by the convention should arrange for the constitution to be sent to the presidents of the alumnae associations, with the message that they submit it to their respective societies, and in due time, if it be accepted, take the necessary steps toward forming the State unions. As fast as these are organized, the officers of the convention should be notified, and delegates elected to form the national meetings. In States where only one eligible alumnae society may exist, its representation could be provided for until such time as a State union might develop.

As our practical interests will always be small, compared with those of an ethical and educational nature, you all realize that we shall imperatively need a National Code of Ethics, something similar to that of the American Medical Association, to be our one common bond of union, and our one—at present—fixed standard. It is so all-important that this code be universally recognized and adopted, that it might, perhaps, be advisable not to draw it up until at least a majority of the States had formed their State unions, but *before* they had taken out their charters.

The formation of a committee for the purpose of forming a national code would then be less the work of a restricted representation of nurses than it would if undertaken now. If delegates representing all or the greater part of the rank and file of our alumnae societies had a voice in choosing this committee or the president who appoints the committee, there would be a wider interest felt in its work, and a larger sense of ownership and responsibility. After being drawn up and accepted by the national organization, the code of ethics should become the cornerstone of the permanent and incorporate association.

The State unions should embody it in their articles, and then proceed to take out their charters.

State constitutions should lay down quite explicitly the rules under which local societies should form, fix the proportion of representation, and require them to suspend or expel members guilty of unprofessional conduct. State officers should stimulate and supervise the formation and work of the local societies, and see that the code was adopted and enforced by them.

To get a system like this into working order, will, as you well know, take time. It is nearly three years since the first step toward a national organization was taken by the calling of a convention of training school superintendents in Chicago. At that time the outline of this plan was suggested by the chairwoman of the nursing section, and the importance of forming school graduates into alumnae associations as a necessary preliminary, was brought before the convention and clearly recognized, and since then the members of that convention have steadily pursued the work of organizing their graduates. But even yet there are some prominent schools whose alumnae have not been formed into line.

If we take the steps here suggested, it will probably be at least five years before the State unions are ready for incorporation, for it is best not to ask for charters until constitutions are tried and revised, and the machinery in working order.

Similarly, as I am advised, it will be better not to seek a charter for the national body until it is thoroughly organized.

As to charters, it is understood, as mentioned before, that a charter from Congress is not to be obtained. But State laws allow and provide for the incorporation of bodies which are national in scope, and by the comity of States, such a charter taken out in one State is recognized by all. The law requires that the headquarters of the association shall be permanently fixed in the State which gives the charter; and, as New York State contains, I believe, the largest number of training schools, it, in all probability, would be the one chosen.

The legal restrictions and conditions under which charters may be secured, will be found as a rule to be less elaborate as regards "corporations of the first class," or those not intended for profit, than as regards those of the "second class," intended for business and profit. An association of nurses would, of course, come under the former head, and little or no trouble will be found in taking the necessary steps when the time comes. Incorporation of our national association is by no means essential. The American Medical Association is not incorporated, though its branches are. But eminent lawyers counsel incorporation for us, as having many practical advantages. It helps to give stability and continuity to our existence as an association; enables us to hold property, which we may some day be able and willing to do, and confers upon us the right to sue and be sued, an unenviable advantage. Should we form a national union, and should Canada form a national union, the bond between us would have to be the term "International," for there is, unfortunately for us, no way in which a national charter can be made to include two countries. If, however, our branch societies alone are chartered and Canada's societies chartered according to her laws, the formation of a central body, composed of delegates from State and Canadian unions alike, will be simply a process of affiliation, and the name, instead of including the term "International," as it otherwise must, could be similar to that borne by this Superintendents' Association, and in the term "American" cover at once all nurses in the United States and Canada. (See footnote[2]—Mr. McLennan's letter.)

Yet it will probably be considered best to form our two national unions under our respective laws, and to amalgamate as an International Association.

The composition of our forces will need every careful consideration. There are some among you whose opinions are always entitled to respect, who hold the view that a nurses' organization should include members of training school boards in order to carry any weight or exert any influence. The arguments used in support of this proposition are as follows, viz: That most of the future progress of nursing, as well as, to a great extent, the standing of nurses in the eyes of the public, depends upon the policy that obtains in training schools; that a large part of the work of an association will be toward improvements and advances in training school methods; that superintendents of schools, being only salaried officers, have no final authority, and must often, in fact, yield their convictions to the decisions of those in control; that

---

[2]"The proposed associations, assuming that they are for charitable and benevolent purposes, including benefit to the members, could be formed in this Province in accordance with Article 3,096 of the Revised Statutes of Quebec with practically no formality, or letters patent could be obtained from the Dominion for societies in all the Provinces, provided that the work of the society did not include insurance in a form that would bring it into conflict with the insurance act."—*Francis McLennan*.

under such circumstances it is idle for nurses to meet and agree upon what they believe to be best for their work's interests, since they have no power to carry out their ideas, and that the only way to organize a practical, common sense and efficient society, is to include in it representatives of training schools or hospital boards. I have tried to give this argument full weight, for there is so much truth in it, and my respect for those who I know hold it is so great that my first mental attitude toward it was that of assent. But fuller study and reflection have changed that attitude completely, and the advice obtained from experienced and practical physicians as well as laymen, is, not to organize on such a system.

The arguments in opposition are these: First, it is hardly likely that training schools or hospital boards would enter into such a scheme with warmth and enthusiasm, for, from their point of view, there would be no valid reason for doing so, no apparent advantage to be gained thereby, as they naturally suppose that in their board meetings they deal with every question relating to training schools with sufficient thoroughness. But if, we could induce boards of managers to send delegates, these would hardly come empowered with authority to act. If for instance, an assembly of nurses voted for a certain change in, let us say, the course of study or the hours of work, the lay members could not commit themselves, but would have to return and report the matter to their full boards, so that practically nothing would be gained, unless they came in such numbers as to bring authority with them, in which case we should be swallowed up. Beyond this, again, our association would not be intended to represent the training school part of our work alone, but all the interests of a body of self-dependent women. Many questions which will come before us will be entirely away from and outside of training school matters and management, and it seems more fitting, as well as more dignified, that we work out as far as we can our own problems; and, as occasion arises, send our representatives, it may be to school boards, it may be to State Legislatures, to ask, in the name of the association, for such changes and conditions as are believed to be for the best good of the work of scientifically nursing the sick.

Instead of inviting representatives of the training schools to join our forces, I believe we should work to secure graduate representation on the boards of hospitals and training schools. The Associated Alumnae of Vassar College have succeeded in obtaining place for a certain number of graduates—three, I believe—on the Board of Trustees of the college, and the alumnae of the University of California look forward to a like privilege. It does seem eminently fitting that graduate nurses should in time be placed on the managing boards of their *almae matres,* where their practical knowledge might prevent many blunders now made through ignorance.

The question, too, whether the medical profession should have any guiding or controling hand in an organization of nurses should, I believe, be answered in an negative. The Royal British Nurses Association has a council and executive committee upon which stand a large proportion of medical men, but while it is quite possible that such an arrangement is the best one to make in a small and compact State, and under their special conditions, with which I do not assume to be familiar, but which are different from ours, it would undoubtedly not be advantageous or desirable for us, in our circumstances. The same practical difficulty would exist as in the case of lay members. Either they would be present in small number and be uninfluential, or they would be present in large numbers and swamp us. Besides it is not likely that they would care to belong. They would always be kind and ready to help us, but would think it best for us to stand alone. The words of one of the best among them on this point are, "No, make your association exclusively a nurses' concern." It might, however, be provided in our articles that invited members be selected from boards of managers and from the medical profession by specified committees and under specified conditions, to attend State and National meetings. They would have privilege of debate, but no vote. In this way the benefits of a mixed membership might be reached, and the drawbacks avoided.

I would also suggest that it might be a good plan to elect in each State a certain number of medical men (of course with their consent) who would constitute and advisory board.

The enormous distances in this country to be traversed by delegates will be a source of difficulty. As a rule in national associations it will be found that the traveling expenses of delegates are paid from the general fund, and certainly nurses, who are busy women and who cannot make up at one time what they lose from their incomes at another, ought not to be expected to bear their own expenses, if sent as delegates. In time we might obtain special rates from the railroad companies, as other associations do.

I would finally express with much earnestness, though briefly, both the advice received, and my own convictions, on the subject of relief funds, pension funds, annuity funds, or any form of financial aid to members as a part of the work of a national association. Let our work be solely and singly educational and ethical, and our one object the development of higher standards in all departments of our work. Let us differentiate ourselves sharply, right here, from trades unions, and conform in motives and methods to professional and educational bodies. The feeling with which nurses should regard a national association ought to be entirely free from motives of self-interest. If we try too much, we shall make a success of nothing, and to attempt to manage a financial concern, would, I believe, be a great mistake.

Our associated alumnae all attend carefully to providing aid for needy members, and in their hands this work is done in a private and dignified way. Plans for mutual help act as a strong bond between them as between members of a family, and should be left to them.

Rather than undertake a similar line of work, I would suggest that if, in the future, we organize, prosper and find the key to any source of revenue, we do as the collegiate alumnae do, and as alumni of universities have long done; aid, by endowments and gifts, institutions or parts of institutions in which we are deeply interested and whose prosperity we earnestly desire. For instance, nurses' homes are being founded by our alumnae associations; nurses' club buildings are being talked of; nurses' beds in hospitals are being endowed, and nurses' cooperative registries are being formed. The Collegiate Alumnae rejoice in the fact that they have indirectly guided many gifts of money to deserving colleges, and we may rejoice in the future with like reason, if we turn any superfluous energy we may have as an association into similar channels.

I have not spoken with any detail of the different lines of work which we all agree in thinking need developing or reforming, because such discussion hardly seems called for this paper.

An organization of nurses, once thoroughly welded together and practiced in self-government, will learn how to approach and deal with the confusion and trouble arising from dozens of different standards of teaching, hundreds of rudimentary training schools, laxity in moral and educational qualifications, the competition of the untrained or partially trained nurse, as well as other difficulties now unforeseen which will doubtless arise as time goes on.

One thing is certain; if we do not learn to remedy these disadvantages, no one else will do it for us. The present is a good time to begin. We have been well started; as yet we have not crystallized into factions, nor become deeply rooted in bad habits. The great schools of the country are such that we can consider with pride and admiration their past work and present tendencies. The commercial and utilitarian system of sending pupils to private duty has very nearly disappeared, and with the spread of intelligent ideas must entirely disappear. We have not much to tear down, but unlimited scope for building up, and I hope and believe that among us are those gifted with the constructive genius necessary for shaping and perfecting the work of our honored and cherished profession.

(Dock, 1896, pp. 42–60)

Work of Women in Municipal Affairs

By Lillian D. Wald
The Nurses' Settlement, New York City

Such data as I have, I collected at the Settlement dinner table, and of course I cannot in this short address do more than touch upon the subject. I was not quite clear in my mind whether I was to have the compliment of being asked to suggest what women could do in municipal affairs, or to report what they have done. The greater number of things which they have accomplished have, of course, been done in association with men.

There is one association called the Health Protective Association that has succeeded in establishing quite a number of sanitary reforms. It was started by some women who lived on ＿＿＿ Hill, having a charming view of the river, but the best citizens were being driven away by the foul odor from the abattoirs in the neighborhood. One day in 1884 eleven women came together and decided to organize for the protection of the view and to improve the air by removing accumulations of manure which were piled up in the vicinity and the next day they organized with fifteen members and incorporated the organization. They went to work intelligently. They went up to Albany and a bill was introduced which made it a misdemeanor to have such accumulations within the city limits. They succeeded in having the manure removed, though the man who owned it had a brother there who had the "biggest kind of pull." When the butchers and other people who were using the city for that purpose discovered how costly it would be to defeat the bill they accepted the reform. Mrs. Trautman is to be credited with much of the good work that association has accomplished. Since then they have abolished a great many nuisances arising from gas houses in the city and it is largely through their efforts that the signs have been introduced forbidding people to spit on the floor of street cars. They have had some stables removed and they are well known in Albany and by sanitary experts as having done very effective and valuable work.

We have had some women on the State Board of Charities. Mrs. Lowell, for one, has served on that board admirably and she has also served on the Board of Arbitration. She has been interested in tenement house reform and in many things that have related to the health and welfare of the people.

Women are now serving on executive committees of the Recreation League, a nurse among them. That has been formed with the hope of stimulating the public to seeing the need of outdoor recreation for the people. Men and women were sent to the Board of Education and succeeded in getting $15,000 for their work and this was largely given through the influence of a committee of women who showed how reasonable it was to give these children a place for out-of-door recreation. Men and women were asked to be inspectors of the playgrounds and among these was a nurse.

The People's Institute started in New York with a very lofty plan of stimulating responsibility in citizenship and it has perhaps the largest local audiences in New York. It is interested in social improvements, social service, etc. Men and women are on the executive committee and among them is a nurse.

The Women's Municipal League was entirely composed of women and there were two nurses among them.

The Civic Club, of Philadelphia, has the credit throughout the country of having pushed women into offices of responsibility, not on the spoils idea, but because they believe that where women are in such places it will not be for selfish purposes, for the good of all. They have effected reforms of a sanitary nature, have introduced traveling libraries, and have started vacation schools, which have now been taken over by the Board of Education.

In the West more has been done by women in municipal affairs than elsewhere and that is largely because there is a western hospitality to ideas as well as other things and the women have taken up the work in the right sort of way.

The Women's Club, of Chicago, is perhaps the most important club as a whole. It numbers 900 members and has a very definite place in Chicago. Through its influence matrons have been in the police stations, the age of protection has been raised and a great many reforms in county jails have been brought about. One woman in Chicago secured rubber tires for the ambulances of the city. She got one such ambulance at first and it was such a success that they use them now in the entire system.

Vacation schools and playgrounds for children have been secured by women in different cities.

The Women's Alliance secured the appointment of five women as sanitary police for factory and tenement house inspection. One woman was engaged to collect data upon the proper collection and disposal of garbage and proved so efficient that she was appointed inspector and superintendent of the night force and proved the most capable one they ever had. She did it in the most businesslike way. The woman who was appointed to succeed Miss Addams as inspector of street cleaning had taken a scholarship in Sanscrit and was considered the flower of the university where she graduated. The first factory law in Illinois was planned and outlined by a woman, who had been appointed Factory Inspector by Governor Altgeld. In inspecting she found there was so little legislative protection for children that she secured the passage of a protective statute law. But when the law was passed she could not get any lawyer to prosecute and so she studied law and was admitted to the bar so that she might prosecute, and she is now looked on as an expert.

In New York the women on the State Charities Aid Association have been of immense help to the community.

You are doubtless familiar with Miss de Graffenried's work. She is one of Carroll D. Wright's most effective assistants and is accurate and reliable, and she has collected most valuable data upon labor matters and statistics generally relating to people and homes.

Miss Morton, of London, is a nurse who has made a specialty of hygiene. She has been elected to the London School Board and polled more votes than any man. For several years she has been hoping to introduce education and manual training into the prison system and has already given her first lectures there. She has also a nurse's settlement.

The kindergarten in Hartford was started by women as well as in many other cities. In New York there has been medical inspection of the public schools established, and although no nurse has been inspector, the discoveries of some nurses that children who were desquamating from scarlet fever and who were still having diphtheritic throats, were attending the public schools, had some effect in securing the necessary appropriation.

There are now some of the nurses of the city who have the right to use the name of the Board of Health, but it is rather a complimentary relationship and has only a semi-official character. They have been presented with badges on which is borne the name of the Board of Health, showing that it will support them. In the public lectures which are provided for the city by the Board of Education, one nurse has for two years been on the lecture list.

I might go on and tell of individual cases. I think the people as a whole believe very much in the practical work that the trained nurse can do, so that it would be less difficult to urge their appointment on health and education boards than women of almost any other profession. However there is one subject that as citizens we shall have to undertake, in the interest of all as well as for our profession, and that is to help on civil service reform. If the spoils system is the only one by which appointments are made women will not have a chance, but if they are made on the merit system trained nurses will come in for their share. Such further education as they would receive would be the only necessary plea for their appointment.

The one idea I wish above all to bring out is, that among the many opportunities for civic and altruistic work pressing on all sides nurses having superior advantages in their practical training should not rest content with being only nurses, but should use their talents wherever possible in reform and civic movements.

(Wald, 1900, pp. 54–57)

The Duty of this Society in Public Work

By L. L. Dock

A long paper on this subject is, naturally, not to be expected, but a few suggestions arising from the intimate following of the Society's affairs during a period of seven years Secretaryship, may, perhaps, be useful, especially to those members who, from the compulsory absorption of their own urgently pressing duties, have not given special time or attention to the question of the character and efficiency of the Society as a whole.

The question which instantly arises when one considers the Society as an organization, and which arises constantly before the vision of those who conduct its affairs is, "How to make the Society more effective." If we compare, in a historically impersonal manner, the objects of the Society, the women of whom it is composed, the training schools which it represents, and the enormous *latent* power and influence which it possesses in these members—with the actual influence exerted and made manifest, we must confess that the Society is not effective—at least, vastly less effective than might be expected of it. True, it has done some sporadic pieces of good work—it has planted and cultivated the Associated Alumnae, established the Teachers' Course, and assists in various good enterprises as they come along, such as Congresses, etc. But to what extent is the Society an influence? To what extent does it affect the public? How much does it actually guide nursing education? What weight has it with hospital managers and staffs? What amount of force does it bring to bear on its own members in questions of education, ethics, etc.?

An honest searching after true answers to all these questions will inevitably bring the admission that the Society, in all these rather abstract but most important ways, has not done what it might do; has not made itself a moral force; is not a public conscience; takes no position in large public questions; is not feared by those of low standards; allows all manner of new conditions and developments in nursing affairs to arise, flourish, succeed, or fail, without taking any notice whatever of them, apparently not even knowing about them. I am speaking—let me repeat—of the Society as a body, not of individual members. Yet this Society, as one body, would often be astonished at the actual extent and weight of its influence, if its whole latent and, at present unsuspected power, were actually to be systematically exerted in an intelligent and energetic manner.

In the past, no committee on current events—as one might call it— has ever existed, and the Secretary has never been empowered to speak for the Society, as it were, on public questions. Yet several occasions have arisen in which your ex-Secretary did, upon her own responsibility undertake to speak for the Society—the matters being such that she felt certain of the Society's position, and the tone of replies strikingly demonstrated the fact that the Society possesses a latent strength which it does not wield often enough.

The present Secretary can mention one or two instances which will illustrate. A practical suggestion seems to be—that a small standing committee, carefully chosen, might be authorized to watch public events as related to nursing, and to make the voice of the Society constantly heard, whether in criticism, in commendation, in warning, or in petition. Many important developments are looming up: A complete revolution in methods of teaching nurses seems to be imminent. A quite determined movement on the part of certain elements of our masculine brothers to seize and guide the helm of the new teaching is also most undeniably in progress. Several of these same brothers have lately openly asserted themselves in printed articles as the founders and leaders of that nursing education, which, so far as it has gone, we all know to have been worked out by the brains, bodies and souls of the women to whom this paper is addressed, and who have often had to win their points in clinched opposition to the will of these same brothers, and solely by dint of their own personal prestige as women.

The different State laws now in progress all vitally affect the nursing education of the future. This Society ought beyond a doubt to make itself heard on all principle-involving points arising in these legislative acts. It has also, for some time been a vexed question in the mind of your ex-Secretary whether glaring professional injustice and indignities suffered by its members at the hands of political jobbers, or overbearing medical or lay managers, should be allowed to pass in silence, or whether the Society should not, to some extent at least, resent or take cognizance of such incidents, and exert some slight degree of protection to its members.

There is also the very delicate question of ethics to one another which has been suggested to the writer by more than one active member, and that is, how far a member of the Society may feel justified in following another in a position where some question of principle was involved, without first making it clear that the principle must be upheld?

These and other points I commend to the Society in the hope that it may truly become an effective public force.

(Dock, 1904, pp. 77–79)

Resolution

"WHEREAS, In order to keep the moral and social status of the nursing body on a high plane and to preserve the Educational basis of professional training intact, it is absolutely essential that the first principle laid down by Florence Nightingale be adhered to whereby alone nursing can be maintained as a high calling—this first principle being, namely, That the authority over pupil and ward nurses and the control of nursing staffs in educational and disciplinary matters, be placed in the hands of women heads, themselves trained nurses; and

"WHEREAS, there is and has been from the outset of nursing reform a strong and well defined determination on the part of a certain element among men to take this authority away from women and so regain their former control over the discipline of nursing staffs, and as the injurious effects of such control may be plainly seen in many foreign hospitals and are beginning to be evident in some of our own in the lowering of educational standards, lengthening of working hours, and disregard of entrance requirements and practical work (such as dietetics, obstetrics, etc.), be it

"*Resolved,* That this Society should assert Miss Nightingale's first principle with courage and maintain it with firmness, doing all in its power as a corporate body to encourage its members to insist upon its recognition, and

"WHEREAS, the struggle of individual training school heads to maintain this principle is and has been occasionally nullified by the readiness of their successors to accept an inferior status with loss of authority, be it further

"*Resolved,* That the ethical sense of this Society suffers a shock when women accept training school positions with deprivation of their rightful control over the nursing staff, and when their predecessors may have sacrified their positions to their principles, and that such action, being regarded as harmful to the highest interests of the nursing profession, meets the moral and ethical disapprobation of this Society."

(Resolution, 1910, pp. 90–91)

The Power of the Professional Press

By Sophia Palmer

It is a surprising fact that an adequate history of journalism had never been written. A meager account of the establishment of newspapers seems to have been the only effort made in this direction. The development of magazines, and especially of professional journals, has been given practically no consideration, excepting where brief mention may have been made in addresses or essays bearing on other subjects. I will give you such facts as I have been able to glean from many sources.

Passing over in review the beginnings of the first general newspapers and magazines published in the English language, we will consider very briefly the development of medicine in this country and the rise of the professional press. medical science was not new when our ancestors crossed the Atlantic, but the country had been settled 150 years before the medical profession came into form as an organization. There seems to have been very little to tempt physicians of high standing to join the early colonies. In 1608 it is recorded, that a Dr. Walter Russell came over to Jamestown, Virginia, and being of a daring and adventurous spirit, accompanied John Smith on many of his expeditions. There is no record of there having been a physician on board the *Mayflower*, but the clergymen coming with the early settlers were required to attend a course of lectures in physic, that they might be able to give medical as well as spiritual care to members of their congregations.

Harvard College was established in 1638, but for many years the men who were properly prepared for the practice of medicine graduated first from Harvard and then went to Europe for their medical education. A number of these men were presidents of Harvard in the early days. During this time all kinds of quakery developed in the colonies. Ignorance and superstition prevailed among the people to an exaggerated degree and have not been altogether eradicated yet.

The Massachusetts Medical Society was organized in 1781, with a special charter from the legislature, granting to it the right to examine and license physicians, and it is interesting to note that, even at that early date, the proper preparation for the practice of medicine for the protection of the people was recognized. In 1782, a Department of Medicine was established at Harvard, one year after the organization of the Massachusetts Medical Society, but it was not until 1810 that it was made a separate department, with a special building and independent faculty. The Massachusetts Medical Society established a magazine, the first official organ of the kind of which I find record, in 1797, and during the next 20 years, the development of state medical organizations and the establishment of medical journals in 20 or more states followed.

Medical journals seems to have passed through many phases, the commercial element being conspicuous from the beginning, just as it has been in the nursing and dental profession. Dentists have not yet succeeded in establishing a journal of their own, but are dependent upon the trade magazines, which are the property of the manufacturers of dental implements. Thacher, writing in 1826, states that medical progress at that time had not kept pace with the progress of wealth and population in the country, that while there were 10,000 regular graduates in medicine, there were 15,000 practitioners who were practically without medical education, that medical schools were too numerous, too greatly under the domination of commercial interests, and he asks if the public would not be better served if the schools were fewer in number, but with higher standards. He spoke also, at this time, of the establishment of medical journals as calling forth the talent of physicians in all parts of the country and as giving great impetus to medical education.

I am sure you see the similarity between the development of nursing and medicine in this country, but with this difference—that nursing progress has been much more rapid than medical progress. We have covered in 48 years practically what the medical profession was accomplishing in 134 years. Nursing schools have multiplied in the same lawless way that medical schools did and have, and in the same way been commercialized. Organization has been the great compelling force in rectifying the faults of the pioneer period in nursing as in medicine. Since the establishment of our own official magazines we have gone forward with really marvelous rapidity. The pioneers have laid a foundation upon which the nurses of the future may, if they choose, build a great profession. The National League of Nursing Education was organized in 1893 and now numbers 500 individual members and 13 state league affiliations. The American Nurses' Association was established in 1897 and now has a membership of more than 30,000. The course in Nursing and Health at Columbia University was opened in 1900, and has graduated more than 300, 6 of whom have this year received college degrees.

The *American Journal of Nursing* was established in the same year, the first number seeing the light in October, 1900. State legislation began in 1903 and now covers 42 states of the Union. The National Organization for Public Health Nursing was organized in 1912, and already numbers 1400 members.

The *British Journal of Nursing* is the oldest of the strictly professional nursing journals and in all of those foreign countries where nursing is making definite progress and where there are national organizations of nurses, we find nursing magazines owned and managed by nurses themselves.

It will take many years of constant effort to overcome the defects that are a part of all pioneer work, especially where such work has fallen under the dominion of commercialism, but when we see what has been accomplished, not only in medicine but in all of the other professions and departments of education which are engaged in practically similar reforms as those necessary in the development of nursing, we may feel satisfied that our efforts have not been misdirected.

In all departments of educational and philanthropic reforms we recognize the power of the professional press. Not only in medicine and nursing, but in law and in all the subdivisions of education, philanthropy and religion, certain magazines are recognized as authoritative. Professional journals became necessary because of the commercialism of the general press. Thacher, writing in 1828, in Boston, and Disraeli, in 1830, in London, deplore the loss of power of the press of those times through such interests. We know that the power of the press in its aggregate force is steadily increasing. At the same time, a great deal of its influence is lost through the lack of proper restraint, the disregard for personal privacy, and the placing of financial gain before all other considerations. Our popular magazines and newspapers spare no expense in gathering news and information of affairs in which all mankind is interested, but the placing of the making of money before the moral welfare of society is bringing each year into greater prominence those magazines which are established on a strictly professional basis. We know that reforms to be lasting must come from within and conditions usually become intolerant before such reforms are undertaken, and already we find recognition of a need of such reforms in popular journalism. Formerly preparation for journalism was only to be obtained through the field of experience. This year the first class received degrees at Columbia University from the first school of journalism to be established, where the students are prepared by the same methods as are used in the education of the members of the other professions, with ideals and standards for the advancement of society which, it is expected, will, in time, counteract the commercial domination of the general press.

It is not necessary in speaking to an audience of this character to dwell more in detail upon the work of the past. All of the subdivisions of our educational work which I have touched upon are imperfect and unfinished. It will take many generations of nurses to complete them all. Such progress as has been made would have been impossible without the power of our own professional journals. But there is one great work which I wish to place before this body and which must be carried to completion through the influence of the professional press—that is the complete reorganization of the manner and method of the training of nurses. A plan has been discussed by the older members, which has been approved by those whose work among us has ended, but which is so tremendous that we have not yet had the courage to undertake it, namely, the establishment of central schools for the preliminary and theoretical training of the nurse, where candidates shall be prepared in all of the departments which do not require actual hospital experience, relieving the hospital of all responsibility of training with the exception of those things which require actual bed-side experience, where pupils for all hospitals, large and small, general and private and for the insane, shall receive the same preparation, just as the physician is prepared for a medical school, only making an adequate term of service in the hospital compulsory before the granting of a diploma by the college and a certificate of registration by the state. To bring about such a complete change, the public must be educated: the hospital public, the medical public and the general public. This could easily be accomplished if we could secure the coöperation of the leading medical journals, the *Modern Hospital* and the *Survey* with our own official organs. Once the idea is accepted, suitable endowments, either state or private, for the establishment of such colleges, at reasonable distances over the country, and the detail of their management could be arranged.

Each year, we know, will bring new problems to be solved, for which we shall have greater need for our professional magazines, our national organ, the *American Journal of Nursing,* our western associate, the *Pacific Coast Journal,* and the *Public Health Nurse Quarterly,* with all of the smaller alumnae and state magazines which are owned, edited and managed by our own members and which exist as a medium through which our ideals and standards may be communicated to the world at large, unrestricted and unrestrained by any other body of workers. The danger which we must guard against is the establishment of so many of such magazines that they will not be sufficiently supported to do the most efficient work. Our national magazine has had a unique history and has come into existence through the loyalty and unselfishness of a small group of members of the American Nurses' Association who financed it and carried it as a trust for a dozen years, until the national body was sufficiently organized and developed to assume its entire responsibility. Today it stands as the property of all the members of the national association, the youngest member sharing equally in its ownership and the responsibility for its future, with the older members who established it and have borne the burden in the past.

Through our professional journals we are recording our history step by step, and we are leaving for those who are to follow us a record of our experiences which will enable them to go forward in a new environment and to fill a larger place in the world-wide scheme of civilization than we have been able to do.

(Palmer, 1915, pp. 148–152)

The Importance of Securing for the Superintendent Powers Equal to Her Responsibilities

By Miss Parsons
Massachusetts General Hospital

Miss Parsons. Superintendents of training schools have in so many instances been seriously handicapped in their work of educating nurses and maintaining a high standard in their schools by their inability to secure the cooperation of the authority superior to them, that it is'nt [sic] strange that there should be a desire to discuss the possibility of securing power commensurate with their responsibilities.

It seems almost superfluous to describe the conditions to this audience that arise when the power is inadequate, because I doubt if there is any superintendent in this room who hasn't had illustrative personal experience.

There are the schools where the superintendents are unable to obtain sufficient appropriation to supply paid instructors and she has to rely upon the voluntary efforts of busy doctors to give the lectures to the nurses, not only that but we haven't had enough properly qualified instructors for the practical nursing. How many of us have sat in the lecture room waiting patiently for the lecturer and were finally dismissed because he had been suddenly called away on a case, and there, at a stroke, without warning, was a week lost out of the careful program made out by the superintendent. How many lectures far too technical or much too superficial have we listened to, and yet were powerless to criticise. All sorts of educational deficiencies and inconsistencies exist owing to the fact that each school is a law unto itself.

One of the most trying conditions is where the community represented by the training school committee demands that the school shall

329

be a source of revenue by sending the nurses out to private families while training. Usually the superintendent of nurses knows that such an arrangement is detrimental to the proper administration of the ward work and the education of the nurses but is powerless to stem the tide of popular sentiment and precedent.

There are no doubt several superintendents of schools who believe that the reduction of a three years' course to a two years' course with the present day requirements is most damaging to the schools and yet they are obliged to submit to that condition if they work in hospitals that have decreed the two year system. Last, but not least, of the discouraging conditions to be mentioned is the school where the superintendent is not supported in the disciplinary measures she believes necessary to maintain high moral standards, and this in its extreme manifestation is where nurses who are morally defective are retained through the influence of some one member of the board of hospital staff. In contrast to the schools such as just referred to are some that have made enviable reputations on account of the excellence of the training given their pupils and because of the character and ability of their graduates. These, at least I can speak of three of them, are so organized that the superintendents are as independent as is possible considering the affiliation with the hospital and the fact that the hospital in involved in any error or criticism concerning the nursing department. In these schools the superintendent of nurses may drop any probationer or pupil during the first six months in the hospital without consultation. After that she may suspend any nurse, and dismiss her if she convinces the superintendent of the hospital and whoever composes the training school committee that her reasons are just. She studies her problems and makes her recommendations as to the policy to be persued all affairs pertaining to the school. In these schools I believe the superintendents have had no serious difficulty in adjusting the welfare of the school to the requirements of the hospital so far as there have been funds to carry on the work.

In other ways I believe there is getting to be an almost unanimous agreement among the organized superintendents of hospitals and the superintendents of training schools concerning the desirability of a three year's course, of paid instructors, of graduate nurses in positions of responsibility, of the eight hour system, and a high educational requirement for candidates.

My personal feeling is that schools for nurses were started in an unfortunate way, although I do not presume to say that under the existing conditions it could have been done better; but it seems to me that instead of burdening the nurses with all the manual work of cleaning the wards and lavatories which in the first few years took about four-fifths of the time, the pupils might have been given the care of the patients with only enough house cleaning to teach them proper methods. If they had been required to pay for the privilege of instruction, we should not still be staggering under the burdens of old traditions that make our efforts so difficult towards emancipation, from the almost purely manual to the proper blend of manual experience and educational standards.

It is of course useless to speculate on what might have been the present situation if beginnings had been different. We have the problem of the training school for nurses as a part of some hospital system, each interdependent, and slowly but surely I believe order is being established out of chaos.

Not only are the hospital and school becoming more reasonably identified but the interdependence of different hospitals and schools is being established in a way that is bringing about better mutual understanding and coöperation which is resulting in greater uniformity of education for the trained nurse whether she be from the large general hospital or the small special hospital. All who wish to see the kind of school that can be developed in a small special hospital should study the system of the childrens' hospital here in Boston.

The ever increasing demands for the well educated and well trained nurse and the process of state registration is surely educating the public to the fact of the duty of the hospital to give an educational equivalent to the pupil in return for her services and time. When the public appreciates that this education is necessary there will logically result *endowments* for the department for nurse education as well as for the scientific and other departments.

Let us also hope that it will result in the establishment of preparatory courses for nurses in the sciences that relate to nursing, all over the country in the public educational institutions. Teachers and Simmons Colleges have initiated a good work in this line.

The ability of the superintendent of nurses to convince her superintendent, her training school committee, or board of trustees, as the case may be, must always depend somewhat on the personal equation of the superintendent and the people with whom she works. Every time an immature, inexperienced person is thrust into such a position the work must suffer, because if the superintendent does not know the needs of her department sufficiently well to *guide* the policy of her school rather than to be led, she is sure to land in great difficulties.

In conclusion I would say that power is not so much a matter of rule as it is of knowledge. So when we are conscious of lack of power to realize our ideals, let us look within and see where we can elevate resourcefulness, let us inform ourselves more about the psychology of the environment in which we find ourselves. Do we perceive the point of view of those who differ from us? If we do, and are still convinced that what we strive for is right and feasible, let us attack the weak spot in the opposition and win our adversary by logic and reason.

Sometimes a field must be abandoned but surely not until every effort has been made to succeed in the work which we have undertaken.

(Parsons, 1911, pp. 55–59)

Standardizing Agencies and State Boards of Nurse Examiners

By Phoebe M. Kandel, R.N.

Head, Department of Nursing Education, Colorado State Teachers College, Greeley, Colorado

In spite of the fact that a well known professor of English disapproves of the use of introductory remarks and calls the introducton to a paper a "doormat," I am going to make use of a "doormat" to my subject, Standardizing Agencies and State Boards of Nurse Examiners.

The bibliography reveals that the topic has been discussed numerous times over a period of about forty years, from the point of view of legislation, registration, functions of state boards of nurse examiners, and the effect and value of standardization programs. Since no previous study of the composition of the state board of nurse examiners was found, it seemed to me timely that we assemble certain information through questionnaires to determine the readiness of our board of nurse examiners to work with the existing academic and professional standardizing agencies, as well as to know more adequately of their ability to be of help to the schools of nursing.

The following are some of the academic and professional standardizing agencies:

Academic:

North Central Association of Colleges and Universities

Association of Colleges and Secondary Schools in the Middle States and Maryland

Association of Colleges and Secondary Schools in the Southern States

Northwest Association of Secondary Schools and Schools of
   Higher Education
American Association of Teachers' Colleges
American Association of University Women

Professional:

American Medical Association (Council on Medical Education)
   Federation of State Boards of Medical Examiners
   National Board of Medical Examiners
American College of Surgeons
American Pharmaceutical Association
American Dental Association
American Dietetic Association
American Library Association
American Psychiatric Association (accredits schools of nursing in
   psychiatric institutions).

The people who are selected to serve on the standardization programs of the above organizations, have at least the minimum of four
years of academic preparation, as well as varied experience. The representative assigned to visit the institutions will have had, in most
instances, the academic preparation equal to that of the president of
the institution.

Let us briefly examine the influences that have contributed to the
standardization of our schools of nursing. Almost forty years ago about
"a baker's dozen" of our ablest leaders advocated nurse registration
laws. Among this group was Miss Sophia Palmer, who presented the
subject to the New York Federation of Women's Clubs. To quote from
the paper presented by Miss Palmer at this meeting, November 9,
1899:

The greatest need in the nursing profession today is a law that shall
place training schools for nurses under the supervision of the University
of the State of New York. Such a law would require every training school
to bring its standard up to a given point . . . would require every woman
who wished to practice nursing to obtain a diploma from a training
school recognized by the University, to pass a Regents' examination,
and to register her license to practice. . . . It is of vital importance that

examining boards shall be selected from among nurses in practically the same manner that medical boards are chosen from physicians, that pharmacists, dentists, and teachers are examined, each by members of their own profession.

It is safe to assume that many of the members of the New York Federation of Women's Clubs shared in the development of the first modern school of nursing at Bellevue Hospital, New York, and that that interest helped in the attainment of the earliest standards for nurses in the United States. They passed resolutions endorsing the formation of a board of examiners chosen by the state society of nurses, and included in their recommendations that nursing be listed with the other professions and be supervised by the New York Board of Regents.

Several months after legal status for nurses was initiated, Mrs. Isabel Hampton Robb and Miss Palmer discussed the points imminent to legislation. They said, "The fullness of time brings us to the vital questions of registration for nurses. . . . When we come to organize a state society, the principal motive being to influence legislation, we take an entirely new departure from the motives actuating us in upbuilding our associations for educational and social purposes. We go before the legislature, not as graduates of any one school, but as citizens of the state."

Early in the year 1901, the nurses of New York State organized their forces and entered upon the struggle for standards through legislation. Here, as in their earlier efforts, the nurses did not work single-handed, but they secured the support of the Regents, and public-spirited laymen. The nursing profession owes much of its progress to Mrs. Whitelaw Reid, who quietly used her very great influence with public men in behalf of the Nurses Bill. Mrs. Reid gave much thought, time, energy, and money to the better understanding of tuberculosis nursing by promoting and supporting the school of nursing at Trudeau Sanitarium, Trudeau, New York.

It is tempting to quote more of the history of the steps for legislation and registration which brought about the first standardizing agency for our schools of nursing. "The attack on the Nurses Bill concentrated on the provision creating a board of nurse examiners nominated by the nurses' society and appointed by the Regents." Women prominent on training school boards strongly favored and supported the measure that nurses manage their own educational affairs, with the result that the nurses secured their own board of examiners. In order to determine standards, the Regents have their inspectors. So the New York bill counted for more than showed at first glance because of the powers of the Regents. By the placing of the schools under the Regents, they have become a part of an almost unique educational system. The regulations governing the education of the nurse are, therefore, in the hands of educational experts, and such regulations must accord with the regulations governing all of the other professions. After the nurses' examining board was appointed, the members were authorized to work out a practical and theoretical syllabus for the schools, and in 1906 they selected a nurse inspector for appointment by the Regents. This step marks the beginning of individual assistance within the schools and the development of standards of subject matter and clinical services for the instruction of undergraduate nurses.

The first course in universities for graduate nurses was established in 1899, Teachers College, Columbia University, under the title of Hospital Economics. To meet the increasing demands of the nurses for preparation in teaching, supervision, and administration in institutional and public health nursing work, the name of the course was changed and enlarged under the title of Department of Nursing Education. In 1910, Mrs. Helen Hartley Jenkins became the benefactress of the department. This represented the first endowment for the university education of nurses, and laid the foundation for the training of nurses for community health service. This department represents the mother-house for academic preparation in nursing education.

The national Curriculum for Schools of Nursing, which expresses the best ideas of the Education Committee of the National League of Nursing Education, was edited in 1917. This Curriculum was to be used as a guide in the organization of the theoretical and clinical program, living conditions and hours of duty, the selection of student nurses, and the teaching-supervisory personnel. At the opening of each school year, a faculty conference hour given to the reading and discussion of the "Conditions Essential in the Education of Nurses," written by the Honorary Chairman of the Committee on Education, Miss Mary Adelaide Nutting, which appears in the Curriculum, would restimulate all nurses who share in the instruction and supervision of student nurses. The use of the Curriculum by all schools of nursing is written into the rules and regulations of many state boards for registration of nurses.

Institutes, summer schools and extension courses have met a real demand, not only for instructors and superintendents of nurses, but for the supervisors and head nurses. The lectures, as well as group discussions, are conducted by experts, and each is of permanent value in helping to develop better attitudes in teaching, supervision, and administration. Summer schools and extension courses are usually found in colleges and universities, and this assures a sympathetic attitude of the administration toward the special group of students. All these have a far-reaching influence in our schools of nursing. In one state this year, Colorado, at the request of a large number of nurses in service, the Educational Committee of the League, encouraged the establishment of classes in Teaching and Supervision Applied to Nursing Education, also History of Nursing. These subjects were offered through the Extension Department of the Colorado State Teachers College, and the classes were composed of head nurses, supervisors, instructors, and superintendents of nurses, and several home-makers. The classes, held in Denver, Colorado Springs, and Pueblo, have been conducted by the Head of the Department of Nursing Education of the College, with a total registration of one hundred and forty-three. Of this number there were two deaconesses and forty-seven nuns.

A large organization to have a weighty indirect influence on the standards of clinical instruction, is the American Red Cross Nursing Service. The eligibility requirements for membership into this organization are very definite, and it is the ambition of many nurses on graduation to indicate their readiness to serve, when needed, by applying for membership.

The Digest of Laws Requiring Registration for Nurses issued by the American Nurses' Association is most illuminating in showing up all discrepancies and differences in the minimum educational requirements for registration. The length of the course varies in different states from two to three years; the hospital requirements vary from twenty to seventy beds; and the daily average number of patients from twelve to fifty.

The two hospital accrediting agencies which have a standardizing effect on schools of nursing are the American Medical Association and the American College of Surgeons. The American Medical Association devotes one whole issue of its Journal annually to what is called the Hospital Number, which includes data about the accredited schools connected with registered hospitals. Copies of this report are sent to the state boards of nurse examiners, to the hospital executives, medical colleges, medical libraries, and other selected places and people. The 1931 report shows that of the 7,259 hospitals and allied institutions in the United States, there are 540 that are not registered or approved by the American Medical Association. In the 540 non-registered hospitals there are 13,315 beds, including 588 bassinettes. Also in the 540 non-registered hospitals there are about fifteen schools of nursing. It is unfortunate that it is possible for schools to continue in hospitals not accredited by the American Medical Association.

The hospital standardization program of the American College of Surgeons, directed by Dr. Malcolm McEachern of the Hospital Activities Committee, affects the standards of every department of the hospital. May I refer you to the main requirements for the approval of hospitals, also to the section of the report that discusses the nursing service. All of their suggestions tend to raise the standards of the school of nursing. To the American Medical Association, the American College of Surgeons, and the American and Catholic Hospital Associations, we record our appreciation of the individual and collective assistance of their influence in the improvement of the standards in nursing education.

With the close of the World War, history repeated itself in advancing the improvement of qualifications in nursing service. The pressing need for more and for better nurses in the field of public health prompted the desirability of an investigation. At the invitation of the Rockefeller Foundation, a conference of persons interested in the development of public health nursing in the United States was called in New York. The scope of the inquiry included general nursing education. The study revealed that the essential qualifications of the public health nurse were formed in the fundamental training, or undergraduate nursing course, and that well-qualified teachers and supervisors were necessary to attain the educational standards embodied in the legislation of the more progressive states. Among the mass of collected data in the report, "Nursing and Nursing Education in the United States," the committee considered of fundamental importance the further development and strengthening of university schools of nursing of a high grade, for the training of leaders and teachers, to whom must be entrusted the development and standardizing of procedures for all nursing schools; for permeating influence which will give inspiration and balance, and gradually improve the efficiency of every institution for the training of nurses. The observations of inadequate teaching equipment, and the universal waste and misuse of the student's time led the Committee to conclude that the period of three years now required in the majority of schools is not necessary.

Following the above study and report, "Nursing and Nursing Education in the United States," a copy of which should be in every school of nursing library, another important plan was projected by the National League of Nursing Education. A committee was composed of twenty-one men and women representing nursing, hospitals, medical, and public health associations, with additional members in the field of general and public education. Dr. William Darrach was selected chairman, Dr. May Ayres Burgess was chosen to direct the study, and the title used to designate the work was Committee on the Grading of Nursing Schools. The objective of the Committee was to help raise the standards of nursing education in the schools of nursing. Early in 1928, the Committee on the Grading of Nursing Schools was authorized to publish the findings covering the first three years of their work. The introduction of the report, "Nurses, Patients and Pocketbooks," prefaces the study by defining the program of grading. It is appropriate that we reacquaint ourselves with the Committee's definition of grading.

> "Grading implies the ultimate adoption of certain minimum standards which must be met if the school is to harvest crops of graduates properly prepared for nursing. It is impossible to decide what these minimum standards are until we know what qualities the graduates should have; and we cannot know that until we know what they will be called upon to do. So we come back again to the decision . . . that grading must be founded upon and accompanied by a careful inquiry into the underlying facts of nursing employment."

The effect that this and subsequent reports from the Grading Committee has had on the improvement of the educational programs and selection of personnel in our schools of nursing can be observed by thoughtful study of the graphs on display in the booth of the Grading Committee at this convention.

The direct effect of the first grading has been the raising of the entrance requirements of schools of nursing to high school graduation, that is fifteen or sixteen units, as the states' requirement may be. Mr. James G. Pentz, Director, Credentials Division, Department of Public Instruction, Pennsylvania, presented interesting data on high school entrance requirements in the March, 1932, issue of the *American Journal of Nursing*.

> In 1928 the schools requiring four years of high school work for admission was 13.2 per cent, while in 1930 the number of schools requiring

four years of high school work for admission had increased to 54.3 per cent, a gain of approximately 300 per cent.

The indirect effect, if this term may be used with grading, has been the discontinuance of schools of nursing, both small and large, distributed over the United States. The discontinuance of the schools of nursing was probably not motivated by the unemployment situation, but by the cost entailed in the development of acceptable class and laboratory facilities, and the provision of clinical instruction in the four required services: medical, surgical, obstetrical and pediatric.

The Committee on Accrediting Schools of Nursing of the National League of Nursing Education have given much deliberation to the subject of criteria which would be helpful in attaining higher standards. Quoting them, "This list should include hours of study, amount and kinds of practical experience, qualifications of instructors and directors of schools, entrance requirements for students, the kind of school records to be kept, methods of examination and requirements for graduation. The requirements for placing a school on such a list must not be the personal opinion of a committee, but must come from a much wider range of experts in the field, whose findings and judgments in the matter shall be collected and made available by the Committee on Accrediting."

In various articles, over a period of years, Miss Adda Eldredge, Director of Nursing Education in the State of Wisconsin, has called our attention to the dangers of too rapidly demanding high school as an entrance requirement when many of our nursing faculty are not high school graduates. As will be recalled, the findings of the Grading Committee disclosed the information that 42 per cent of the faculty of our schools were not high school graduates. This is not to construe the impression that the educational standards of admission should not be high school graduation, fifteen or sixteen units, but it does mean that the administrative and teaching personnel within our schools, many of whom have done, and are doing, constructive work, should avail themselves of additional educational preparation applied to nursing education.

Now that we have our setting, by review, and we are to consider the state boards of nurse examiners in relation to other standardizing agencies, it may be timely to look into the composition of the membership of the state boards of nurse examiners. Questionnaires were sent to all of the states. Because of the necessary time consumed in sending material about, it is very gratifying to have heard from twenty-six. Since some of the questions asked were not answered by all, only the information on educational preparation and experience will be given. The information was not secured to be destructively critical, but to determine how nearly ready our state boards of nurse examiners are to take their place with other existing standardizing agencies of secondary education, colleges, and universities. The findings as they relate to the educational preparation of the entire group of the nurse members of the boards, which includes the persons definitely appointed to inspect or evaluate the schools, show that of the 106 members of the board of the 26 states heard from, twenty-three have had from one to three years of high school, and eighty-three are high school graduates. Fourteen have had from one to three years of college and ten have had from four to five years of college. Nine have had instruction in state supervision of nursing education. The experience is distributed as follows: 24 have had head nurse experience, 29 supervision, 39 teaching of nursing procedures or sciences, 35 have been or are now superintendent of nurses, and 17 have been or are now superintendents of hospitals. Fifteen have had supervision in public health nursing and allied interests. Of the sixteen inspectors, educational directors, or evaluators studied, all are high school graduates. Four have had one to three years of college; five have had four years of college, and four have had five years of college. Eight have had instruction in state supervision of nursing education. The data revealed that not all of the educational directors are considered a part of the state boards of nurse examiners.

The work accomplished by our state boards of nurse examiners is very commendable, for some of them have worked under many handicaps. Quoting from the questionnaire returned by one state board, "The influence of politics in our schools of nursing definitely retards any progress schools might make. When one realizes how limited our requirements and what minimum requirements a school needs to meet to be really accredited, one is amazed, and certainly such status is responsible for the thick strata of mediocrity that is so apparent in the nursing profession." Continuing the quotation, "I have thought many times of the inadequacy of our present system of standardization. For example: the curriculum that we publish if followed out in detail really requires as a basic education four years of high school, yet the law in this state requires much less high school education."

From another state, "While our law is inadequate in providing the number of people necessary to give the amount of supervision which we should like to do in this state, still our situation is not as bad as it might appear upon the surface. Our training schools always support enthusiastically any program of the Board of Registration and we are overloaded with urgent calls asking us to visit them and check upon their progress, but as this has to be done, in my case, on Saturday afternoons or Sundays, we are able to visit only those places that we feel must be brought up to the minimum standard."

In conclusion, may I suggest the following recommendations. The first two have been made at this and previous meetings.

1. A National Council on Nursing Education of the League cooperating with the American Nurses' Association.
2. The formation of a National Accrediting Association with intrastate relationships comparable to the existing academic and professional standardizing agencies.

Until these come into being, the following recommendations will help to bring about a better recognition of the quality of instruction in our schools of nursing.

3. The selection of nurses, if possible, with some academic preparation for state board of nurse examiners, as well as experience in teaching, supervision and administration. I believe that one of the members on the board should be a public health nurse. I also believe that each member of the board should take formal class work to acquire the attitude of the student.
4. Legislative changes in those states that prohibit the appointment of school of nursing faculty to serve as state board of nurse examiners.
5. The selection of an educational director whose academic preparation at least approximates that of the head of the school of nursing in the state presenting the highest qualifications for her work. Some experience in teaching, supervision, and administration is essential to be a helpful counsellor.
6. A closer working relationship between state boards of nurse examiners and the state educational director of schools of nursing than exists in several states.

All of these recommendations, if accepted, will make for a better understanding of the school problems and school programs, and provide for greater confidence between the faculty of the schools of nursing and state boards of nurse examiners. Furthermore, the policy of standardization will be more in keeping with the policies of the existing academic and other professional accrediting agencies.

(Kandel, 1932, pp. 221–230)

The New Scutari

By Shirley C. Titus, R.N.

Dean, School of Nursing, Vanderbilt University, Nashville, Tennessee

If a text were necessary for the remarks which I have been asked to make relative to the subject of nursing education, especially as it relates to the future, I think I should offer as this text the following quotation:

> There is a tide in the affairs of men,
> Which, taken at the flood, leads on to fortune;
> Omitted, all the voyage of their life
> Is bound in shallows and in miseries.
> On such a full sea are we now afloat;
> And we must take the current as it serves
> Or lose our ventures.

Throughout the long centuries that have marked the tortuous and weary journey of man toward that unknown goal, the future, there seems to have been recurring intervals where the tide of social change sweeps to the flood, engulfing, obliterating, and even destroying, the old familiar landscape of social and cultural life. And always upon the ruins of the old, verdant fields have arisen which cultivated by a new and hopeful people have been productive of another and richer social harvest.

That we of this generation have been appointed to live through one of these great flood tides of social change there seems little doubt, for already we have experienced an acceleration in social change that no previous generation, so it is claimed, has witnessed. Whitehead in his remarkable essay, "On Foresight," in commmenting on this accleration states that whereas in the past the time-span between notable changes in social customs was considerably longer than a single life, today it is distinctly shorter. Therefore, he goes on to state, while it was possible for each past generation to assume with certainty that it would live substantially amid conditions governing the lives of its fathers and that these same conditions would mold with equal force the lives of their children, our generation may cherish no such assumption.

Because of this shortening of the time-span, because of this violent acceleration in social change, we of this generation have seen the passing of that world in which our forefathers lived and we shall most probably see the birth of a complete new social order. It is already clearly recognized that the new highly integrated social order which promises to take the place of the loose, individualistic democracy of our forefathers can be no laissez-faire growth, that only a rational, conscious, deliberate direction of human affairs will preserve our civilization.

Such thinking has found expression in certain new phrases, phrases which already have grown stale to the ear because of excessive repetition in their use. However stale the phrases—"a planned society," "social planning," etc.—may grow, let us not overlook the preëminent importance of the thought giving rise to them. Walter Lippman says that the idea that a social order can and should be *planned* and managed has taken root amongst the peoples of the world and such thinking constitutes a revolution in the outlook of mankind. "In the magnitude of its implication it is like the discovery of reason in ancient Greece, like the intuition of the sanctity of human life among the sages and the mystics, like the revival of interest in the natural world during the Renaissance."

I hear you ask—"But what has all this to do with nursing education?" Indeed it has much to do with nursing education, very, very much indeed. Nursing, like every form of life activity, is a part of the warp and woof of the whole social fabric. Nursing cannot be an isolated, separated thing-in-itself; the flow, the interplay of social forces inevitably as day follows the night exerts an effect on nursing and nursing education. "Divine Omnipotence itself cannot ordain that effect should not be effect; it cannot change the earth to what it was a thousand years ago."

The most striking attribute of the standard pattern of nursing education today is its social ineffectualness. The lack of correlation between the production and utilization of graduate nurses has become increasingly great with the passing of the years. That this is true is not a matter of wonder for the curriculum of the nursing school is substantially the same today as it was twenty or thirty years ago, although during these two or three decades the social changes have occurred so rapidly, and have been of such magnitude, that one might with complete truth say we have already lived through a social revolution.

No deep and searching analysis is necessary to determine the reasons why nursing has ceased to be a truly effective social instrument. A fixed and rigid curriculum in a changing world is accountable for the fact that the nurse no longer is adequately prepared to meet properly the varying nursing needs of the community and is likewise accountable for the fact that the nursing school today is an educational anomaly and an anachronism.

The rigidity and stereotyped nature of the nursing curriculum is attributable to the fact that the school of nursing, unlike other vocational and professional schools which are created and maintained for the sole purpose of serving educational ends exclusively, is not free to make changes in its curriculum in accordance with changing social needs. It has not been able to do so because of its organization setting and the economic basis on which it rests.

For the sake of brevity and clarity, I shall ask you to visualize for a moment a superstructure resting on a double foundation. The superstructure is the educational program of the school, and the two foundations which support it are:

1. The Organization of the School—
     that is, the school of nursing is an integral part of a hospital, an institution which is created and maintained for the purpose of caring for the sick and not for the purpose of carrying on the business of education.

2. The Apprenticeship[1] System of Nursing—
     that is, the student nurse is an employee of the hospital as well as being a student in the school of nursing.

Now the thesis which I wish to postulate is that the two foundations on which the educational program of the nursing school rests not only influence its development but *actually* determine it—that, in fact, no other educational program than the one now offered by the standard school of nursing has been possible, or ever will be possible, as long as the program rests on either one or both of the foundations that now support it. This is to say, that in my opinion, if conditions are to be

---

[1]The economic aspect of the apprenticeship system alone is referred to at this point.

made such that nursing and the nurse may properly serve society in a complete and satisfactory way, we as a profession must anticipate the establishment not only of an entirely new curriculum but the establishment of a new pattern or system of nursing education. New foundations as well as a new superstructure must be erected if the school of nursing is to properly prepare nurses for the varying nursing needs of the modern community.

However, we may shrink from it, how impossible, how colossal it may seem to us, the fact remains that today nurses—*all* nurses—are confronted with a task that they cannot ethically avoid. It is our lot, it is our fate, to serve destiny in a period of creation; we as a group face a second and more tremendous Scutari. This hour seems pregnant with the power to influence and determine the future course of nursing and to restore it once more to the social effectiveness that has distinguished it in former centuries. Let us not beguile ourselves into believing that a laissez-faire attitude is any longer possible, that somehow or other blind chance will come to the rescue of nursing. Can we doubt that change is necessary, that action is needed, when bleak and stark before us lies that grim reality, that paradoxical situation, an everincreasing army of unemployed nurses and an undernursed community? As I see it—

On such a full sea are we now afloat;
And we must take the current as it serves
Or lose our ventures—

But how shall we take the current? Well, why not face our problems as others are facing world problems, others who realizing that no longer may human affairs be safely left to the blind interplay of social forces, that man must become master, rather than victim of destiny if civilization is to endure, dare to pit human intelligence against so-called "natural law." Social planning is no more nor no less than the bending of natural law to human will, and logic rather than experience promises to be the essence of the new social order.

Perhaps no group has been more passionately devoted to their profession than have nurses; we nurses have literally fought and sacrificed and died for our profession and its standards. But we as a group must face the fact that our efforts in behalf of our profession have been diffuse rather than concentrated; we have acted individually rather than as a group, and we have dealt with our problems largely in an emotional way rather than a rational way.

If ever a group needed to conceive and to establish a plan of practical action—a conscious, deliberate, purposeful, intelligent plan of action— we are that group. I myself am led to believe that nursing will never become truly socially effective, that it will never become the dynamic force it should be in this great program of social reconstruction that now challenges the peoples of the earth, unless we as a group avail ourselves of this latest form of social engineering, the social plan. If we do not, our profession without doubt will continue to be the victim of destiny it has been during these past two or three decades, and the affairs of nursing will continue to be directed by those who, blind to the true social import and value of nursing, have demanded a program of nursing education which could successfully serve only the lesser social need, the providing of a nursing service at lowest cost to the hospital sick, rather than a program of nursing education which would successfully meet the larger, and preëminently more important social need, namely the need of the community at large for a skilled and adequate nursing service.

Therefore, "if I were king," to ape our good friend Dr. Lyons, I would call my wisest councilors together and immediately draft a social plan for nursing. As I see such a plan it would probably consist of three parts. First, I would instruct these councilors to determine the basic, central problem of nursing—the prima mobile, so to speak, of all our problems—and I would instruct them on pain of death to reduce this problem to the simplest possible formula and to set it forth in simple, clear language so that all might understand it.

One of the singular, almost incredible, facts about nursing is that the true nature of our professional difficulties is not known or appreciated by the large majority of nurses. How often do we spend our energies attacking the related rather than basic, central problem itself; how often we think we are treating the disease when in reality we are only taking the patient's history or ascertaining the ravages of the disease that besets our profession. For example, we are prone to believe that time-studies offer a solution to the basic problems of nursing. Unfortunately, the time-study, like any other assembling of facts, can only measure for us the extent, the depth, and the redness of the sore; it cannot eradicate it. Time-studies cannot give us a plan, a method, for removing the conditions which give rise to our difficulties.

It has been said that insight and foresight are necessary to the making of any social plan. This is to say, there must be a clear understanding of the present before any understanding may be reached as to how the future may be gauged and controlled. Only by means of a thorough-going study and analysis of the present, and a determination of the real connection and significance of the facts so disclosed—that is, only through a study of *cause* as well as effect—may any plan of action for "the masterful administration of the unforeseen" be made.

The past eight years have seen nursing engaged in the very worth while occupation of gathering facts about itself. There has been, in my estimation, however, a considerable lag between the assembling of facts and the determination of the connection or significance of these facts, and the causes giving rise to them. It does seem that by this time sufficient facts have been assembled so that the basis of the ills of nursing could be determined and a plan formulated for the solving of our difficulties.

We may blame ourselves that the public so little understands the problems of nursing and has given so little support to us in our struggles to meet more adequately the nursing needs of the modern community. We may blame ourselves that, with three or four notable exceptions, no nursing school has been the recipient of any of those great monetary gifts which so characterize the history of education in this country. Is it possible that with the deeply intimate, personal relationships nurses have with all kinds and varieties of people, our profession should have been so passed over, so isolated and so unsupported in its struggles, if the individual nurse had thoroughly understood the problems beset-ting her profession and had been able clearly to indicate to the public wherein and by what means the cause of nursing could be supported and assisted?

The first step in making a social plan for nursing as you see deals, so to speak, with the general problem of "how and why nursing got this way"; the second step should logically deal with the problem of "what are we going to do about it." Now, "if I were king" and held the power of authority, I should direct the councilors to prepare forthwith a scheme or plan by which nursing could seek state support for schools of nursing.

While we may hope that as years go on more of our schools may become privately endowed, the salvation of nursing does not lie in this direction. Even if the gods proved most kind, we may anticipate at best that only a small number of the total number of nursing schools might become endowed.

Neither may we hope that through any process of enlightenment, or through the development of mere good will, will the hospitals of this country give up the goose which has laid for them so golden an egg. Money is money and we may never hope that our schools of nursing will be removed from their present organization setting until we as a profession find a way by which a new system could be substituted for the apprenticeship system of nursing, a system which would necessitate no increase in the cost of nursing service to the hospital over and beyond what it now must meet with the operation of the apprenticeship system of nursing.

The basic problem of nursing—the prima mobile of all the problems of nursing—has been the revenue bearing aspects of the apprenticeship system. I have already indicated in a previous part of this paper that it is my belief that nursing can never become really socially effective as long as nursing education rests on its present foundations. The way out, it would seem, is to place schools of nursing on a full fee paying basis (by "full fee paying basis," I mean student nurses should be required to pay both maintenance and instructional fees), and to have the state assume the responsibility for operating the school of nursing in precisely the same way as it does for its junior colleges, normal schools, and universities. Then and then only will the school of nursing become as other vocational and professional schools, namely, entirely free to serve educational ends exclusively, and entirely free to modify its curriculum in the light of social needs.

I can hear you say, "A wonderful dream—but only a dream." I do not believe this idea is Utopian; I do not think it is impossible to realize. Nothing is impossible to achieve if intelligence backs the scheme and the goal is the true improvement of social welfare, the effective meeting of a basic human need.

It would seem that this period of depression would be the time to move forward with a plan for a change in the pattern of nursing education. Why do not those schools who boast of long waiting lists make efforts to establish themselves on a full-paying basis (not, of course, increasing the revenue of the hospital, but automatically reducing the service hours rendered by the student in proportion to the maintenance and instructional fees charged). Why do we not in this period of depression lay our plans to tap state resources when boom times return again, or shall we again let a golden opportunity—golden both literally and figuratively—slip through our fingers as we did the prosperity period of 1920–1929?

If any indictment could be drawn against nursing it is that we have been most derelict in this matter of thinking through a plan or scheme by which state support for schools of nursing could be sought. The scheme I have in mind is not a scheme for actually getting money out of a legislature; it is a scheme for the organization and administration of a school of nursing which would operate under the auspices of the state system of education. I draw your attention to the fact that at the present moment if some Mussolini were to approach us and say, "I'll back your schools of nursing—just tell me how to do it," we could not tell him how it could be done!

On the Pacific coast there are several schools of nursing which are affiliated with junior colleges, but we need not look to them for organization suggestions for a state supported, fee-paying school of nursing for such schools are still an integral part of a hospital organization and the junior college does not come into the problem of the education of the nurse except during the preclinical period. The management of the preclinical period under such conditions is simple; the management of the clinical education of the nurse is the real problem.

The plan I have in mind conceives of a thoroughgoing reorganization of the school of nursing and its educational program. Such a reorganization is necessarily a most complex, technical problem and would require the most intensive and intelligent thinking of the best experts in nursing education. Such thinking, it is my firm belief, should be going on in an official way at the present time, for without such a scheme in hand we may never hope to secure state support for our schools of nursing. Without state support, I repeat again, the present pattern of nursing education will necessarily continue, and with it will continue this social waste which cannot in any way be justified or excused, namely, an increasing army of unemployed nurses and an undernursed community.

And so I pass to the third part of a king's social plan for nursing. This part has to do with leadership.

In Plato's beautiful Allegory of the Cave, it is told, as you will no doubt remember, that there was a great cave in which a large group of people sat chained in such a way that their backs were to the doorway of the cave and they faced its posterior way. Outside of the cave there ran an elevated roadway, and back of this roadway burned a large fire so that as people and objects passed up and down the roadway their shadows fell upon that wall of the cave which the chained prisoners faced. Now the prisoners, never having been outside the cave and never having seen aught else than the shadows of the world without, mistook appearance for substance; they believed the shadows to be real objects.

The story goes on to tell how one of the prisoners, a philosopher, escaped from his chains and went forth into the outer world and how he returned to the cave again and pleaded with his former companions to break their chains and to go with him out into the glory and wonder of the world of reality. The prisoners, knowing nothing else than that which they had experienced, could not conceive of anything different or better, so they laughed at the philosopher, and hugging their chains the tighter, refused to accompany him.

If Plato's philosopher had been able to persuade any of his former companions to shake off their chains and to go out into the world of real and true things, I am confident it would have been the youngest, not the oldest of the group. The nearer the person is to the coming generation, the shorter the period of time he is taught to think of appearance as substance, the more readily he will adjust himself to new conditions and thoughts and the less satisfied he will be that the world in which he lives is "the best of all possible worlds." Each generation is caught in the pattern of thought of its own generation and may progress only within the limits of this thinking.

Around the council boards of nursing the younger generation or generations are missing. While I do not advocate that gray hair shall not be found at these boards, I do state that a balanced or dynamic leadership for nursing in this rapidly changing world will alone be possible if we avail ourselves of the thinking of the younger generations of nurses.

So, "if I were king," I could command a revamping of our lines of professional organization and would definitely provide for the inclusion of a certain proportion of younger nurses on our boards of directors and the appointment of some of these nurses to certain important committees. These younger women being born as they were amid different social and cultural conditions, possessing as they do a different standard of values, and thinking as is their wont in an entirely different manner from the older generation, could and would make, without doubt, a peculiarly valuable contribution to the sum total of thinking that is clearly needed if nursing once more is to be restored to its old and honored position in the hearts and affection of mankind.

This hour seems pregnant with the power to influence and determine the future course of nursing and to restore it once more to the social effectualness that has distinguished it in former centuries. May this hour bring forth a conscious, deliberate, purposeful effort on the part of our profession to meet the great challenge that clearly confronts us. Then, like Simeon upon the temple steps, one may say, "Lord, lettest thou thy servant depart in peace."

(Titus, 1933, pp. 232–240)

Epilogue

Epilogue

Over the 40-year period, 1894–1933, nursing, like the nation, underwent considerable change. Industrialization, the growth of cities, scientific and technological advances, and the emphasis on progress affected the health of people and health care as a business enterprise. Nursing as an acceptable career for women grew in importance as did the need for nurses in all dimensions of health and illness.

In reviewing events of the period, organization of the Superintendents' Society emerges as one of the more significant undertakings by nurses for nursing. Although some historians might be critical of the tendency to overpraise the activities of the pioneer leadership group, when examining the contributions of the Superintendents' Society and the NLNE, there emerges a chronicle of accomplishments impressive in its scope. The implementation of a standard curriculum, an eight-hour work day, a national nurses' association, legislation that credentialed nurses, accreditation of programs, and the movement of nurses into schools of higher learning can be traced to the efforts and influence of the early leaders. Irrespective of their lack of higher education, the absence of suffrage for women, and little public acknowledgement of the value of women's work, they were able to place nursing on a professional course at a critical time in its history.

Adelaide Nutting, as an active participant, described in detail advances made during the first 30 years of organization. Her presentation is included here because of its clarity, its content, and its relevance to the evolution of the profession.

Thirty Years of Progress in Nursing

By Adelaide Nutting, R.N.

New York, New York

I am asked to tell you something of the progress made in nursing during the thirty years since this society was established, and I must acknowledge frankly at the outset that the task is attempted with some hesitation. For the idea of progress is the subject of much discussion these days, and we are not nearly as sure about it as we used to be. What is progress? Is it that kind of improvement which can be measured by statistics? This was the prevailing idea during the last century, says Dean Inge.

It was obvious to many of our grandparents that the nation which travels sixty miles an hour must be five times as civilized as one which travels only twelve. I am inclined to think that this would still seem an obvious measure of progress to many of the grandchildren of those grandparents.

Or is progress a spiritual thing? There are those who believe this, and think that human betterment can only come through the development of our spiritual capacities and that all other things should serve as means to this end. And then there are numerous other ideas about it, from those of Wells, who sees only mental progress—a clearing and enlargement of ideas—to others who think progress can come only through science, or through education, or through new forms of social organization.

In trying, therefore, to show some of the ways in which nursing has grown to its present stature, I do so with no certainty as to how far such growth is evidence of real progress. It is obvious that at certain stages of our journey changes were made which seemed to lead in the right direction, but some of the results as we now see them do little to satisfy us of the wisdom of the course then taken. Moreover, we are,

I am sure, quite too near the past thirty years in which most of us have lived and worked to be able to secure any adequate perspective of our field of labor, of the part we have played in it. It would be difficult to bring a dispassionate judgment to bear upon matters with which we have been so intimately concerned. But we can at least trace the main lines of development and follow the sequence of events, for such appraisal as we can bring to them.

The past thirty years in nursing show a period of intense activity, of rapid and continuous development in old and in new fields of work, of a consequent phenomenal growth in numbers and of many new and complex problems arising within the work itself and in the various relationships outside of it.

The earliest schools of nursing in this country were created independently of hospitals by boards or committees with power and freedom to develop the education of nurses as they would. From the beginning that responsibility was largely given over to the hospitals and eventually transferred wholly to them. What one surveys then in looking back over the developments in nursing is a period of nearly fifty years of almost unrestricted experiment with a system of education in which the School has existed as an integral part of the hospital, created and conducted to serve its needs, with the education of the nurse becoming thereby and inevitably a by-product of her service to the hospital.

Offering as these early schools did a new field of training and occupation for women at a time when such fields were rare, they attracted a large number of students, some of whom were women of rather exceptional ability. The result of their labors was that reform of hospital nursing to which must undoubtedly be attributed in considerable degree the extraordinary growth of hospitals which has characterized the past thirty years.

At the first convention held by this Society thirty years ago there were present 44 heads of training schools in Canada as well as the United States. As the entire number of such schools was then about 70 this was a good representation. Thirteen states were represented, 9 of them by a single member only. Today there are Schools of Nursing in every state and a great many in several of them. There are Schools of Nursing also in the Philippines, in Hawaii, in Porto Rico and in Cuba, built up by American nurses. I see that there are now 75 trained nurses at work in far Alaska. So I suppose that schools will soon be on their way there—perhaps, indeed, they are there already.

Altogether there are now recorded about 1800 schools of nursing which have grown up in the rapidly multiplying hospitals of the country during the past thirty years. A picture of their rate of growth is interesting. In the ten years between 1890 and 1900 there were over 400 schools of nursing established in connection with hospitals which arose during that period; in the next ten years, about 700 more schools were created in newly erected hospitals; and in the last ten years just ended there are recorded a further 600 schools of nursing of similar origin. In all of these hospitals the first imperative need was a good nursing service, and no one saw any way of providing this except by creating schools whose students could form the nursing staff. Of course, the continuous demand for nurses in such large numbers who were capable of organizing schools and of directing their work was obviously an entirely impossible one to meet. These new schools had to be built up in various sections of the country out of whatever material was available for the purpose, and the results of that period of hasty growth form a part of our educational problem in nursing today. Think what it meant to a young profession just beginning to develop its educational structure, and to work out its standards of practice to be forced into such abnormal growth as the swiftly multiplying hospitals of the period required. Careful study of the situation will show these schools adjusting themselves more and more completely to the hospitals with which they were connected, more and more absorbed in efforts to meet their manifold and constantly increasing needs. Whichever way hospitals grew, their schools as a matter of course, followed. Never, probably, in history, has any institution, philanthropic or otherwise, had so useful and flexible an instrument of service at its command. Seldom does history record a service of purer devotion, than that which schools of nursing have rendered to hospitals.

Naturally, during the greater part of this period there has not been much opportunity for educational development, both because the entire energies of the schools were absorbed in meeting the working demands of the moment and for other reasons which will be considered later. Yet educational advances have been made and some of them are noteworthy.

It is in the direction of numbers and of enlargement in fields of nursing that the most remarkable advances have been made. Numerically indeed nursing is moving on with a swift and apparently increasing momentum which nothing in sight seems likely to check.

Shortly before this Society was formed in 1893, there were not 500 graduate nurses in the whole country. The last census shows about 150,000 graduate nurses, trained and registered and it is of interest to note that a very large proportion (80 per cent) of the whole increase of women in all professional service was found in just two pursuits—nursing and teaching. It is of further interest for us to realize clearly that we have now reached a stage where we are graduating approximately 15,000 nurses annually, and that the certainty of increasing the existing number by 150,000 at the end of the current ten year period offers something to think about. Even with any degree of depreciation that seems likely to occur, there is more than a reasonable outlook that we may all live to hear the last faint echo of the final cry of a shortage of nurses.

The expansion of the field of nursing has been extraordinary and is still going on. Its extent and diversity can only be roughly indicated here. Within each field there is found a good deal of elaboration and specialization, most notable perhaps in hospitals and training schools where the single official who formerly directed the nursing service and was the only teacher there has given place to a whole hierarchy of assistants, supervisors (one hospital has three distinct types of supervisors), instructors, and special workers. The Bureau of Occupations at Nursing Headquarters listed 30 different kinds of work for which nurses with some form of special training or experience were required.

Medicine is steadily transferring to nursing, duties and procedures hitherto performed only by physicians. The giving of anesthetics, for instance, has been in some places turned over entirely from physicians to nurses despite the fact that laws in other sections have been enacted forbidding it.

A recent article by Dr. Goldwater proposes the passing over to nurses of an entirely new range of duties now the province of the medical interne, and shows how in certain hospitals this transfer is already going on, such nurses becoming known as clinic assistants.

In public health work, which offers a new and apparently almost limitless field of activity for nurses, there are several quite distinct branches of work calling for special preparation, such as school nursing, maternity and infant protection, rural nursing, industrial nursing, etc.

The public health movement did not create the public health nurse, it found her at work in her district nursing the sick, watching over their families and the neighborhood, and teaching in the homes those sanitary practices, those measures of personal and home hygiene, which do much to prevent disease and to promote health. Such visiting nurses whose teaching was a cardinal principle of their work were occupied in 50 communities when the public health campaign was set in motion.

But forty years before this date the work had its origin in England as one of the first results of the reform in nursing then taking place. The duty of inculcating hygienic habits in home life was always as incumbent upon the district nurse in England as her actual care of the sick. The importance of this kind of teaching is hardly understood until one sees it in the light of the modern public health movement and realizes that it has become a cornerstone of that whole structure. The nurse familiar with the ravages of disease becomes your zealous crusader against it.

There are now about 12,000 nurses engaged in some form of public health work and the usefulness of their efforts so far has created a steady demand for more of them and for the kind of preparation which will enable them to contribute more fully and effectively to the growing needs of the most promising field which nurses have as yet entered.

A most important phase of progress has been the development of nursing associations. The formation of the Society of Superintendents was the recognition of problems common to all nurses, which could not be handled by any isolated effort, and called for their united energies. One of its avowed purposes was to foster the creation of a National Association of Trained Nurses. A few Training School Alumnae Associations were already in existence, and within a few years there arose, first, the Nurses Associated Alumnae, which later became the American Nurses Association. Then there followed in rapid succession the organization of State Nurses Associations which within a comparatively brief period were formed in every state. With these organizations began in 1903 the first attempt through appropriate legislation to bring order out of the chaos in educational standards, methods and ideals, which had resulted from the rapid and uncontrolled growth of Training Schools for Nurses, over a long period of years.

The laws secured are very modest in all of their requirements, and most of them are as yet permissive only. Their educational standard is a moderate one—in most states one or two years of High School followed by two years of hospital training as a rule accompanied by a slender body of formal instruction.

The entire profession of nursing is now organized very much after the fashion of the medical and other professions. Every state has its body of practicing nurses, its schools for training them, its associations of nurses, its laws regulating the practice of nursing and in some small degree the preparation for it. There are three National Associations and an International Council of Nurses of which 14 countries are members and which has held conferences in London, Paris, Cologne, and San Francisco. It is now gathering itself together following the suspension of work during the war, and holds its next congress at Helsingfors, Finland in 1925.

Nursing has also developed something in the way of a literature. Thirty years ago there were but one or two very elementary books on nursing, now several eminent publishing houses vie with each other in ministering to the needs of student nurses. One of the generous contributions of medicine to nursing is the array of text-books for nurses written by physicians, especially those on the sciences.

There are two or three excellent nursing periodicals of national scope, and several state and alumnae publications.

Thus roughly reviewing the general growth and development in nursing, we reach the most important element in the situation—the School of Nursing. Contrasting the conditions in our leading schools today with those of the past we may well feel that great advances have been made. Measuring them by the changing need in the large and growing field of work occupied by nurses, or by any generally accepted standards of professional education, they seem relatively small. It is little wonder, however, that they seem large to those who have labored to secure them, and know how slow and difficult the process has been, and how precarious often the gains made. For against suitable educational and other requirements for admission the hospital sets its imperative need for large numbers of workers irrespective of the fine shades of qualifications; against reasonable hours of duty for student nurses, it holds up the undeniable necessity of the sick, for nursing service. There is a clearly discernible tradition in most hospitals that every hour the nurse spends in class room or study is taken away from the patients to whom by right it belongs. Against the indispensable costs in any deserving scheme of education the hospital opposes its lack of resources for such purposes. But costs must be placed somewhere. They are incurred in a measure for every act, and are as inevitable as death. Somebody always pays. And Schools of Nursing which in the very nature of things should be a matter of constant and appreciable expense, have been for years through the services of their students contributors to hospital incomes.

In a sense the Superintendent of a School of Nursing is ever at war with herself. She is not only the director of the School but of the Nursing Service and her desire to take good care of the sick is presumably as great as to provide adequate training for her students. In her battlefield, which the hospital is, the balance between them is struck with difficulty. Hospitals should be placed in a position to pay for such nursing and other services as they require, and the value of the services of students should not enter into the situation. A sort of haunting nightmare of every superintendent of nurses is I suppose something like this—How shall I be able to secure enough applicants to form a class of students to enter next September, which will be large enough to take care of this hospital full of sick persons—but this should never be her real problem.

Of genuine and permanent improvements the most outstanding would probably be found in the quality of teaching and supervision, and in the enlargement and wider range of instruction. The employment of trained teachers in schools has now been going on for about ten years, and is steadily increasing, and this, together with the introduction in 1914 of a curriculum for schools of nursing has helped to strengthen teaching in nearly every subject.

The preliminary courses which offered something in the way of a reform twenty years ago are now found in most schools of good standing, and they have done much to ensure at least a minimum of sound teaching in the sciences.

Hours of duty are still a most serious problem. With the exception of the State of California in which student nurses in hospitals come under the provisions of the eight hour law, the eight hour day has made slow headway in hospitals generally. A nine hour day is still the working day for students in the majority of hospitals, and twelve hours the all but universal system for night duty.

There is no one condition which stands more squarely in the path of progress in nursing than this survival of long hours for student nurses in hospitals. It is difficult to refrain from asking why they should be longer tolerated in institutions devoted to the saving of human life and health. One would naturally expect the whole purpose and spirit of hospitals to find appropriate expression in measures for conserving and safeguarding the strength and energies of those whom it employs.

The difficulty in giving the desired amount and variety of instruction within the two year course led to the extension of that course to three years. This was begun with the highest hopes of effecting numerous improvements in the whole scheme of training; but as time went on, it became increasingly clear that the third year was of great importance to the hospital but of most uncertain benefit to the students as a body. The third year was virtually swallowed up by the hospital and became largely an added year of experience often in services in which the student had already spent her required number of months.

Those with some promise of executive ability were placed in charge of wards or other departments, spending from six to ten months in this capacity. The length of the period of night duty, already too long, was extended, sometimes to ten or eleven months, as was also almost universally the length of the period of service in the private wards either on general or special duty. Except in a few instances, no new branches of training were available and no resources to develop new courses of instruction or to find adequately qualified teachers for them. The amount of theory offered in the third year is sometimes less than half of the amount given in the first and second years, and the School is evidently put to it to find either subjects or teachers to fill this period creditably with instruction. The work of the third year must either be required or elective. If required, then the training and instruction given must offer equal opportunity for all. Now the electives offered are few, suited only to the capacities of a small number, and are chiefly in the form of experience unaccompanied by instruction.

Eventually after a trial of years it seemed evident that a proper use of the students' time was probably impossible, and that the attempt to improve the education of nurses by thus lengthening the course of training was not under the existing system a sound or just policy. To me, at least, it finally became entirely clear that we had not made the best possible use of the two year period of training before embarking upon the third year, and that what we now must do was to retrace our steps and study carefully the whole of the two year course with the view of finding out just what could be done to make the best possible use of the students' time. It is because I take the ground as the report does, that the training school must remain for some time to come within the hospital, as it now is (though I hope with increasing freedom to pursue its work) that I am willing to see the three-year course to which I looked forward years ago with highest hopes reduced to a period which can be properly used within the hospital. It is not against three years of training (in itself), but three years in the hospital that one finds oneself opposed. The appeal made by this Society of Superintendents of Schools of Nursing to the Carnegie Foundation in 1911 to make a study of the work in schools of nursing testifies to our growing anxiety over our educational problems which we seemed powerless to solve unaided. Upon the school of nursing in the final analysis all true progress in nursing must depend. Its standards and methods and its ideals are matters of serious moment, not only to nurses, but to all who are or may be concerned with sickness or the safeguarding of health—in a word, the entire public.

The education of nurses has long been a favorite study for controversy, but it is not always realized that schools of nursing hold a peculiar relationship to hospitals, whose needs and interests they have universally been created to serve. They have not therefore either the freedom, the power, or the resources to deal adequately with their very complex educational problem, or to develop their schools beyond a certain point. This should always be remembered in any discussion of their work. Ten years later, however, such a study was in progress. The developments in the field of nursing had reached a stage where a serious study of the method of training had become imperative and financed by the Rockefeller Foundation, directed by a Committee representing medicine, nursing and the laity, the entire system of education in nursing has been subjected to careful scrutiny and impartial evaluation. The study has occupied three years, was conducted by experts in various branches of education, and guided by a trained investigator of eminence in her particular field—Josephine Goldmark. This study with the full report which has just been published is an event of the first magnitude—and it is difficult to estimate in any adequate way the effect which it will have upon the whole nursing situation. Already it has clarified to the public mind a number of obscure or complex issues, and has served to set in motion that discussion and consideration of the desired changes in method which is the first step toward their realization. Every nurse should not only study this report, but should bring it to the attention of as large a number of others outside of nursing as can be reached. The report should be in the hands of all hospital trustees and of physicians concerned with the education of nurses.

There is one point in the report which we must not overlook. Nursing had always cut a wide swathe in its own conception of its task, and has brought thereby within the range of its efforts much that had little to do with nursing, and a good many patients whose ailments were not such as to require the skilled care of a trained nurse. Having accepted the idea that trained attendants are necessary in the care of certain mild forms of sickness, it is incumbent upon us to live squarely up to our convictions. We shall need to apply the same zeal, energy and resourcefulness in our efforts to train attendants that we apply to our other problems. There should be a committee at work on this matter in every state, selecting suitable places for training, working out appropriate ways of finding a suitable supply of applicants, advising and guiding every step of their training, and continuing to safeguard their practice and working lives in every practicable way in order not only that those who employ them, but that these workers themselves may be protected.

Surveying the course of events during the years in which we have been struggling with our educational problems, one is tempted to wonder if the decisive moment in our educational progress may not have come unseen and unrecognized on the day when some part of the education of nurses passed out beyond the hospital and into the University—when some institution became interested in the education of nurses which did not need or desire to profit by their services—the day when Isabel Hampton with the support of this Society prevailed upon the Dean of Teachers College to open her doors of that Department of Columbia University to graduate nurses. For within a few years an organized body of instruction for nurses was built up there, a professorship in nursing established, and the first endowment for the University education of nurses received through which the College was enabled to lay the foundation for the training of public health nurses. Within a few more years, that valorous friend of nursing, Dr. Beard, had brought about the establishment of a University School of Nursing in Minnesota, and how this has been followed by similar schools in other states, you all know. The past few weeks have seen another step forward, in the founding of two more schools of nursing, on a distinctly new basis. These are the Schools at Western Reserve University, Cleveland, endowed by Mrs. Chester Bolston, and at Yale University by the Rockefeller Foundation. Greatly as we have rejoiced in every new link which connects nursing with the University we have here cause for deeper satisfaction. Schools of nursing in the past have all lacked two great essentials, first, adequate funds for their support; second, an administrative body charged with the responsibility of conducting educational work. What sets this new school at Yale University far in advance of any other in its possibilities is that it has seen these two conditions as fundamental to the proper education of nurses. The School is to have its own funds (I deliberately put these first), its own Dean, faculty, buildings and equipment. Although the plans are not fully formulated, there is little reason to doubt that the school at Western Reserve University will follow a somewhat similar plan.

So at last we have reached the stage where these things,—the every day conditions of other forms of professional education are now to be applied to the education of nurses. The school at Yale University is avowedly committed to an experiment, a much needed and most important one in our educational field. Our Miss Goodrich, who has undertaken this task is by temperament and habit a pioneer and a resolute and adventurous one.

she has no fear of treading any new path. Her capacity for brilliant leadership is well known, and her long and richly varied experience in administrative tasks in nursing will enable her to make the fullest possible use of the inspiring opportunities and resources before her. The loss at Teachers College of her devoted work for our students is very great. There is no one who can take her place. There never in fact could be anybody to do that. But our interest in the important educational experiment she is courageously attacking is almost as great as her own—our anxiety to help forward new things in nursing, is a part of our very being.

The picture of the growth of nursing as I have tried to sketch it outlines only main factors in our progress and not all probably even of them. How coldly bare and formal it all sounds in the mere recital, how full in actual life it has been of warm devotion and of splendid energy of heroic tasks carried through with unfaltering courage and of common daily tasks patiently and faithfully fulfilled. Our golden age, however, is not in the past, it is in the future, and the best inheritance we can carry over from the past is the spirit which has brought us through these difficult years, with undiminished courage and unshaken faith in the beliefs and principles for which we have striven.

That spirit leads one to seek ever a better way; leads one to question, to grope for the right solution to the difficult problem. Following where it leads one may falter, may fall if need be, but the spirit which giveth life survives error, survives even failure. It alone leads to progress.

(Nutting, 1923, pp. 101–111)

Epilogue continued

Although many of nursing's goals failed to be achieved to the extent desired, the stage was set for the ongoing growth and refinement of the profession. Leaders looked to the future with determination and optimism. Besides the National League of Nursing Education, the American Nurses' Association, and individual state nurses' associations, a number of equally important organizations like the National Organization for Public Health Nursing and the National Association for

Colored Graduate Nurses formed during the years of focus. Those organizations contributed significantly to the early work of the Superintendents' Society, and confirmed nursing's social commitment.

Despite the need to accommodate to the political realities of the time, educational standards were put in place and suitable criteria for admission to schools of nursing were established. Affiliation with university schools, expansion of the concepts of health promotion and disease prevention, and specialization in nursing practice were additional positive outcomes that are validated in the annual convention proceedings. Change also can be noted with respect to the quality of the papers themselves; they became more scientific and scholarly over time, with frequent citing of references and the use of professional credentials.

Nursing's leaders of that time spoke to concerns that survive to the present. Topics such as holism, pay equity, downward substitution of personnel, women's rights, and other gender-related matters of relevance today, recur with conspicuous regularity in the early literature. The relationship between issues of the past and those of the present is striking. Educational problems remain unresolved as nursing continues to debate the value of university preparation as a basic requirement; control of practice is still problematic as nurses try to achieve independence in advanced roles; recruitment remains a concern as nursing declines in its attractiveness as a career option; ethical dilemmas persist but now include those generated by a highly technical practice environment; questions surrounding nursing's image persevere particularly in relation to professional status; and the struggle for power endures as nursing strives to attain equity, autonomy, and prestige.

The proceedings of the annual conventions of the Superintendents' Society and the NLNE, during the years 1894–1933, provide a history that merits intensive study. This book highlights issues and events that the authors consider most relevant. As the 40-year era concluded, nursing confronted new challenges that included unemployment generated by a growing financial depression, an increase in the incidence of communicable disease, and the initial rumblings of unrest abroad. However, shaping of the profession continued as nursing matured.

The first 40 years left a legacy that changed the profession and had a profound impact on health care in America.

References

Allerton, E. (1898). How far are training schools responsible for the lack of ethics among nurses. *Fifth Annual Convention of the ASSTSN* (pp. 45–47). Harrisburg, PA: Harrisburg Pub.; and reprinted in Reverby, S. (Ed.). (1985). *Annual Conventions 1893–1899 ASSTSN.* New York: Garland Pubishers.

Alline, A. (1907). The supply and demand of students in the nurse training-schools. *Proceedings of the Thirteenth Annual Convention of the ASSTSN* (pp. 29–36). Baltimore: J. H. Furst.

Anderson, A. (1910). Preparation of the teacher for the training school. *Proceedings of the Sixteenth Annual Convention of the ASSTSN* (pp. 139–144). Baltimore: J. H. Furst.

Beecroft, L. A. (1910). Ethics to be observed between training schools. *Proceedings of the Fifteenth Annual Convention of the ASSTSN* (pp. 53–57). Baltimore: J. H. Furst.

Bolton, F. (1925). The responsibility of the university school of nursing to the individual student, the hospital, and the community. *Proceedings of the Thirtieth Annual Convention of the NLNE* (pp. 131–142). Baltimore: Williams & Wilkins.

Brennan, A. S. (1897). Comparative value of theory and practice in training nurses. *First and Second Annual Conventions of the ASSTSN* (pp. 64–66). Harrisburg, PA: Harrisburg Publishers; and reprinted in Reverby, S. (Ed.). (1985). *Annual Conventions 1893–1899 ASSTSN.* New York: Garland Publishers.

Burgess, M. A. (1928). *Nurses, Patients, and Pocketbooks.* New York: Report of A Study of the Economics of Nursing Conducted by the Committee on the Grading of Nursing Schools.

Clayton, S. L. (1916). The purpose and place of ethics in the curriculum. *Proceedings of the Twenty-second Annual Convention of the ASSTSN* (pp. 252–256). Baltimore: Williams & Wilkins.

Davis, M. E. P. (1907). What we are overlooking of fundamental importance in the training of the modern nurse. *Proceedings of the Thirteenth Annual Convention of the ASSTSN* (pp. 104–107). Baltimore: J. H. Furst.

Dock, L. L. (1896). A national association for nurses and its legal organization. *Proceedings of the Third Annual Convention of the ASSTSN* (pp. 42–60). Harrisburg, PA: Harrisburg Publishers; and reprinted in Reverby, S. (Ed.). (1985). *Annual Conventions 1893–1899 ASSTSN.* New York: Garland Publishers.

Dock, L. L. (1897). Directories for nurses. *First and Second Annual Conventions of the ASSTSN* (pp. 57–60). Harrisburg, PA: Harrisburg Pub.; and reprinted in Reverby, S. (Ed.). (1985). *Annual Conventions 1893–1899 ASSTSN.* New York: Garland Publishers.

Dock, L. L. (1904). The duty of this society in public work. *Proceedings of the Tenth Annual Convention of the ASSTSN* (pp. 77–79). Baltimore: J. H. Furst.

Foley, E. (1922). Main issues in public health nursing. *Proceedings of the Twenty-seventh Annual Convention of the NLNE* (pp. 221–226). Baltimore: Williams & Wilkins.

Gillette, H. (1915). How to help pupil nurses to study. *Proceedings of the Twenty-first Annual Convention of the NLNE* (pp. 115–122). Baltimore: Williams & Wilkins.

Gladwin, M. (1929). Address. *Proceedings of the Thirty-fifth Annual Convention of the NLNE* (pp. 28–34). New York: National Headquarters.

Goodrich, A. (1912). A general presentation of the statutory requirements of the different states. *Proceedings of the Eighteenth Annual Convention of the ASSTSN* (pp. 212–222). Springfield, MA: Thatcher Art Printery.

Goodrich, A. (1930). The new epoch in nursing. *Proceedings of the Thirty-sixty Annual Convention of the NLNE* (pp. 84–89). New York: National Headquarters.

Grant, L. M. (1927). Teaching of ethics and ethical problems. *Proceedings of the Thirty-third Annual Convention of the NLNE* (pp. 229–230). New York: National Headquarters.

Gray, C. (1917). The relation of the private duty nurse to the public as an educator. *Proceedings of the Twenty-third Annual Convention of the NLNE* (pp. 267–272). Baltimore: Williams & Wilkins.

Gray, C. (1919). The results of organized publicity in interesting the public in nursing. *Proceedings of the Twenty-fifth Annual Convention of the NLNE* (pp. 197–203). Baltimore: Williams & Wilkins.

Haasis, B. (1919). The present conditions of supply and demand. *Proceedings of the Twenty-fifth Annual Convention of the NLNE* (pp. 207–215). Baltimore: Williams & Wilkins.

Hampton, I. A. (1897). Introduction. *First and Second Annual Conventions of the ASSTSN* (pp. 3–5). Harrisburg, PA: Harrisburg Pub.; and reprinted in Reverby, S. (Ed.). (1985). *Annual Conventions 1893–1899 ASSTSN.* New York: Garland Publishers.

Harmer, B. (1925). Teaching and learning through experience. *Proceedings of the Thirty First Annual Convention of the NLNE* (pp. 124–132). New York: National Headquarters.

Hodgkins, M. (1932). *Through improvements in the educational process* (pp. 198–206). New York: National Headquarters.

Kandel, P. (1932). Standardizing agencies and state boards of nurse examiners. *Proceedings of the Thirty-eighth Annual Convention of the NLNE* (pp. 221–230). New York: National Headquarters.

McKechnie, M. W. (1904). What has been accomplished in the way of legislation for nurses. *Proceedings of the Tenth Annual Convention of the ASSTSN* (pp. 62–65). Baltimore: J. H. Furst.

Nutting, M. A. (1911). Report of the committee on education. *Proceedings of the Seventeenth Annual Convention of the ASSTSN* (pp. 70–75). Baltimore: J. H. Furst.

Nutting, M. A. (1923). Thirty years of progress. *Proceedings of the Twenty-ninth Annual Convention of the NLNE* (pp. 101–111). Baltimore: Williams & Wilkins; Nutting, M. A. (1926). *A sound economic basis for schools of nursing and other addresses.* New York: G. P. Putnam's

Sons; and Nutting, M. A. (1926). *A sound economic basis for schools of nursing and other addresses.* Reprinted in S. Reverby (Ed.). (1985). *The History of American Nursing.* New York: Garland Publishers.

Olmstead, K. (1920). The recruiting of student nurses. *Proceedings of the Twenty-sixth Annual Convention of the NLNE* (pp. 289–294). Baltimore: Williams & Wilkins.

Pahl, H. W. (1915). The eight hour law for pupil nurses in California after one and one-half years practical demonstration in a general hospital of one hundred beds. *Proceedings of the Twenty-First Annual Convention of the NLNE* (pp. 178–183). Baltimore: Williams & Wilkins.

Palmer S. (1897). Training school alumnae associations. *First and Second Annual Conventions of the ASSTSN* (pp. 52–56). Harrisburg, PA: Harrisburg Pub.; and reprinted in Reverby, S. (Ed.). (1985). *Annual Conventions 1893–1899 ASSTSN.* New York: Garland Publishers.

Palmer, S. (1915). The power of the professional press. *Twenty-First Annual Convention of the NLNE* (pp. 148–152). Baltimore: Williams & Wilkins.

Parsons, S. (1911). The importance of securing for the superintendent powers equal to her responsibilities. *Proceedings of the Seventeenth Annual Convention* (pp. 55–59). Baltimore: J. H. Furst.

Parsons, S. (1916). The training school prospectus and its educational possibilities. *Proceedings of the Twenty-second Annual Convention* (pp. 171–174). Baltimore: Williams & Wilkins.

Perry, C. M. (1913). Nursing ethics and discipline. *Proceedings of the Nineteenth Annual Convention of the NLNE* (pp. 87–93). Baltimore: Williams & Wilkins.

Powell, L. (1911). How the training school for nurses benefits by relation to a university. *Proceedings of the Seventeenth Annual Convention* (pp. 150–154). Baltimore: J. H. Furst.

Powell, L. M. and Clayton, S. L. (1923). Report of the committee on ethical standards. *Proceedings of the Twenty-eighth Annual Convention* (pp. 27–29). Baltimore: Williams & Wilkins.

Resolution. (1910). *Proceedings of the Fifteenth Annual Convention of the ASSTSN* (pp. 90–91). Baltimore: J. H. Furst.

Robb, I. H. (1897a). The three years' course of training in connection with the eight hour system. *First and Second Annual Conventions of the ASSTSN* (pp. 33–40). Harrisburg, PA: Harrisburg Pub.; and reprinted in Reverby, S. (Ed.). (1985). *Annual Conventions 1893–1899 ASSTSN.* New York: Garland Publishers.

Robb, I. H. (1897b). Nursing in the smaller hospitals and in those devoted to the care of special forms of disease. *Fourth Annual Convention of the ASSTSN* (pp. 59–68). Harrisburg, PA: Harrisburg Pub.; and reprinted in Reverby, S. (Ed.). (1985). *Annual Conventions 1893–1899 ASSTSN.* New York: Garland Publishers.

Smith, E. F. S. (1913). Factors of elimination in schools for nurses. *Proceedings of the Nineteenth Annual Convention of the NLNE* (pp. 54–59). Baltimore: Williams & Wilkins.

Snively, M. A. (1897). Report of the committee on a uniform curriculum for training schools for nurses. *First and Second Annual Conventions of the ASSTSN* (pp. 24–30). Harrisburg, PA: Harrisburg Pub.; reprinted in Reverby, S. (Ed.). (1985). *Annual Conventions 1893–1899 ASSTSN* New York: Garland Publishers.

Stewart, I. (1913). Report of the committee for approaching women's colleges. *Proceedings of the Nineteenth Annual Convention of the NLNE* (pp. 35–38). Baltimore: Williams & Wilkins.

Stewart, I. (1929). Professional school or trade school? *Proceedings of the Thirty-fifth Annual Convention of the NLNE* (pp. 131–137). New York: National Headquarters.

Taylor, E. J. (1929). Interprofessional relationships from the viewpoint of the superintendent of nurses. *Proceedings of the Thirty-fifth Annual Convention of the NLNE* (pp. 208–213). New York: National Headquarters.

Taylor, E. J. (1931). Preparation for administrative positions in schools of nursing. *Proceedings of the Thirty-seventh Annual Convention of the NLNE* (pp. 154–168). New York: National Headquarters.

Titus, S. (1933). The new scutari. *Proceedings of the Thirty-ninth Annual Convention of the NLNE* (pp. 232–240). New York: National Headquarters.

Tucker, K. (1916). The training school's responsibility in public health nursing. *Proceedings of the Twenty-second Annual Convention of the NLNE* (pp. 113–117). Baltimore: Williams & Wilkins.

Urch, D. D. (1932). Through better selection of students. *Proceedings of the Thirty-eighth Annual Convention of the NLNE* (pp. 185–191). New York: National Headquarters.

Wald, L. D. (1900). Work of women in municipal affairs. *Proceedings of the Sixth Annual Convention of the ASSTSN* (pp. 54–57). Harrisburg, PA: Harrisburg Pub.; and reprinted in Reverby, S. (Ed.). (1985). *Annual Conventions 1893–1899 ASSTSN.* New York: Garland Publishers.

Walker, L. (1900). How to prepare nurses for the duties of the alumnae. *Proceedings of the Sixth Annual Convention of the ASSTSN* (pp. 44–48). Harrisburg, PA: Harrisburg Pub.; and reprinted in Reverby, S. (Ed.). (1985). *Annual Conventions 1893–1899 ASSTSN.* New York: Garland Publishers.

Wheeler, C. (1930). The selection of students for schools of nursing and problems of adjustment. *Proceedings of the Thirty-sixth Annual Convention of the NLNE* (pp. 120–129). New York: National Headquarters.

Wolf, A. (1928). How can general duty be made more attractive to graduate nurses. *Proceedings of the Thirty-fourth Annual Convention of the NLNE* (pp. 209–217). New York: National Headquarters.